Rotator Cuff Tear

Medicine and Sport Science

Vol. 57

Rotator Cuff Tear

Volume Editor

Nicola Maffulli London

40 figures, 18 in color, and 5 tables, 2012

KARGER

Basel · Freiburg · Paris · London · New York · New Delhi · Bangkok · Beijing · Tokyo · Kuala Lumpur · Singapore · Sydney

Medicine and Sport Science
Founded 1968 by E. Jokl, Lexington, Ky.

Prof. Nicola Maffulli
Centre for Sports and Exercise Medicine
Barts and The London School of Medicine and Dentistry
Mile End Hospital, 275 Bancroft Road
London E1 4DG (UK)

Library of Congress Cataloging-in-Publication Data

Rotator cuff tear / volume editor, Nicola Maffulli.
p. ; cm. -- (Medicine and sport science, ISSN 0254-5020 ; v. 57)
Includes bibliographical references and index.
ISBN 978-3-8055-9814-9 (hard cover : alk. paper) -- ISBN 978-3-8055-9815-6 (e-ISBN)
1. Shoulder join--Rotator cuff--Wounds and injuries. 2. Shoulder join--Rotator cuff--Surgery. I. Maffulli, Nicola. II. Series: Medicine and sport science ; v. 57. 0254-5020
[DNLM: 1. Rotator Cuff--injuries. 2. Rotator Cuff--surgery. 3. Orthopedic Procedures. 4. Shoulder Joint--injuries. 5. Shoulder Joint--surgery. W1 ME649Q v.57 2011 / WE 810]
RD557.5.R685 2011
617.1'57--dc23

2011027927

Bibliographic Indices. This publication is listed in bibliographic services, including Current Contents®.

www.karger.com
Printed in Switzerland on acid-free and non-aging paper (ISO 9706) by Reinhardt Druck, Basel
ISSN 0254–5020
ISBN 978–3–8055–9814–9
e-ISBN 978–3–8055–9815–6

Contents

List of Contributors

W. Ben Kibler
Shoulder Center of Kentucky, Lexington, Ky., USA

Alessandra Berton
Campus Bio-Medico University, Rome, Italy

Fabrizio Campi
D. Cervesi Hospital, Cattolica/Rimini, Italy

Francesco Caranzano
Mauriziano Hospital, Turin, Italy

Michael R. Carmont
Princess Royal Hospital, Telford, UK

Brian J. Cole
Rush University Medical Center, Chicago, Ill., USA

Scott J. Deering
University of Kentucky, Lexington, Ky., USA

Angelo Del Buono
Campus Bio-Medico University, Rome, Italy

Vincenzo Denaro
Campus Bio-Medico University, Rome, Italy

Nicholas R. Forsyth
Keele University Medical School, Stoke on Trent, UK

Francesco Franceschi
Campus Bio-Medico University, Rome, Italy

Stefano Gatti
University of Siena School of Medicine, Siena, Italy

Vasili Karas
Rush University Medical Center, Chicago, Ill., USA

Christian Lattermann
University of Kentucky, Lexington, Ky., USA

Umile Giuseppe Longo
Campus Bio-Medico University, Rome, Italy

Nicola Maffulli
Centre for Sports and Exercise Medicine
Barts and the London School of Medicine and Dentistry, London, UK

Scott D. Mair
University of Kentucky, Lexington, Ky., USA

Andrea Marinozzi
Campus Bio-Medico University, Rome, Italy

Omer Mei-Dan
Meir University Hospital, Kfar Saba, Israel

Francesco Oliva
University of Rome 'Tor Vergata' School of Medicine, Rome, Italy

Leonardo Osti
Campus Bio-Medico University, Rome, Italy

Paolo Paladini
D. Cervesi Hospital, Cattolica/Rimini, Italy

Alessio Palumbo
Campus Bio-Medico University, Rome, Italy

Rocco Papalia
Campus Bio-Medico University, Rome, Italy

Nicola Papapietro
Campus Bio-Medico University, Rome, Italy

Giuseppe Porcellini
D. Cervesi Hospital, Cattolica/Rimini, Italy

Garrett M. Snyder
University of Kentucky, Lexington, Ky., USA

Sebastiano Vasta
Campus Bio-Medico University, Rome, Italy

Vincent M. Wang
Rush University Medical Center, Chicago, Ill., USA

Biagio Zampogna
Campus Bio-Medico University, Rome, Italy

Preface

Basic Science and Rotator Cuff Repair: Where Have We Arrived?

The history of rotator cuff tendinopathy probably started in 1834 when Dr. Smith attributed shoulder pain to 'rupture of the rotator cuff tendon'. One century later, in 1934, Dr. Codman showed that most lesions occur on the articular side of the cuff tendons, in agreement with the hypothesis that Dr. Charles S. Neer would develop in 1972, when he wrote that 'the coraco-acromial ligament and the anterior third of the acromion are responsible for a characteristic syndrome of disability of the shoulder'. However, the pathogenetic mechanisms leading to rotator cuff tendinopathy are still debated. Intrinsic causes, such as changes in vascularity and cellular metabolisms related to ageing, and extrinsic causes, such as subacromial impingement or microtrauma in repetitive overhead movements, are currently considered as the main aetiological factors [1–3]. The rotator cuff tendons play an important role in stabilizing the humeral head. When a massive cuff tear is present, superior migration of the glenohumeral rotation centre occurs during abduction, and a decreased ability of glenohumeral elevation may occur, given the importance of the supraspinatus tendon in beginning the glenohumeral abduction [4, 5]. The long head of the biceps brachii (LHB) stabilizes the glenohumeral joint limiting abnormal translations. LHB may be affected by a wide range of pathologies, from instability (with tendon subluxation) to tenosynovitis to tendon rupture [6]. Rotator cuff tears (RCTs) and tendinopathy of the LHB are the leading causes of shoulder pain with a prevalence for RCTs of 20% in the general population. This prevalence increases with age [7], and RCTs negatively affect patients' quality of life [8].

RCTs have been divided into full- and partial-thickness tears, and several classifications are available for both of these conditions. The importance of classifications resides in the fact that for each specific degree of rotator cuff pathology, a specific treatment should be indicated. However, this is still not well established. Although conservative measures are the first-line therapy, there is evidence for poor spontaneous tendon healing based on histological data [1]. As a consequence, partial-thickness RCTs may progress to full-thickness tears, and pain and dysfunction may persist; in a similar fashion, conservatively managed full-thickness tears can be the cause of discomfort in high-demanding subjects, such as athletes or people who need a wide shoulder range of motion for working activities. Surgical management has developed over time, especially thanks to arthroscopic assisted surgery. Full-thickness tears are generally repaired placing one or two rows of anchors to re-attach the ruptured tendon to its footprint. A great debate is still ongoing about the advantages of using a single- or double-row anchor construct. Biological, biomechanical, and clinical studies have been conducted to establish the superiority of one technique over the other, but no clinical differences have been found, and currently there seems to be little clinical evidence in favour of using a double-row technique, which requires more time and is more expensive and technically demanding [9]. Augmentation with acellular soft tissues could be a possible method to increase tendon function for massive RCTs, but there are contrasting data on its effectiveness in improving functional outcome and, although uncommon, there is the risk for infectious or non-infectious inflammatory response [10]. Platelet-rich plasma is a recent technique developed to speed up tendon healing and to reduce pain. However, its mechanism of action is still unclear, and its long-term effectiveness needs to be assessed [11].

Partial-thickness tears may be surgically addressed with different techniques. Debridement with or without acromioplasty may be a valid option reaching favourable results in tears involving less than 50% of the tendon thickness, while a formal tendon repair is generally advocated for tears involving more than 50% of the cuff thickness. Many options are available to repair the ruptured tendon (conversion to full-thickness and subacromial repair, transtendon repair, or tranosseous repair) and all techniques lead to a relatively high rate of good to excellent results [12]. The tendon of LHB must be accurately assessed, being responsible for many of the symptoms. Tenotomy is related to a greater incidence of cosmetic deformity, but it is does produce satisfactory results. However, there is no univocal consensus regarding which technique should be preferred [13, 14].

Although we purport to know more about the pathogenesis, diagnosis and management of rotator cuff pathology, we are far from the target. Our efforts should be directed at trying to find the treatment that best fits the specific need of each patient. For this reason, the need for randomized trials is mandatory, and the continuing research for the golden treatment should be a must.

Nicola Maffulli, London

References

1 Thompson WO, et al: A biomechanical analysis of rotator cuff deficiency in a cadaveric model. Am J Sports Med 1996;24:286–292.

2 Longo UG, et al: Light microscopic histology of supraspinatus tendon ruptures. Knee Surg Sports Traumatol Arthrosc 2007;15:1390–1394.

3 Longo UG, et al: Histopathology of the supraspinatus tendon in rotator cuff tears. Am J Sports Med 2008;36:533–538.

4 Tétreault P, et al: Passive contribution of the rotator cuff to abduction and joint stability. Surg Radiol Anat 2011 (Epub ahead of print).

5 Elser F, et al: Anatomy, function, injuries, and treatment of the long head of the biceps brachii tendon. Arthroscopy 2011;27:581–592.

6 Yamamoto A, et al: Prevalence and risk factors of a rotator cuff tear in the general population. J Shoulder Elbow Surg 2010;19:116–120.

7 Gartsman GM, et al: Self-assessment of general health status in patients with five common shoulder conditions. J Shoulder Elbow Surg 1998;7:228–237.

8 Fukuda H: The management of partial-thickness tears of the rotator cuff. J Bone Joint Surg Br 2003; 85:3–11.

9 Saridakis P, Jones G: Outcomes of single-row and double-row arthroscopic rotator cuff repair: a systematic review. J Bone Joint Surg Am 2010;92: 732–742.

10 Labbé MR: Arthroscopic technique for patch augmentation of rotator cuff repairs. Arthroscopy 2006;22:1136.e1–6.

11 Castricini R, et al: Platelet-rich plasma augmentation for arthroscopic rotator cuff repair: a randomized controlled trial. Am J Sports Med 2011;39: 258–265.

12 Papalia R, et al: Results of surgical management of symptomatic shoulders with partial-thickness tears of the rotator cuff. Br Med Bull 2010 (Epub ahead of print).

13 Hsu AR, et al: Biceps tenotomy versus tenodesis: a review of clinical outcomes and biomechanical results. J Shoulder Elbow Surg 2011;20:326–332.

14 Frost A, Zafar MS, Maffulli N: Tenotomy versus tenodesis in the management of pathologic lesions of the tendon of the long head of the biceps brachii. Am J Sports Med 2009;37:828–833.

Maffulli N (ed): Rotator Cuff Tear. Med Sport Sci. Basel, Karger, 2012, vol 57, pp 1–9

Epidemiology, Genetics and Biological Factors of Rotator Cuff Tears

Umile Giuseppe Longo[a,b] · Alessandra Berton[a,b] · Nicola Papapietro[a,b] · Nicola Maffulli[c] · Vincenzo Denaro[a,b]

[a]Department of Orthopaedic and Trauma Surgery and [b]Centro Integrato di Ricerca (CIR), Campus Bio-Medico University, Rome, Italy; [c]Centre for Sports and Exercise Medicine, Queen Mary University of London, Barts and The London School of Medicine and Dentistry, Mile End Hospital, London, UK

Abstract

Rotator cuff disease is among the most common musculoskeletal disorders with high direct and indirect costs in industrialized countries. Not all rotator cuff tears are symptomatic. Genetics has recently been investigated as a factor involved in the pathogenesis of rotator cuff pathology. Genetic factors seem to be involved in symptom presentation and tear progression. As rotator cuff disease is multifactorial, no single gene is directly involved in the pathology. Phenotypic expression of genetic susceptibility manifests at the level of ultrastructure of the tendon. Predisposing genes may also operate through apoptosis and regenerative capacity. Studies on cellular and molecular biology are more numerous, but still incomplete, and recently have focussed on the role of apoptosis in tendinopathy, analyzing its key mediators and cellular changes. Oxidative stress is responsible for reduction of collagen synthesis. Biological investigations have identified recently new risk factors. Preliminary reports introduced the possible role of glucose as a risk factor for rotator cuff tear. Further studies are required to fully clarify the genetic and biological factors involved in rotator cuff tears.

Epidemiology

Rotator cuff disease is among the most common musculoskeletal disorders [1–4]. It is the third cause of musculoskeletal disease (16%), after the back (23%) and the knee (19%) [5]. Its relevance is correlated not only to its high prevalence rate, but also to the fact that it is disabling, causing high direct and indirect costs in industrialized countries [6, 7].

The incidence of cuff tears ranges from 5% [8] to 39% [9]. It increases in the elderly population [9–19], being approximately 6 and 30% in those under and over 60 years, respectively [18, 19]. Partial thickness tears are more frequent than full thickness, with a prevalence of 13 versus 7% [13]. Symptomatic disease is generally localized in the dominant arm, and in 28% of patients in the non-dominant shoulder only. Bilateral disease is present in 36% of patients [20].

Not all rotator cuff tears are symptomatic, thus influencing the reported incidence of the disease [9]. Moreover, several patients with shoulder problems do not require medical consultation and/or treatment. Different methods have been used to study apparently healthy shoulders, including arthrography [21], ultrasonography [22] and MRI [23]. They showed an increased incidence of rotator cuff tears with aging, particularly partial thickness, concluding that rotator cuff lesions are a natural correlate of ageing. Several asymptomatic tears can progress clinically [20, 24]. The onset of pain and reduced ability to perform activities of daily living [20, 24] can occur over a mean of 2.8 years [24] and may be associated with enlargement of the tear. Given the natural history of cuff tears, it has been proposed that monitoring tears size and pain should be applied to realize a secondary prevention intervention [24, 25].

Rotator cuff disease is particularly common in the working population [26], causing high healthcare costs in Western industrialized countries [6] and relevant costs for workers' compensation systems [7].

Epidemiological data on the association between mechanical overuse and cuff tearing are inconclusive. The prevalence rate of rotator cuff syndrome in workers range between 29% in those highly exposed to repetitive work, and 16% in those weakly exposed to repetitive work [27]. However, other studies show that 70% of patients with full-thickness tears undertake light work only [28].

Epidemiologic studies have helped to identify factors potentially associated with rotator cuff disease.

Genetics

Genetics has recently been investigated as a factor involved in the pathogenesis of rotator cuff pathology [29–32]. Different studies show its potential role in cuff disease, but investigations are still incomplete [33].

A familiar predisposition towards rotator cuff disease has been noted [20, 34–36]. Yamaguchi et al. [20] observed a strong trend between family history of rotator cuff tear (10.9% compared with 6.9%; p = 0.06) and risk of rotator cuff tear, in 586 patients who underwent diagnostic shoulder ultrasound for shoulder pain. Harvie et al. [35] compared the relative risk of full-thickness tears in siblings and spouses of 205 patients diagnosed as having full-thickness rotator cuff tears by ultrasound. Genetic susceptibility was demonstrated by the higher risk of full-thickness tears in siblings (2.42 compared with controls, 95% confidence interval 1.77–3.31). Moreover, siblings had a higher risk of experiencing symptoms (4.65 compared with controls, 95% confidence interval 2.42–8.63). The analysis of relatedness from a population-based, multigenerational level study show significantly elevated risks for first- and second-degree relatives [37]. It is particularly evident in relatives of young patients, who represent the best group to study genetic predisposition [37]. Accordingly, patients stratified by family history and matched for age, gender and environmental conditions show a different prevalence of rotator cuff tears [36].

Genetic factors also seem to be involved in symptom presentation [35, 36, 38, 39] and tear progression [36]. The relative risk of painful tear is 1.44 in siblings of symptomatic patients, compared to 1 in control subjects [36]. Heritable components of pain may present at any point of the sensorineural pathway of the cuff [35]. Pain may be associated with enlargement of the tear. The tendency of tear size to progress has been observed to be greater in siblings of patients over a period of 5 years [36]. Tear size was increased in 16.1% of siblings, compared with 1.5% of the control group [36].

Specific gene abnormalities have not been identified [34]. As rotator cuff disease is a multifactorial condition [40–51], it is difficult to select a single gene involved in its pathology. The main difficulty in genetic studies is to understand the interactions between gene products with each other and with the environment.

The phenotypic expression of genetic susceptibility may manifest in the ultrastructure of the tendon. Genetic factors have been hypothesized to influence structural components of the tendon. There is an association of Achilles tendon injuries with polymorphisms of tenascin C and collagen type Vα1 [50, 52–60]. Similar mechanisms may act in the pathogenesis of rotator cuff disease. Predisposing genes may also operate through apoptosis and regenerative capacity. Recently, a differential expression of members of the glutamate signalling cascades has been demonstrated in a rat model [61]. Glutamate has a proapoptitic effect in cultured tendon fibroblasts, and directly regulates the expression of apoptosis-related genes. Glutamate is upregulated in bone subjected to mechanical loading [62], and it seems to allow long-term changes in response to short-term mechanical stresses [63]. Overexcitation of these signalling mechanisms can cause tendinopathy.

Identification of predisposing genes may be helpful to define individuals at risk and to develop specific treatment for rotator cuff pathology.

Biological Factors

The study of cellular and molecular biology of tendon is increasing [64, 65], but still incomplete. Biological data integrate anatomical and physiological ideas on rotator cuff disease, leading to a comprehensive view of the condition [46, 47, 66–70]. Recent studies focus on the role of apoptosis in tendinopathy [71], analyzing its key mediators and cellular changes [72–76].

Apoptosis is a process of programmed cell death [77, 78]. It is induced by different chemical signals, such as glucocorticoids, growth factor withdrawal, reactive oxygen species, and cytokine [79], and is mediated by the interaction of caspases with intracellular substrates. Some evidence shows the potential contribution of apoptosis in tendinopathy, including rotator cuff disease [71, 80, 81]. The number of apoptotic cells in the torn edges of rotator cuff tendons is twice that of normal tendons [71]. Apoptotic cells are mainly fibroblast-like cell [71]. Chemical mediators of apoptosis are increased at the torn edges of tendons. Such mediators include caspases 3 and 8, belonging to a group of cysteine proteases for aspartic acid residues, which activate oxidative stress-induced apoptosis in human tendon fibroblasts [72]. There are also anti-apoptotic mediators that attempt to limit the degree of cellular death. cFLIP (cellular FLICE-inhibitory protein) blocks the recruitment and processing of caspase [73]. Hsp (heat-shock proteins) interfere with the caspase-driven apoptotic pathways [76]. Specifically, Hsp-27 inhibits cytochrome c and ATP-triggered activity of caspase 9. Hsp-70 prevents Apaf-1 interaction with the caspases. Moreover, they modulate intracellular glutathione [82], protect cells from heat stress [83], from the cytotoxic effects of TNF-α [84], and from nitric oxide [85].

Pro-inflammatory cytokines are upregulated in rat and human models of rotator cuff tendinopathy [75]. They are closely related to apoptosis, particularly in that induced by oxidative stress. In cyclically-loaded tenocytes, increased cytokine expression leads to the formation of highly reactive oxygen species, protein kinases and apoptotic mediators which cause cell apoptosis [86].

Oxidative stress is responsible for reduction of collagen synthesis. It leads to phosphorylation of JNK (c-Jun N-terminal protein kinase) that induces an apoptotic pathway and upregulates MMP1 that degrades tendon matrix. Following the early observations of high levels of MMP1 in the granulation tissue of the torn supraspinatus tendon in patients with a partial or total supraspinatus tendon rupture [87], subsequent studies showed strong phosphorylated JNK activity, accompanied by increased MMP1 activity in torn human supraspinatus tendon in vivo [74]. Chemical inhibitors of JNK could be considered a potential therapeutic agent in the failed healing response shown in tendinopathy.

This biomolecular evidence suggests a pathogenetic pathway secondary to exercise-induced oxidative stress. It could lead to apoptosis and weakened collagenous matrix, predisposing to tendinopathy and increased risk of tendon rupture.

Biological investigations have recently concerned new identified risk factors. Preliminary reports introduced the possible role of glucose as a risk factor for rotator cuff tear. Statistically significant higher fasting plasma glucose levels within the normoglycaemic range have been found in non-diabetic patients undergoing arthroscopic rotator cuff repair compared with patients of a similar age undergoing arthroscopic meniscectomy [88]. The non-enzymatic glycosylation processes changes collagen cross-links [89–91], and may have a causative role in tendinopathy. However, the role of this process in the pathogenesis of rotator cuff tears needs to be demonstrated. If further studies were to confirm the association between glucose and cuff disease, new approaches to the prevention and management of rotator cuff tears could be applied.

Some studies analyzed the correlation between serum levels of lipids and rotator cuff tears [92, 93]. The interest on this relationship arises from data of a possible role of high serum lipid concentration in complete rupture of the Achilles tendon [94–96]. Moreover, BMI has been considered a possible risk factor for rotator cuff pathology [97]. It would decrease vascularity through elevated cholesterol [98], atherosclerosis [99], diabetes, hypertension, metabolic syndrome and decreased physical activity [100]. Studies analyzing serum levels of lipid in patients with rotator cuff tears are discordant [92, 93]. A prospective study of patients with rotator cuff tendon tears showed higher levels of total cholesterol, triglycerides, low-density lipoprotein cholesterol, and lower levels of high-density lipoprotein cholesterol compared with patients with shoulder pain but without tears [92]. This data was not confirmed by histological/pathological evidence of cholesterol deposition. Another study found no statistically significant difference in serum triglyceride and total cholesterol concentrations between a group of patients undergoing arthroscopic rotator cuff repair and a group of patients of a similar age undergoing arthroscopic meniscectomy [93]. There was no evidence of fatty degeneration in tendon samples from the rotator cuff and the long head of the biceps tendon. More information is needed to clarify the topic. Actually no definitive conclusion on the role of serum cholesterol and triglyceride concentration in the pathogenesis of rotator cuff tears can be made.

Conclusions

Even though rotator cuff tears are frequent and several techniques have been developed for its management [101–119], there are no definitive data on epidemiology, genetics and biological factors in this field. An enhanced understanding of these factors holds the promise of new approaches to the prevention and management of these common conditions. Further studies are necessary to better clarify these aspects of rotator cuff disease.

References

1 Maffulli N, Longo UG, Gougoulias N, Loppini M, Denaro V: Long-term health outcomes of youth sports injuries. Br J Sports Med 2010;44:21–25.

2 Maffulli N, Longo UG, Gougoulias N, Caine D, Denaro V: Sport injuries: a review of outcomes. Br Med Bull 2011;97:47–80.

3 Maffulli N, Longo UG, Spiezia F, Denaro V: Sports injuries in young athletes: long-term outcome and prevention strategies. Phys Sportsmed 2010;38:29–34.

4 Maffulli N, Longo UG, Spiezia F, Denaro V: Aetiology and prevention of injuries in elite young athletes. Med Sport Sci 2011;56:187–200.

5 Urwin M, Symmons D, Allison T: Estimating the burden of musculoskeletal disease in the community. Ann Rheum Dis 1998;57:649–655.

6 Meislin RJ, Sperling JW, Stitik TP: Persistent shoulder pain: epidemiology, pathophysiology, and diagnosis. Am J Orthop (Belle Mead NJ) 2005;34:5–9.

7 Hegmann K, Moore J: Common neuromusculoskeletal disorders; in King PM (ed): Sourcebook of Occupational Rehabilitation. New York, Plenum Press, 1998, pp 30–32.

8 Neer CS 2nd: Impingement lesions. Clin Orthop Relat Res 1983;173:70–77.

9 DePalma A, Callery G, Bennett G: Variational anatomy in degenerative lesions of the shoulder joint. Instr Course Lect 1949;6:255–281.

10 Codman EA, Akerson IB: The pathology associated with rupture of the supraspinatus tendon. Ann Surg 1931;93:348–359.

11 DePalma A, White J, Callery G: Degenerative lesions of the shoulder joint at various age groups which are compatible with good function. Instr Course Lect 1950;7:168–180.

12 Fukuda H, Hamada K, Yamanaka K: Pathology and pathogenesis of bursal-side rotator cuff tears viewed from en bloc histologic sections. Clin Orthop Relat Res 1990:75–80.

13 Fukuda H, Mikasa M, Yamanaka K: Incomplete thickness rotator cuff tears diagnosed by subacromial bursography. Clin Orthop Relat Res 1987: 51–58.

14 Grant J, Smith G: Age incidence of rupture of the supraspinatus tendon. Anat Rec 1948;100:666.

15 Keyes E: Anatomic observations on senile changes in the shoulder. J Bone Joint Surg Am 1935;17:953–960.

16 Meyer A: Further evidences of attrition in the human body. Am J Anat 1924;34:241–267.

17 Quiniann E, Sinert R: Rotator cuff injury (available at http://wwwemadicinecom/emerg/tople512htm).

18 Keyes EL: Observations on rupture of the supraspinatus tendon: based upon a study of seventy-three cadavers. Ann Surg 1933;97:849–856.

19 Lehman C, Cuomo F, Kummer FJ, Zuckerman JD: The incidence of full-thickness rotator cuff tears in a large cadaveric population. Bull Hosp Jt Dis 1995;54:30–31.

20 Yamaguchi K, Ditsios K, Middleton W, Hildebolt C, Leesa M, Galatz, Teefey S: The demographic and morphological features of rotator cuff disease. A comparison of asymptomatic and symptomatic shoulders. J Bone Joint Surg Am 2006;88:1699–1704.

21 Petersson CJ: Ruptures of the supraspinatus tendon. Cadaver dissection. Acta Orthop Scand 1984;55: 52–56.

22 Milgrom C, Schaffler M, Gilbert S, Van Holsbeeck M: Rotator cuff changes in asymptomatic adults. The effect of age, hand dominance and gender. J Bone Joint Surg Br 1995;77-B:296–298.

23 Sher JS, Uribe JW, Posada A, Murphy BJ, Zlatkin MB: Abnormal findings on magnetic resonance images of asymptomatic shoulders. J Bone Joint Surg Am 1995;77:10–15.

24 Yamaguchi K, Tetro A, Blam O, Evanoff B, Teefey S, Middleton W: Natural history of asymptomatic rotator cuff tears: a longitudinal analysis of asymptomatic tears detected sonographically. J Shoulder Elbow Surg 2001;10:199–203.

25 Yamaguchi K, Lashgari C: Natural history of rotator cuff disorders and non-surgical treatment; in Norris TR (ed): Orthopaedic Knowledge Update: Shoulder and Elbow ed 2. Rosemont/IL, American Academy of Orthopaedic Surgeons, 2002, pp 155–162.

26 Roquelaure Y, Ha C, Leclerc A, Touranchet A, Sauteron M, Melchior M, Imbernon E, Goldberg M: Epidemiologic surveillance of upper-extremity musculoskeletal disorders in the working population. Arthritis Rheum 2006;55:765–778.

27 Leclerc A, Franchi P, Cristofari MF, Delemotte B, Mereau P, Teyssier-Cotte C, Touranchet A: Carpal tunnel syndrome and work organisation in repetitive work: a cross-sectional study in France. Study group on repetitive work. Occup Environ Med 1998;55:180–187.

28 Harryman DT 2nd, Hettrich CM, Smith KL, Campbell B, Sidles JA, Matsen FA 3rd: A prospective multipractice investigation of patients with full-thickness rotator cuff tears: the importance of comorbidities, practice, and other covariables on self-assessed shoulder function and health status. J Bone Joint Surg Am 2003;85:690–696.

29 Lippi G, Longo UG, Maffulli N: Genetics and sports. Br Med Bull 2010;93:27–47.

30 Longo UG, Fazio V, Poeta ML, Rabitti C, Franceschi F, Maffulli N, Denaro V: Bilateral consecutive rupture of the quadriceps tendon in a man with BstUI polymorphism of the COL5A1 gene. Knee Surg Sports Traumatol Arthrosc 2010;18:514–518.

31 Longo UG, Lamberti A, Maffulli N, Denaro V: Tendon augmentation grafts: a systematic review. Br Med Bull 2010;94:165–188.

32 Longo UG, Lamberti A, Maffulli N, Denaro V: Tissue engineered biological augmentation for tendon healing: a systematic review. Br Med Bull 2011;98:31–59.

33 Magra M, Maffulli N: Genetic aspects of tendinopathy. J Sci Med Sport 2008;11:243–247.

34 September AV, Schwellnus MP, Collins M: Tendon and ligament injuries: the genetic component. Br J Sports Med 2007;41:241–246.

35 Harvie P, Ostlere SJ, Teh J, McNally EG, Clipsham K, Burston BJ, Pollard TC, Carr AJ: Genetic influences in the aetiology of tears of the rotator cuff. Sibling risk of a full-thickness tear. J Bone Joint Surg Br 2004;86:696–700.

36 Gwilym SE, Watkins B, Cooper CD, Harvie P, Auplish S, Pollard TC, Rees JL, Carr AJ: Genetic influences in the progression of tears of the rotator cuff. J Bone Joint Surg Br 2009;91:915–917.

37 Tashjian RZ, Farnham JM, Albright FS, Teerlink CC, Cannon-Albright LA: Evidence for an inherited predisposition contributing to the risk for rotator cuff disease. J Bone Joint Surg Am 2009;91:1136–1142.

38 Foulkes T, Wood JN: Pain genes. PLoS Genet 2008; 4:e1000086.

39 Buskila D: Genetics of chronic pain states. Best Pract Res Clin Rheumatol 2007;21:535–547.

40 Denaro V, Ruzzini L, Longo UG, Franceschi F, De Paola B, Cittadini A, Maffulli N, Sgambato A: Effect of dihydrotestosterone on cultured human tenocytes from intact supraspinatus tendon. Knee Surg Sports Traumatol Arthrosc 2010;18:971–976.
41 Denaro V, Ruzzini L, Barnaba SA, Longo UG, Campi S, Maffulli N, Sgambato A: Effect of pulsed electromagnetic fields on human tenocyte cultures from supraspinatus and quadriceps tendons. Am J Phys Med Rehabil 2011;90:119–127.
42 Longo UG, Franceschi F, Ruzzini L, Rabitti C, Morini S, Maffulli N, Forriol F, Denaro V: Light microscopic histology of supraspinatus tendon ruptures. Knee Surg Sports Traumatol Arthrosc 2007; 15:1390–1394.
43 Longo UG, Franceschi F, Ruzzini L, Rabitti C, Morini S, Maffulli N, Denaro V: Histopathology of the supraspinatus tendon in rotator cuff tears. Am J Sports Med 2008;36:533–538.
44 Longo UG, Oliva F, Denaro V, Maffulli N: Oxygen species and overuse tendinopathy in athletes. Disabil Rehabil 2008;30:1563–1571.
45 Longo UG, Franceschi F, Ruzzini L, Rabitti C, Morini S, Maffulli N, Denaro V: Characteristics at haematoxylin and eosin staining of ruptures of the long head of the biceps tendon. Br J Sports Med 2009;43:603–607.
46 Longo UG, Forriol F, Campi S, Maffulli N, Denaro V: Animal models for translational research on shoulder pathologies: from bench to bedside. Sports Med Arthrosc 2011 (in press).
47 Longo UG, Berton A, Khan WS, Maffulli N, Denaro V: Histopathology of rotator cuff tears. Sports Med Arthrosc 2011 (in press).
48 Maffulli N, Longo UG, Franceschi F, Rabitti C, Denaro V: Movin and Bonar scores assess the same characteristics of tendon histology. Clin Orthop Relat Res 2008;466:1605–1611.
49 Maffulli N, Franceschi F, Longo UG, Ruzzini L, Denaro V: Clinical evidence for suture anchor repair of rotator cuff tears does add up: some just do not want to see it. Arthroscopy 2010;26:1568–1570.
50 Maffulli N, Longo UG, Denaro V: Novel approaches for the management of tendinopathy. J Bone Joint Surg Am 2010;92:2604–2613.
51 Maffulli N, Longo UG, Berton A, Loppini M, Denaro V: Biological factors in rotator cuff tears. Sports Med Arthrosc 2011 (in press).
52 Mokone GG, Schwellnus MP, Noakes TD, Collins M: The COL5A1 gene and Achilles tendon pathology. Scand J Med Sci Sports 2006;16:19–26.
53 Mokone GG, Gajjar M, September AV, Schwellnus MP, Greenberg J, Noakes TD, Collins M: The guanine-thymine dinucleotide repeat polymorphism within the tenascin-C gene is associated with Achilles tendon injuries. Am J Sports Med 2005;33: 1016–1021.
54 Longo UG, Ronga M, Maffulli N: Achilles tendinopathy. Sports Med Arthrosc 2009;17:112–126.
55 Longo UG, Ronga M, Maffulli N: Acute ruptures of the Achilles tendon. Sports Med Arthrosc 2009;17: 127–138.
56 Maffulli N, Ajis A, Longo UG, Denaro V: Chronic rupture of tendo achillis. Foot Ankle Clin 2007;12: 583–596, vi.
57 Maffulli N, Longo UG, Loppini M, Denaro V: Current treatment options for tendinopathy. Expert Opin Pharmacother 2010;11:2177–2186.
58 Maffulli N, Longo UG, Maffulli GD, Rabitti C, Khanna A, Denaro V: Marked pathological changes proximal and distal to the site of rupture in acute Achilles tendon ruptures. Knee Surg Sports Traumatol Arthrosc 2011;19:680–697.
59 Maffulli N, Longo UG, Maffulli GD, Khanna A, Denaro V: Achilles tendon ruptures in diabetic patients. Arch Orthop Trauma Surg 2011;131: 33–38.
60 Maffulli N, Longo UG, Maffulli GD, Khanna A: Achilles tendon ruptures in elite athletes. Foot Ankle Int 2011;32:9–15.
61 Molloy TJ, Kemp MW, Wang Y, Murrell GA: Microarray analysis of the tendinopathic rat supraspinatus tendon: glutamate signaling and its potential role in tendon degeneration. J Appl Physiol 2006;101:1702–1709.
62 Skerry TM: Identification of novel signaling pathways during functional adaptation of the skeleton to mechanical loading: the role of glutamate as a paracrine signaling agent in the skeleton. J Bone Mineral Metabol 1999;17:66–70.
63 Spencer GJ, Genever PG: Long-term potentiation in bone – a role for glutamate in strain-induced cellular memory? BMC Cell Biol 2003;4:9.
64 Castricini R, Longo UG, De Benedetto M, Panfoli N, Pirani P, Zini R, Maffulli N, Denaro V: Platelet-rich plasma augmentation for arthroscopic rotator cuff repair: a randomized controlled trial. Am J Sports Med 2011;39:258–265.
65 Forriol F, Longo UG, Concejo C, Ripalda P, Maffulli N, Denaro V: Platelet-rich plasma, rhOP-1 (rhBMP-7) and frozen rib allograft for the reconstruction of bony mandibular defects in sheep. A pilot experimental study. Injury 2009;40(suppl 3):S44–S49.
66 Longo UG, Buchmann S, Berton A, Maffulli N, Denaro V: Arthroscopic knots and strength sutures for rotator cuff repair. Sports Med Arthrosc Rev 2011 (in press).
67 Longo UG, Berton A, Alexander S, Maffulli N, Wallace AL, Denaro V: Biological resurfacing for early osteoarthritis of the shoulder. Sports Med Arthrosc 2011 (in press).
68 Longo UG, Vasta S, Maffulli N, Denaro V: Scoring systems for the functional assessment of patients with rotator cuff pathology. Sports Med Arthrosc 2011 (in press).

69 Longo UG, Lamberti A, Khan WS, Maffulli N, Denaro V: Synthetic augmentation for massive rotator cuff tears. Sports Med Arthrosc 2011 (in press).
70 Khan WS, Longo UG, Ahrens PM, Denaro V, Maffulli N: A systematic review of the reverse shoulder replacement in rotator cuff arthropathy, rotator cuff tears and rheumatoid arthritis. Sports Med Arthrosc 2011 (in press).
71 Yuan J, Murrell GA, Wei AQ, Wang MX: Apoptosis in rotator cuff tendonopathy. J Orthop Res 2002;20: 1372–1379.
72 Yuan J, Murrell GA, Trickett A, Wang MX: Involvement of cytochrome c release and caspase-3 activation in the oxidative stress-induced apoptosis in human tendon fibroblasts. Biochim Biophys Acta 2003;1641:35–41.
73 Tran SE, Meinander A, Holmstrom TH, Rivero-Muller A, Heiskanen KM, Linnau EK, Courtney MJ, Mosser DD, Sistonen L, Eriksson JE: Heat stress downregulates flip and sensitizes cells to fas receptor-mediated apoptosis. Cell Death Differ 2003;10:1137–1147.
74 Wang F, Murrell GA, Wang MX: Oxidative stress-induced c-Jun N-terminal kinase (JNK) activation in tendon cells upregulates MMP1 mRNA and protein expression. J Orthop Res 2007;25:378–389.
75 Millar NL, Wei AQ, Molloy TJ, Bonar F, Murrell GA: Cytokines and apoptosis in supraspinatus tendinopathy. J Bone Joint Surg Br 2009;91:417–424.
76 Millar NL, Wei AQ, Molloy TJ, Bonar F, Murrell GA: Heat-shock protein and apoptosis in supraspinatus tendinopathy. Clin Orthop Relat Res 2008;466: 1569–1576.
77 Cohen JJ: Apoptosis. Immunol Today 1993;14:126–130.
78 White E: Life, death, and the pursuit of apoptosis. Genes Dev 1996;10:1–15.
79 Tsan MF, Gao B: Cytokine function of heat-shock proteins. Am J Physiol Cell Physiol 2004;286: C739–C744.
80 Lian O, Scott A, Engebretsen L, Bahr R, Duronio V, Khan K: Excessive apoptosis in patellar tendinopathy in athletes. Am J Sports Med 2007;35:605–611.
81 Scott A, Khan KM, Heer J, Cook JL, Lian O, Duronio V: High strain mechanical loading rapidly induces tendon apoptosis: an ex vivo rat tibialis anterior model. Br J Sports Med 2005;39:e25.
82 Leeuwenburgh C, Hollander J, Leichtweis S, Griffiths M, Gore M, Ji LL: Adaptations of glutathione antioxidant system to endurance training are tissue and muscle fiber specific. Am J Physiol 1997;272:R363–R369.
83 Mosser DD, Caron AW, Bourget L, Denis-Larose C, Massie B: Role of the human heat-shock protein hsp70 in protection against stress-induced apoptosis. Mol Cell Biol 1997;17:5317–5327.
84 Jäättelä M, Wissing D, Bauer PA, Li GC: Major heat-shock protein hsp70 protects tumor cells from tumor necrosis factor cytotoxicity. EMBO J 1992;11: 3507–3512.
85 Bellmann K, Jäättelä M, Wissing D, Burkart V, Kolb H: Heat-shock protein hsp70 overexpression confers resistance against nitric oxide. FEBS Lett 1996;391:185–188.
86 Nguyen MT, Lue H, Kleemann R, Thiele M, Tolle G, Finkelmeier D, Wagner E, Braun A, Bernhagen J: The cytokine macrophage migration inhibitory factor reduces pro-oxidative stress-induced apoptosis. J Immunol 2003;170:3337–3347.
87 Gotoh M, Hamada K, Yamakawa H, Tomonaga A, Inoue A, Fukuda H: Significance of granulation tissue in torn supraspinatus insertions: an immunohistochemical study with antibodies against interleukin-1β, cathepsin D, and matrix metalloprotease-1. J Orthop Res 1997;15:33–39.
88 Longo UG, Franceschi F, Ruzzini L, Spiezia F, Maffulli N, Denaro V: Higher fasting plasma glucose levels within the normoglycaemic range and rotator cuff tears. Br J Sports Med 2009;43:284–287.
89 Reddy GK: Glucose-mediated in vitro glycation modulates biomechanical integrity of the soft tissues but not hard tissues. J Orthop Res 2003;21:738–743.
90 Reddy GK, Stehno-Bittel L, Enwemeka CS: Glycation-induced matrix stability in the rabbit Achilles tendon. Arch Biochem Biophys 2002;399: 174–180.
91 Bai P, Phua K, Hardt T, Cernadas M, Brodsky B: Glycation alters collagen fibril organization. Connect Tissue Res 1992;28:1–12.
92 Abboud JA, Kim JS: The effect of hypercholesterolemia on rotator cuff disease. Clin Orthop Relat Res 2010;468:1493–1497.
93 Longo UG, Franceschi F, Spiezia F, Forriol F, Maffulli N, Denaro V: Triglycerides and total serum cholesterol in rotator cuff tears: do they matter? Br J Sports Med 2010;44:948–951.
94 Mathiak G, Wening JV, Mathiak M, Neville LF, Jungbluth K: Serum cholesterol is elevated in patients with Achilles tendon ruptures. Arch Orthop Trauma Surg 1999;119:280–284.
95 Ozgurtas T, Yildiz C, Serdar M, Atesalp S, Kutluay T: Is high concentration of serum lipids a risk factor for Achilles tendon rupture? Clin Chim Acta 2003;331:25–28.
96 Ames PR, Longo UG, Denaro V, Maffulli N: Achilles tendon problems: not just an orthopaedic issue. Disabil Rehabil 2008;30:1646–1650.
97 Wendelboe AM, Hegmann KT, Gren LH, Alder SC, White GL Jr, Lyon JL: Associations between body-mass index and surgery for rotator cuff tendinitis. J Bone Joint Surg Am 2004;86-A:743–747.

98 Kim K, Owen W, Williams D, et al: A comparison between BMI and conicity index on predicting coronary heart disease: The Framingham Heart Study. Ann Epidemiol 2000;10:424–431.
99 Hubert HB, Feinleib M, McNamara PM, Castelli WP: Obesity as an independent risk factor for cardiovascular disease: a 26-year follow-up of participants in The Framingham Heart Study. Circulation 1983;67:968–977.
100 Siervogel RM, Wisemandle W, Maynard LM, Guo SS, Chumlea WC, Towne B: Lifetime overweight status in relation to serial changes in body composition and risk factors for cardiovascular disease: The Fels Longitudinal Study. Obes Res 2000;8:422–430.
101 Franceschi F, Longo UG, Ruzzini L, Rizzello G, Denaro V: Arthroscopic management of calcific tendinitis of the subscapularis tendon. Knee Surg Sports Traumatol Arthrosc 2007;15:1482–1485.
102 Franceschi F, Ruzzini L, Longo UG, Martina FM, Zobel BB, Maffulli N, Denaro V: Equivalent clinical results of arthroscopic single-row and double-row suture anchor repair for rotator cuff tears: a randomized controlled trial. Am J Sports Med 2007;35: 1254–1260.
103 Franceschi F, Longo UG, Ruzzini L, Rizzello G, Maffulli N, Denaro V: The Roman bridge: a 'double pulley-suture bridges' technique for rotator cuff repair. BMC Musculoskelet Disord 2007;8:123.
104 Franceschi F, Longo UG, Ruzzini L, Papalia R, Rizzello G, Denaro V: To detach the long head of the biceps tendon after tenodesis or not: outcome analysis at the 4-year follow-up of two different techniques. Int Orthop 2007;31:537–545.
105 Franceschi F, Longo UG, Ruzzini L, Rizzello G, Maffulli N, Denaro V: Arthroscopic salvage of failed arthroscopic Bankart repair: a prospective study with a minimum follow-up of 4 years. Am J Sports Med 2008;36:1330–1336.
106 Franceschi F, Longo UG, Ruzzini L, Morini S, Battistoni F, Dicuonzo G, Maffulli N, Denaro V: Circulating substance p levels and shoulder joint contracture after arthroscopic repair of the rotator cuff. Br J Sports Med 2008;42:742–745.
107 Franceschi F, Longo UG, Ruzzini L, Rizzello G, Maffulli N, Denaro V: No advantages in repairing a type II superior labrum anterior and posterior lesion when associated with rotator cuff repair in patients over age 50: a randomized controlled trial. Am J Sports Med 2008;36:247–253.
108 Franceschi F, Longo UG, Ruzzini L, Rizzello G, Maffulli N, Denaro V: Soft tissue tenodesis of the long head of the biceps tendon associated to the Roman bridge repair. BMC Musculoskelet Disord 2008;9:78.
109 Longo UG, Franceschi F, Spiezia F, Marinozzi A, Maffulli N, Denaro V: The low- profile Roman bridge technique for knotless double- row repair of the rotator cuff. Arch Orthop Trauma Surg 2011; 131:357–361.
110 Longo UG, Ramamurthy C, Denaro V, Maffulli N: Minimally invasive stripping for chronic Achilles tendinopathy. Disabil Rehabil 2008;30:1709–1713.
111 Khanna A, Friel M, Gougoulias N, Longo UG, Maffulli N: Prevention of adhesions in surgery of the flexor tendons of the hand: what is the evidence? Br Med Bull 2009;90:85–109.
112 Franceschi F, Marinozzi A, Papalia R, Longo UG, Gualdi G, Denaro E: Intra- and juxta-articular osteoid osteoma: a diagnostic challenge: misdiagnosis and successful treatment: a report of four cases. Arch Orthop Trauma Surg 2006;126:660–667.
113 Maffulli N, Longo UG, Gougoulias N, Denaro V: Ipsilateral free semitendinosus tendon graft transfer for reconstruction of chronic tears of the Achilles tendon. BMC Musculoskelet Disord 2008;9:100.
114 Maffulli N, Walley G, Sayana MK, Longo UG, Denaro V: Eccentric calf muscle training in athletic patients with Achilles tendinopathy. Disabil Rehabil 2008;30:1677–1684.
115 Longo UG, Rittweger J, Garau G, Radonic B, Gutwasser C, Gilliver SF, Kusy K, Zieliński J, Felsenberg D, Maffulli N: No influence of age, gender, weight, height, and impact profile in achilles tendinopathy in masters track and field athletes. Am J Sports Med 2009;37:1400–1405.
116 Maffulli N, Longo UG: Conservative management for tendinopathy: is there enough scientific evidence? Rheumatology 2008;47:390–391.
117 Maffulli N, Longo UG: How do eccentric exercises work in tendinopathy? Rheumatology 2008;47: 1444–1445.
118 Maffulli N, Longo UG, Ronga M, Khanna A, Denaro V: Favorable outcome of percutaneous repair of achilles tendon ruptures in the elderly. Clin Orthop Relat Res 2010; 468:1039–1046.
119 Longo UG, King JB, Denaro V, Maffulli N: Double-bundle arthroscopic reconstruction of the anterior cruciate ligament: does the evidence add up? J Bone Joint Surg Br 2008;90:995–999.

Nicola Maffulli, MD, MS, PhD, FRCS(Orth)
Centre for Sports and Exercise Medicine
Barts and The London School of Medicine and Dentistry
Mile End Hospital, 275 Bancroft Road, London E1 4DG (UK)
Tel. +44 20 8223 8839, E-Mail n.maffulli@qmul.ac.uk

Maffulli N (ed): Rotator Cuff Tear. Med Sport Sci. Basel, Karger, 2012, vol 57, pp 10–17

Biomechanics of the Rotator Cuff: European Perspective

Umile Giuseppe Longo[a,b] · Alessandra Berton[a,b] · Nicola Papapietro[a,b] · Nicola Maffulli[c] · Vincenzo Denaro[a,b]

[a]Department of Orthopaedic and Trauma Surgery and [b]Centro Integrato di Ricerca (CIR), Campus Bio-Medico University, Rome, Italy; [c]Centre for Sports and Exercise Medicine, Queen Mary University of London, Barts and The London School of Medicine and Dentistry, Mile End Hospital, London, UK

Abstract

The rotator cuff has an important role in the stability and function of the glenohumeral joint. To understand the biomechanical proprieties of the rotator cuff, it is essential to understand the pathogenesis and effects of rotator cuff tears. The rotator cuff provides a stabilizing effect to the shoulder, because of compression of the humeral head against the glenoid cavity. The wide range of motion of the shoulder is allowed by the variety of rotational moments of the cuff muscles. Rotator cuff muscles action must be precisely coordinated to obtain the desired movement. Rotator cuff tendons are subjected to complex tension loads. The rotator cuff is also subjected to compressive loads. Upwardly directed humeral load squeezes the cuff between the humeral head and the coracoacromial arch. Extrinsic factors have always been considered among causes of cuff tears. However, evidence shows that acromial impingement is not the primary cause of rotator cuff tears. Tears of the rotator cuff change load distribution and determine a pattern that induces tear progression and extension. Progressive tears of the rotator cuff compromise glenohumeral stability and determine superior translation of the humeral head.

Biomechanical Properties of the Rotator Cuff

The rotator cuff has an important role in the stability and function of the glenohumeral joint. Understanding the biomechanical proprieties of the rotator cuff is essential to understand the pathogenesis and effects of rotator cuff tears.

The rotator cuff has different functions. It provides a stabilizing effect of the shoulder, because of compression of the humeral head against the glenoid cavity [1, 2]. This mechanism, known as 'concavity compression', is allowed by the antagonistic forces of the subscapularis anteriorly, and infraspinatus and teres minor posteriorly

[3–6]. Studies have demonstrated superior glenohumeral instability when rotator cuff paralysis was simulated [7].

The humeroscapular articulation can be considered as consisting of two concentric spheres: the spherical proximal humeral convexity, constituted by the tuberosities and the superficial surface of the rotator cuff tendons, that articulates with the undersurface of the coracoacromial arch, and the spherical humeral articular surface, that articulates with the glenoid. The rotator cuff serves as a spacer that determines the different radius of the two spheres. This geometrical conformation enhances shoulder stability and scapulohumeral load transfer. Degeneration of cuff tendon, tightness of the posterior inferior capsule, and incongruent coracoacromial undersurface cause loss of the concentricity of the spheres, leading the humeral head to anterosuperior translation [8].

The rotator cuff has also the function to rotate the humerus with respect to the scapula. The wide range of motion of the shoulder is allowed by the variety of rotational moments of the cuff muscles, whose tendons insert continuously around the humeral head. The position of the joint influences both the direction and the force of cuff muscles. Depending on the initial position of the arm, the supraspinatus can determine abduction and/or external rotation [9]. At higher glenohumeral angles, the supraspinatus has a major role in elevation, while at lower glenohumeral angles the deltoid contribution to initial elevation is greater [10]. In external and internal humeral rotation, the subscapularis and infraspinatus also play a role in abduction [9]. The force and torque that a muscle can generate vary with the position of the joint. At the extremes of the range of motion, the muscles of the rotator cuff are weaker, because they are fully contracted or extended, while maximal force is in the middle of their excursion.

The action of the muscles of the rotator cuff must be precisely coordinated to obtain the desired movement [11]. As in the shoulder there is not a fixed axis of rotation, muscular functions must be balanced. Shoulder muscles must work together to produce a net torque and neutralize opposed elements. The superior portion of the cuff and the deltoid are needed to neutralize the adduction of the latissimus dorsi when pure internal rotation is required. Conversely, posterior cuff and posterior deltoid muscles are needed to neutralize the internal rotation moment of the same muscle when pure adduction is required. The action of the posterior deltoid and infraspinatus are needed to neutralize cross-body and internal rotation moments of the anterior deltoid when forward elevation without rotation is required [6].

The rotator cuff tendons are subjected to complex tension loads. Concentric tension loads are generated when the direction of the humerus is the same of cuff muscle, as in abduction against resistance. These loads are better tolerated by the cuff insertion which clears the acromion at low angles of elevation, protecting it from impingement by the coracoacromial arch. Eccentric tension loads are produced when humeral motion is opposed to the direction of action of the cuff muscles, as in active resistance to a downward force imposed on the arm. Bending loads continuously stress cuff tendons when the humeral head rotates with respect to the scapula. Cuff elasticity allows it to resist these loads. The tendons of the rotator cuff are also subjected to compressive loads. An upwardly directed humeral load squeezes the cuff between the humeral head and the coracoacromial arch. Tendon compression has been demonstrated in vivo. Subacromial pressure is 8 mm Hg at rest, 39 mm Hg at 45° of flexion, and 56 mm Hg with the arm in an elevated position with 1 kg weight held in the hand [12]. Moreover, a morphologic adaptation of the supraspinatus tendon to mechanical forces has been shown, with fibrocartilaginous areas in regions of compression [13].

Role of Mechanical Factors in Rotator Cuff Tears

The aetiology of rotator cuff tears is multifactorial [14–27]. Extrinsic factors have classically been considered among the causes of rotator cuff tears [27–36]. Their role in the pathogenesis of rotator cuff tears has been better defined and takes alongside to that of intrinsic factors, such as biologic degeneration and no vascularization of tendons [27, 31, 33, 34, 36–39].

The theory of subacromial impingement was first described by Neer and Poppen [40], who observed that 'the area of degeneration and rupture was concentrated on the supraspinatus tendon. On forward elevation this area abutted against the coraco-acromial ligament, the anterior acromion and sometimes the acromio-clavicular joint'. Later, a correlation between acromial shape and cuff disease was hypothesized [41–43]. In a cadaver study, Bigliani et al. [44] found full-thickness tears in 33% of cases. Tears were associated in 73% of cases with a type III acromion (hooked), in 24% of cases with type II (curved) and in 3% with type I (flat). However, acromial impingement is not the primary cause of rotator cuff tears [18–22, 26, 35, 38]. Acromial impingement is associated with changes on the bursal side of the rotator cuff, which is less frequently damaged than the intratendinous or articular side [45]. Acromioplasty does not avoid the occurrence of rotator cuff tears, leading to damage of tendons in 20% of cases [46]. Acromial changes seem to be secondary to pathology of the bursal side of the cuff [47, 48], and a type II and III acromion are acquired rather than developmental [49]. An acromial hook is produced by traction induced by cuff degeneration [42]. It results in a greater load on the coracoacromial arch, producing traction spurs in the coracoacromial ligament [50].

Defects of the deep surface of the rotator cuff are common in throwers, who require to achieve large ranges of external rotation. The mechanism of cuff injury is explained by the abutment of the edge of the glenoid against the deep surface of tendon insertion at the extreme of rotation [51–56]. Magnetic resonance imaging with the arm positioned at the limits of motion can show contact between the acromion and the humerus distal to the cuff insertion, and abutment of the undersurface of the supraspinatus tendon against the superior glenoid fossa.

Effects of Injury

Lesions of the rotator cuff change load distribution and determine a pattern that induces tear progression and extension [57–64]. Rotator cuff tears typically start at the deep surface of the anterior insertion of the supraspinatus, close to the long head of the biceps. This site is subject to greater loads, even at rest. Fibres fail when load exceeds their strength, increasing load on the neighbouring structures. The ability to repair decreases because of weakening of the cuff and subsequent increased loads. Even when scar tissue forms, its strength is not enough to resist subsequent loads. Partial thickness tears predisposes to further damage of the remaining rotator cuff. A tear of 60% of the tendon thickness increases of 23.8% tensile strain in the posterior tendon [65]. Tears of the inferior aspect of the articular side of the tendon increase strain in the middle and superior portions of the supraspinatus [66]. As the risk of failure increases and the degenerative process continues, a full-thickness defect is produced in the anterior supraspinatus tendon. Loads are concentrated at the margin of the tear, facilitating extension of the defect. Lower loads induce additional fibre failure because of a vicious circle correlated with tendon degeneration and inability to heal. Supraspinatus defects propagate posteriorly through the remainder of the supraspinatus and the infraspinatus.

Progressive dissolution of the rotator cuff compromises glenohumeral stability provided by the concavity compression mechanism, and the humeral head translates superiorly [67, 68]. This is a most important biomechanical consequence of rotator cuff tears, and represents the main radiograph signs of massive cuff deficiency [69], with narrowing of the acromiohumeral interval from loss of the interposed superior cuff tendon, a phenomenon known as the 'spacer' effect of the cuff tendon [50]. Different studies demonstrate 6 mm of proximal translation of the humeral head when the cuff tendon is absent [70]. It can result in 'acetabularization' of the undersurface of the acromion. The residual cuff is squeezed between the head and the coracoacromial arch, and traction spurs develop in the coracoacromial ligament. The displaced humeral head erodes the upper glenoid lip and labrum, reducing the superior glenoid concavity, further allowing humeral head translation. These elements further contribute to cuff degeneration.

The dynamic function of the rotator cuff is obviously compromised by tears. External rotation and elevation are primarily decreased [70–73]. Some studies show a decrease of 5% in abduction force after tears of one third and two thirds of the supraspinatus, and of 17% after compete detachment of the tendon. Other simulations show losses of 19, 36, and 58% after retraction of one third, two thirds, and the entire supraspinatus, respectively [74].

Biomechanical Factors in Rotator Cuff Repair

Some biomechanical factors should be taken into account in rotator cuff repair. Superior stability of the shoulder is one of the main problems associated with rotator cuff tears [75]. The action of infraspinatus and subscapularis is more effective than that of the supraspinatus in concavity compression. Thus, they should be repaired whenever possible to prevent humeral head translation and associated problems [76]. A graft can be considered in patients with massive rotator cuff tears [77–80]. Growth factors did not show improvement of tendon healing, even though further studies are required [75, 81]. When the superior glenoid concavity is reduced because of humeral head erosion, the tendency to superior subluxation cannot be reversed by cuff repair surgery. In these patients, shoulder replacement can be an option [82–93].

References

1 Bassett RW, Browne AO, Morrey BF, An KN: Glenohumeral muscle force and moment mechanics in a position of shoulder instability. J Biomech 1990;23:405–415.

2 Karduna AR, Williams GR, Williams JL, Iannotti JP: Kinematics of the glenohumeral joint: influences of muscle forces, ligamentous constraints, and articular geometry. J Orthop Res 1996;14:986–993.

3 Lippitt S, Matsen F: Mechanisms of glenohumeral joint stability. Clin Orthop Relat Res 1993:20–28.

4 Soslowsky LJ, Carpenter JE, Bucchieri JS, Flatow EL: Biomechanics of the rotator cuff. Orthop Clin North Am 1997;28:17–30.

5 Wuelker N, Roetman B, Plitz W, Knop C: Function of the supraspinatus muscle in a dynamic shoulder model (in German). Unfallchirurg 1994;97:308–313.

6 Sharkey NA, Marder RA, Hanson PB: The entire rotator cuff contributes to elevation of the arm. J Orthop Res 1994;12:699–708.

7 Thompson WO, Debski RE, Boardman ND 3rd, Taskiran E, Warner JJ, Fu FH, Woo SL: A biomechanical analysis of rotator cuff deficiency in a cadaveric model. Am J Sports Med 1996;24:286–292.

8 Harryman DT 2nd, Sidles JA, Clark JM, McQuade KJ, Gibb TD, Matsen FA 3rd: Translation of the humeral head on the glenoid with passive glenohumeral motion. J Bone Joint Surg Am 1990;72:1334–1343.

9 Otis JC, Jiang CC, Wickiewicz TL, Peterson MG, Warren RF, Santner TJ: Changes in the moment arms of the rotator cuff and deltoid muscles with abduction and rotation. J Bone Joint Surg Am 1994;76:667–676.

10 Liu J, Hughes RE, Smutz WP, Niebur G, Nan-An K: Roles of deltoid and rotator cuff muscles in shoulder elevation. Clin Biomech (Bristol, Avon) 1997;12:32–38.

11 Rowlands LK, Wertsch JJ, Primack SJ, Spreitzer AM, Roberts MM: Kinesiology of the empty can test. Am J Phys Med Rehabil 1995;74:302–304.

12 Sigholm G, Styf J, Korner L, Herberts P: Pressure recording in the subacromial bursa. J Orthop Res 1988;6:123–128.

13 Okuda Y, Gorski JP, An KN, Amadio PC: Biochemical, histological, and biomechanical analyses of canine tendon. J Orthop Res 1987;5:60–68.

14 Denaro V, Ruzzini L, Longo UG, Franceschi F, De Paola B, Cittadini A, Maffulli N, Sgambato A: Effect of dihydrotestosterone on cultured human tenocytes from intact supraspinatus tendon. Knee Surg Sports Traumatol Arthrosc 2010;18:971–976.

15 Denaro V, Ruzzini L, Barnaba SA, Longo UG, Campi S, Maffulli N, Sgambato A: Effect of pulsed electromagnetic fields on human tenocyte cultures from supraspinatus and quadriceps tendons. Am J Phys Med Rehabil 2011;90:119–127.

16 Franceschi F, Longo UG, Ruzzini L, Morini S, Battistoni F, Dicuonzo G, Maffulli N, Denaro V: Circulating substance P levels and shoulder joint contracture after arthroscopic repair of the rotator cuff. Br J Sports Med 2008;42:742–745.

17 Lippi G, Longo UG, Maffulli N: Genetics and sports. Br Med Bull 2010;93:27–47.

18 Longo UG, Franceschi F, Ruzzini L, Rabitti C, Morini S, Maffulli N, Forriol F, Denaro V: Light microscopic histology of supraspinatus tendon ruptures. Knee Surg Sports Traumatol Arthrosc 2007;15:1390–1394.

19 Longo UG, Franceschi F, Ruzzini L, Rabitti C, Morini S, Maffulli N, Denaro V: Histopathology of the supraspinatus tendon in rotator cuff tears. Am J Sports Med 2008;36:533–538.
20 Longo UG, Oliva F, Denaro V, Maffulli N: Oxygen species and overuse tendinopathy in athletes. Disabil Rehabil 2008;30:1563–1571.
21 Longo UG, Franceschi F, Ruzzini L, Rabitti C, Morini S, Maffulli N, Denaro V: Characteristics at haematoxylin and eosin staining of ruptures of the long head of the biceps tendon. Br J Sports Med 2009;43:603–607.
22 Longo UG, Franceschi F, Ruzzini L, Spiezia F, Maffulli N, Denaro V: Higher fasting plasma glucose levels within the normoglycaemic range and rotator cuff tears. Br J Sports Med 2009;43:284–287.
23 Longo UG, Franceschi F, Spiezia F, Forriol F, Maffulli N, Denaro V: Triglycerides and total serum cholesterol in rotator cuff tears: do they matter? Br J Sports Med 2010;44:948–951.
24 Longo UG, Forriol F, Campi S, Maffulli N, Denaro V: Animal models for translational research on shoulder pathologies: from bench to bedside. Sports Med Arthrosc 2011 (in press).
25 Longo UG, Berton A, Alexander S, Maffulli N, Wallace AL, Denaro V: Biological resurfacing for early osteoarthritis of the shoulder. Sports Med Arthrosc 2011 (in press).
26 Longo UG, Berton A, Khan WS, Maffulli N, Denaro V: Histopathology of rotator cuff tears. Sports Med Arthrosc 2011 (in press).
27 Maffulli N, Longo UG, Franceschi F, Rabitti C, Denaro V: Movin and Bonar scores assess the same characteristics of tendon histology. Clin Orthop Relat Res 2008;466:1605–1611.
28 Maffulli N, Longo UG: Conservative management for tendinopathy: is there enough scientific evidence? Rheumatology (Oxford) 2008;47:390–391.
29 Maffulli N, Longo UG: How do eccentric exercises work in tendinopathy? Rheumatology (Oxford) 2008;47:1444–1445.
30 Maffulli N, Franceschi F, Longo UG, Ruzzini L, Denaro V: Clinical evidence for suture anchor repair of rotator cuff tears does add up: some just do not want to see it. Arthroscopy 2010;26:1568–1570.
31 Maffulli N, Longo UG, Loppini M, Denaro V: Current treatment options for tendinopathy. Expert Opin Pharmacother 2010;11:2177–2186.
32 Maffulli N, Longo UG, Gougoulias N, Loppini M, Denaro V: Long-term health outcomes of youth sports injuries. Br J Sports Med 2010;44:21–25.
33 Maffulli N, Longo UG, Gougoulias N, Caine D, Denaro V: Sport injuries: a review of outcomes. Br Med Bull 2011;97:47–80.
34 Maffulli N, Longo UG, Spiezia F, Denaro V: Sports injuries in young athletes: long-term outcome and prevention strategies. Phys Sportsmed 2010;38: 29–34.
35 Maffulli N, Longo UG, Spiezia F, Denaro V: Aetiology and prevention of injuries in elite young athletes. Med Sport Sci 2011;56:187–200.
36 Maffulli N, Longo UG, Berton A, Loppini M, Denaro V: Biological factors in rotator cuff tears. Sports Med Arthrosc 2011 (in press).
37 Maffulli N, Longo UG, Maffulli GD, Rabitti C, Khanna A, Denaro V: Marked pathological changes proximal and distal to the site of rupture in acute Achilles tendon ruptures. Knee Surg Sports Traumatol Arthrosc 2011;19:680–687.
38 Maffulli N, Longo UG, Denaro V: Novel approaches for the management of tendinopathy. J Bone Joint Surg Am 2010;92:2604–2613.
39 Rizzello G, Franceschi F, Longo UG, Ruzzini L, Meloni MC, Spiezia F, Papalia R, Denaro V: Arthroscopic management of calcific tendinopathy of the shoulder – do we need to remove all the deposit? Bull NYU Hosp Jt Dis 2009;67:330–333.
40 Neer C, Poppen N: Supraspinatus outlet. Orthop Trans 1987;11:234.
41 Bigliani LU, Ticker JB, Flatow EL, Soslowsky LJ, Mow VC: The relationship of acromial architecture to rotator cuff disease. Clin Sports Med 1991;10:823–838.
42 Neer CS 2nd: Anterior acromioplasty for the chronic impingement syndrome in the shoulder: a preliminary report. J Bone Joint Surg Am 1972;54:41–50.
43 Bigliani L, Norris T, Fischer J: The relationship between the unfused acromial epiphysis and subacromial impingement lesions. Orthop Trans 1983;7:138.
44 Bigliani L, Morrison D, April E: The morphology of the acromion and rotator cuff impingement. Orthop Trans 1986;10:228.
45 Schneeberger AG, Nyffeler RW, Gerber C: Structural changes of the rotator cuff caused by experimental subacromial impingement in the rat. J Shoulder Elbow Surg 1998;7:375–380.
46 Hyvonen P, Lohi S, Jalovaara P: Open acromioplasty does not prevent the progression of an impingement syndrome to a tear. Nine-year follow-up of 96 cases. J Bone Joint Surg Br 1998;80:813–816.
47 Ozaki J, Fujimoto S, Nakagawa Y, Masuhara K, Tamai S: Tears of the rotator cuff of the shoulder associated with pathological changes in the acromion. A study in cadavera. J Bone Joint Surg Am 1988;70:1224–1230.

48 Fukuda H, Hamada K, Nakajima T, Tomonaga A: Pathology and pathogenesis of the intratendinous tearing of the rotator cuff viewed from en bloc histologic sections. Clin Orthop Relat Res 1994: 60–67.

49 Yazici M, Kopuz C, Gulman B: Morphologic variants of acromion in neonatal cadavers. J Pediatr Orthop 1995;15:644–647.

50 Flatow EL, Soslowsky LJ, Ticker JB, Pawluk RJ, Hepler M, Ark J, Mow VC, Bigliani LU: Excursion of the rotator cuff under the acromion. Patterns of subacromial contact. Am J Sports Med 1994;22: 779–788.

51 Ferrari JD, Ferrari DA, Coumas J, Pappas AM: Posterior ossification of the shoulder: The Bennett lesion. Etiology, diagnosis, and treatment. Am J Sports Med 1994;22:171–176.

52 Jobe CM: Posterior superior glenoid impingement: expanded spectrum. Arthroscopy 1995;11:530–536.

53 Liu SH, Boynton E: Posterior superior impingement of the rotator cuff on the glenoid rim as a cause of shoulder pain in the overhead athlete. Arthroscopy 1993;9:697–699.

54 Rossi F, Ternamian PJ, Cerciello G, Walch G: Posterosuperior glenoid rim impingement in athletes: the diagnostic value of traditional radiology and magnetic resonance (in Italian). Radiol Med 1994;87:22–27.

55 Tirman PF, Bost FW, Garvin GJ, Peterfy CG, Mall JC, Steinbach LS, Feller JF, Crues JV 3rd: Posterosuperior glenoid impingement of the shoulder: findings at MR imaging and MR arthrography with arthroscopic correlation. Radiology 1994;193: 431–436.

56 Walch G, Liotard JP, Boileau P, Noel E: Posterosuperior glenoid impingement. Another shoulder impingement (in French). Rev Chir Orthop Reparatrice Appar Mot 1991;77:571–574.

57 Franceschi F, Longo UG, Ruzzini L, Rizzello G, Denaro V: Arthroscopic management of calcific tendinitis of the subscapularis tendon. Knee Surg Sports Traumatol Arthrosc 2007;15:1482–1485.

58 Franceschi F, Ruzzini L, Longo UG, Martina FM, Zobel BB, Maffulli N, Denaro V: Equivalent clinical results of arthroscopic single-row and double-row suture anchor repair for rotator cuff tears: a randomized controlled trial. Am J Sports Med 2007; 35:1254–1260.

59 Franceschi F, Longo UG, Ruzzini L, Rizzello G, Maffulli N, Denaro V: The Roman bridge: a 'double pulley-suture bridges' technique for rotator cuff repair. BMC Musculoskelet Disord 2007;8:123.

60 Franceschi F, Longo UG, Ruzzini L, Papalia R, Rizzello G, Denaro V: To detach the long head of the biceps tendon after tenodesis or not: outcome analysis at the 4-year follow-up of two different techniques. Int Orthop 2007;31:537–545.

61 Franceschi F, Longo UG, Ruzzini L, Rizzello G, Maffulli N, Denaro V: Arthroscopic salvage of failed arthroscopic Bankart repair: a prospective study with a minimum follow-up of 4 years. Am J Sports Med 2008;36:1330–1336.

62 Franceschi F, Longo UG, Ruzzini L, Rizzello G, Maffulli N, Denaro V: No advantages in repairing a type II superior labrum anterior and posterior lesion when associated with rotator cuff repair in patients over age 50: a randomized controlled trial. Am J Sports Med 2008;36:247–253.

63 Franceschi F, Longo UG, Ruzzini L, Rizzello G, Maffulli N, Denaro V: Soft tissue tenodesis of the long head of the biceps tendon associated to the Roman bridge repair. BMC Musculoskelet Disord 2008;9:78.

64 Longo UG, Franceschi F, Spiezia F, Marinozzi A, Maffulli N, Denaro V: The low-profile Roman bridge technique for knotless double-row repair of the rotator cuff. Arch Orthop Trauma Surg 2011;131: 357–361.

65 Yang S, Park HS, Flores S, Levin SD, Makhsous M, Lin F, Koh J, Nuber G, Zhang LQ: Biomechanical analysis of bursal-sided partial thickness rotator cuff tears. J Shoulder Elbow Surg 2009;18:379–385.

66 Bey MJ, Ramsey ML, Soslowsky LJ: Intratendinous strain fields of the supraspinatus tendon: effect of a surgically created articular-surface rotator cuff tear. J Shoulder Elbow Surg 2002;11:562–569.

67 Veeger HE, van der Helm FC: Shoulder function: the perfect compromise between mobility and stability. J Biomech 2007;40:2119–2129.

68 Wuelker N, Plitz W, Roetman B: Biomechanical data concerning the shoulder impingement syndrome. Clin Orthop Relat Res 1994:242–249.

69 Kaneko K, De Mouy EH, Brunet ME: Massive rotator cuff tears. Screening by routine radiographs. Clin Imaging 1995;19:8–11.

70 Poppen NK, Walker PS: Normal and abnormal motion of the shoulder. J Bone Joint Surg Am 1976;58:195–201.

71 Deutsch A, Altchek DW, Schwartz E, Otis JC, Warren RF: Radiologic measurement of superior displacement of the humeral head in the impingement syndrome. J Shoulder Elbow Surg 1996;5: 186–193.

72 Ludewig PM, Cook TM: Translations of the humerus in persons with shoulder impingement symptoms. J Orthop Sports Phys Ther 2002;32: 248–259.

73 Michener LA, McClure PW, Karduna AR: Anatomical and biomechanical mechanisms of subacromial impingement syndrome. Clin Biomech (Bristol, Avon) 2003;18:369–379.
74 Halder AM, O'Driscoll SW, Heers G, Mura N, Zobitz ME, An KN, Kreusch-Brinker R: Biomechanical comparison of effects of supraspinatus tendon detachments, tendon defects, and muscle retractions. J Bone Joint Surg Am 2002;84:780–785.
75 Castricini R, Longo UG, De Benedetto M, Panfoli N, Pirani P, Zini R, Maffulli N, Denaro V: Platelet-rich plasma augmentation for arthroscopic rotator cuff repair: a randomized controlled trial. Am J Sports Med 2011;39:258–265.
76 Halder AM, Zhao KD, Odriscoll SW, Morrey BF, An KN: Dynamic contributions to superior shoulder stability. J Orthop Res 2001;19:206–212.
77 Longo UG, Lamberti A, Maffulli N, Denaro V: Tendon augmentation grafts: a systematic review. Br Med Bull 2010;94:165–188.
78 Longo UG, Lamberti A, Maffulli N, Denaro V: Tissue engineered biological augmentation for tendon healing: a systematic review. Br Med Bull 2011;98:31–59.
79 Longo UG, Vasta S, Maffulli N, Denaro V: Scoring systems for the functional assessment of patients with rotator cuff pathology. Sports Med Arthrosc 2011 (in press).
80 Longo UG, Lamberti A, Khan WS, Maffulli N, Denaro V: Synthetic augmentation for massive rotator cuff tears. Sports Med Arthrosc 2011 (in press).
81 Forriol F, Longo UG, Concejo C, Ripalda P, Maffulli N, Denaro V: Platelet-rich plasma, rhOP-1 (rhBMP-7) and frozen rib allograft for the reconstruction of bony mandibular defects in sheep. A pilot experimental study. Injury 2009;40(suppl 3):S44–S49.
82 Khan WS, Longo UG, Ahrens PM, Denaro V, Maffulli N: A systematic review of the reverse shoulder replacement in rotator cuff arthropathy, rotator cuff tears and rheumatoid arthritis. Sports Med Arthrosc 2011 (in press).
83 Longo UG, Ramamurthy C, Denaro V, Maffulli N: Minimally invasive stripping for chronic Achilles tendinopathy. Disabil Rehabil 2008;30:1709–1713.
84 Longo UG, Ronga M, Maffulli N: Achilles tendinopathy. Sports Med Arthrosc 2009;17:112–126.
85 Khanna A, Friel M, Gougoulias N, Longo UG, Maffulli N: Prevention of adhesions in surgery of the flexor tendons of the hand: what is the evidence? Br Med Bull 2009;90:85–109.
86 Ames PR, Longo UG, Denaro V, Maffulli N: Achilles tendon problems: not just an orthopaedic issue. Disabil Rehabil 2008;30:1646–1650.
87 Franceschi F, Marinozzi A, Papalia R, Longo UG, Gualdi G, Denaro E: Intra- and juxta-articular osteoid osteoma: a diagnostic challenge: misdiagnosis and successful treatment: a report of four cases. Arch Orthop Trauma Surg 2006;126:660–667.
88 Maffulli N, Longo UG, Gougoulias N, Denaro V: Ipsilateral free semitendinosus tendon graft transfer for reconstruction of chronic tears of the Achilles tendon. BMC Musculoskelet Disord 2008;9:100.
89 Maffulli N, Walley G, Sayana MK, Longo UG, Denaro V: Eccentric calf muscle training in athletic patients with Achilles tendinopathy. Disabil Rehabil 2008;30:1677–1684.
90 Longo UG, Rittweger J, Garau G, Radonic B, Gutwasser C, Gilliver SF, Kusy K, Zieliński J, Felsenberg D, Maffulli N: No influence of age, gender, weight, height, and impact profile in achilles tendinopathy in masters track and field athletes. Am J Sports Med 2009;37:1400–1405.
91 Longo UG, Ronga M, Maffulli N: Acute ruptures of the achilles tendon. Sports Med Arthrosc 2009; 17:127–138.
92 Maffulli N, Longo UG, Ronga M, Khanna A, Denaro V: Favorable outcome of percutaneous repair of achilles tendon ruptures in the elderly. Clin Orthop Relat Res 2010;468:1039–1046.
93 Longo UG, King JB, Denaro V, Maffulli N: Double-bundle arthroscopic reconstruction of the anterior cruciate ligament: does the evidence add up? J Bone Joint Surg Br 2008;90:995–999.

Nicola Maffulli, MD, MS, PhD, FRCS(Orth)
Centre for Sports and Exercise Medicine
Barts and The London School of Medicine and Dentistry
Mile End Hospital, 275 Bancroft Road, London E1 4DG (UK)
Tel. +44 20 8223 8839, E-Mail n.maffulli@qmul.ac.uk

Maffulli N (ed): Rotator Cuff Tear. Med Sport Sci. Basel, Karger, 2012, vol 57, pp 18–26

Role of Biomechanics in Rotator Cuff Pathology: North American Perspective

Vasili Karas · Brian J. Cole · Vincent M. Wang

Rush University Medical Center, Chicago, Ill., USA

Abstract

The biomechanical properties of, and mechanical environment surrounding, the rotator cuff continue to be a research area of great interest as injury and failure of these tendons are among the most common of shoulder pathologies, with incidence increasing in older populations. Recent literature has refined our knowledge of the anatomy, the role of the various tendons in movement and shoulder stability, and structural and material properties of the human rotator cuff. Furthermore, animal models have characterized the effects of mechanical loading on rotator cuff properties, the biomechanical interactions among cuff tendons in uninjured and deficient rotator cuffs have been described, and more recent imaging studies have provided novel insights into the function of the rotator cuff in vivo. Research to advance our understanding of the biomechanical factors contributing to rotator cuff disease is needed, as the etiology, prognostic indicators, and reasons for treatment failure are poorly understood. We summarize published biomechanical literature on the rotator cuff to provide a current perspective on potential mechanisms involved in cuff pathology.

Rotator Cuff Failure in Biomechanical Literature

Although the epidemiology of rotator cuff tears is not well established, rotator cuff tears, either symptomatic or asymptomatic, approach a prevalence of 7–30% [1–12]. Moreover, rotator cuff tears pose a challenging problem with regard to clinical management and diagnosis as they can be symptomatic or asymptomatic, and can be accompanied by pain, loss of muscle strength, and range of motion deficits [1, 13–18]. In contrast to the reported dissociation between symptoms and the presence of rotator cuff tears, cadaveric and animal models have shown an alteration in the biomechanics of the shoulder in the presence of tears [8, 19–23].

In a study of the spatially varying material properties of the human supraspinatus tendon, Lake et al. [24] showed a significant difference in the tensile modulus of the posterior portion of the tendon when compared to the medial and anterior portions.

Despite these differences, histological scores of degeneration did not correlate to their biomechanical findings. However, a study of normal versus torn supraspinatus tendons found a significant increase in infiltration of mast cells and macrophages in torn tendons with mild to moderate tendinopathy [25]. This finding contradicts earlier studies that show degeneration of the tendon rather than infiltrate within the tendon [26, 27]. Interestingly, there is a greater cellular and vascular response in small tears of the rotator cuff, while large and massive tears are primarily degenerative in nature [28]. However, it is unclear whether the latter observations are applicable to both partial and full-thickness tears, and whether these findings vary with tear location.

There exists a stress concentration within the articular side of the supraspinatus tendon in a finite element model [29]. This finding has since been corroborated in both physiologic [30–32] and pathologic states [32]. Sano et al. [30] used finite element analysis derived from MRI and histologic data to model the biomechanical properties of intact tendon (fig. 1). They then modeled an articular, bursal, and intratendinous tear and show increased stress concentration at these levels [32]. Despite biomechanical data which suggest strain gradients within the rotator cuff tendon [20, 33], to date, clinical evidence does not demonstrate failure of the tendon proper in a specific location as the primary mechanism of failure. In revision of rotator cuff repairs, the anchor or the suture tendon interface is commonly the focal point of failure [34–36]. In tests of native humerus-tendon-muscle constructs in cadavera, insertion site failure or musculotendinous junction failure occurs before rotator cuff tendon tear [33]. This evidence suggests that, under conditions of uniaxial tension applied along the tendon fibers, in its uninjured state, the rotator cuff tendon proper is biomechanically more robust than its bony insertion on the lateral side and its muscular junction on the medial side. Sano et al. [37] showed a negative correlation between the ultimate tensile strength of the supraspinatus tendon and the tendons' histologic properties at the bony insertion. Sano also concludes that microscopic degeneration is more common at the insertion than in the middle portion (from lateral at insertion to medial at musculotendinous junction) of the supraspinatus. Finally, Fukuda et al. [38] postulated that intratendinous mechanical shear forces may be responsible for early tendon defects. Itoi et al. [39] divided the supraspinatus tendon into thirds and noted that, despite a similar modulus of elasticity between the articular and bursal sides, the anterior portion of the tendon exhibited a significantly higher elastic modulus than that of the middle and posterior thirds.

Impingement: Biomechanical Considerations

Neer and Poppen first described subacromial impingement in an intraoperative study of 400 patients with rotator cuff tears [40]. They postulated that the etiology of the rotator cuff tears in 95% of their patients was subacromial impingement on the cuff

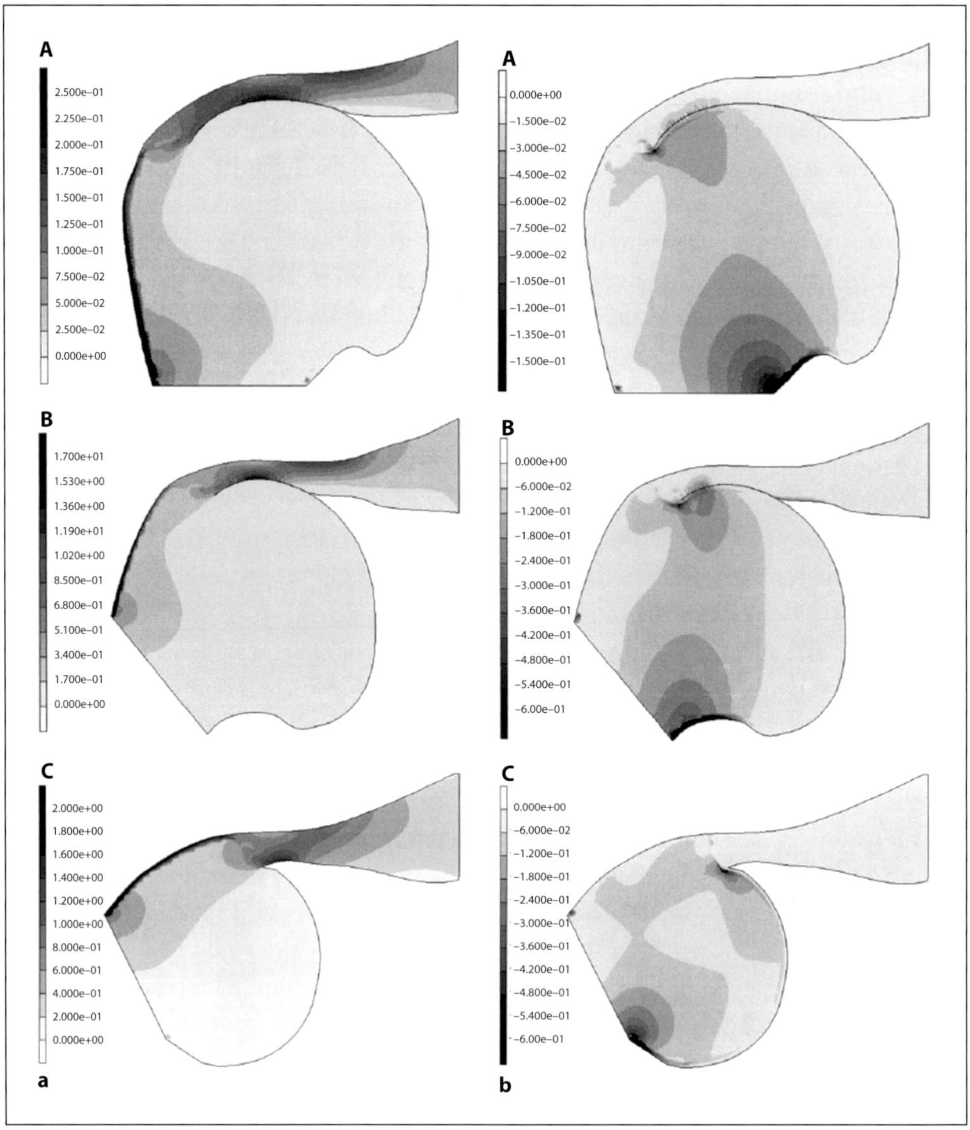

Fig. 1. Finite element results for tensile (**a**) and compressive (**b**) stress at abduction angles of 0° (A), 30° (B), and 60° (C). Darker color denotes greater stress. Reprinted with permission from Elsevier [30].

by the anterior third of the acromion [41]. Subsequently, the shape of the acromion [42], the presence of arthritic changes in the acromioclavicular joint [43], and spurs on the acromion and distal clavicle [44] have been found to result in narrowing of the subacromial space.

It is likely that subacromial contact in and of itself is not detrimental, but a narrowed acromiohumeral distance predisposes an individual to rotator cuff disease [41,

42, 45]. This point was most recently made in a meta-analysis of in vivo imaging of the rotator cuff with ultrasound [45]. Seitz et al. [45] identified five contemporary studies that compared the acromiohumeral space in patients with and without diagnosed rotator cuff tears and impingement. They concluded that patients with full-thickness rotator cuff tears have a significantly smaller acromiohumeral space than those without pathology.

The anatomic shape of the acromion is associated with the severity of rotator cuff disease with type III or hooked acromial shape having the highest penchant for pathology [42, 46, 47]. The slope of the acromion is another measure used to assess acromial shape, and has also been implicated in symptomatic impingement [48] and increased tendon compression [49, 50].

However, it is unclear whether impingement induces cuff damage or whether weakness, dysfunction, and fatigue or overuse of the rotator cuff lead to subacromial impingement (e.g., via the resulting superior humeral translation). Recent cadaveric evidence suggests that non-pathologic contact pressure between 0.04 and 0.11 MPa from 0 to 100° of flexion exists beneath the coracoacromial arch. Similarly, acromial contact pressure reached 0.43 MPa in flexion [51]. Contact occurred in otherwise grossly intact tendons devoid of pathologic changes. Although the authors did not present histologic or biochemical results for the tendons, Yamamoto et al. [51] suggest that contact of the rotator cuff tendons with the coracoacromial arch is not necessarily a pathologic phenomenon. A study evaluating the effect of acromioplasty on glenohumeral translation and rotator cuff contact pressure, even with complete resection of the coracoacromial ligament, showed a pressure of at least 0.02 MPa on the rotator cuff at all times [52].

Mechanical overuse of the supraspinatus was explicitly tested by Soslowsky et al. [53] by examining tendon alterations in a rat model of decline treadmill running. The tendon in their overuse model exhibited an increased cross-sectional area, hypercellularity, and collagen disorganization. Biomechanically, maximum stress and elastic modulus were significantly lower in the overuse group when compared to cage control rats. Impingement of the tendons was not included in the study design, and yet these tendons showed signs of biomechanical and cellular degradation [53].

Schneeberger et al. [54] tested an alternative hypothesis of rotator cuff pathology in an in vivo rat model by producing impingement on the supraspinatus with surgically implanted plates and then analyzing the tendon grossly and histologically. They found that the tendons showed signs of bursal sided degeneration in every instance of simulated impingement, demonstrating that impingement may indeed have a detrimental effect on rotator cuff tendons.

Soslowsky et al. [55] used a combination of the aforementioned approaches by subjecting rats to the overuse model with the addition of simulated subacromial impingement with the use of an Achilles tendon allograft. They examined three groups of rats: an overuse, an impingement, and an overuse + impingement group. The authors found that both impingement and overuse had detrimental effects on the supraspinatus. In addition, the combined group showed a significant increase in cross-sectional area and a significant decrease in maximum stress and elastic modulus when compared to either of the individual groups.

Rotator Cuff Pathology: Age and Symptoms

A prospective clinical study of 411 patients found a tear in 23% of subjects with an increase in incidence that correlated directly with age. Specifically, 38% (52 of 136) of asymptomatic patients older than 70 had full-thickness tears appreciable on ultrasound [12]. This study along with MRI findings by Sher et al. [56] in asymptomatic patients of a younger cohort, suggest that tears in the rotator cuff, especially with advanced age, could be classified as 'normal aging'. Moosmayer et al. [1] found the prevalence of rotator cuff tears to be 7.6% overall, and 15% in ages of 70–79, a smaller prevalence overall yet also an increase with age. Neer et al. [57] described three stages of rotator cuff lesions characterized by age: <25 years for stage I, between 25 and 40 for stage II, and stage III for those >40. The stages correspond to the most common characteristics of impingement, with stage three including rotator cuff tears. Although heavily biased toward impingement as the primary cause of rotator cuff tears, Neer's stages suggest that age is a component to rotator cuff pathology.

As a microscopic correlate, Kumagai et al. [58] found that elderly cadavera without tendon tears (52–90 years) were characterized by calcification, fibrovascular proliferation and microtears in the tendon, and patients in a younger cohort did not demonstrate these histologic findings.

Despite the increasing prevalence of RC tears with age, clinical symptoms do not always accompany a tear [2, 59, 60]. In fact, across all ages, there is still debate as to what factors cause symptoms. Based on imaging studies of symptomatic and asymptomatic patients with rotator cuff tears, size of tear [2, 59, 60] and fatty infiltration [60] are indicators of symptomatic tears.

Karas et al. [3] recently reviewed the biomechanical effects of rotator cuff tears in cadaveric models. The in vivo biomechanics of the shoulder, however, whether in symptomatic or symptomatic patients, are altered in the presence of a rotator cuff tear based on electromyography and kinematics [61, 62]. In confirmed rotator cuff tears, muscle activation is increased when compared with non-pathologic shoulders. In asymptomatic subjects, the subscapularis had increased activity whereas, in symptomatic subjects, the rotator cuff muscles associated with torn tendons had increased activity. Yamaguchi et al. [62] analyzed the three-dimensional kinematics of the glenohumeral joint in patients with symptomatic and asymptomatic rotator cuff pathology and found statistically significant humeral head migration in both groups, which suggests that symptoms do not result from a change in kinematics.

Results from translational scientific studies on the rotator cuff have led to an improved understanding of potential biomechanical mechanisms of cuff injury. The

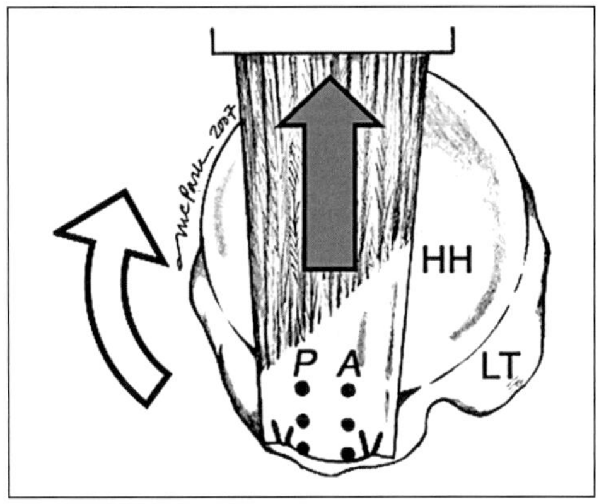

Fig. 2. Schematic of custom testing configuration allowing for dynamic humeral external rotation during cyclic loading of the supraspinatus tendon. The straight arrow represents the vector for tendon loading. The curved arrow represents the direction of rotation. A = Anterior tendon region; P = posterior tendon region; LT = lesser tuberosity; HH = humeral head. Modified from Park et al. [64].

reliability of ongoing and future work to more closely simulate clinically observed pathology will not only provide further insight into the etiology of rotator cuff disease, but also facilitate potential approaches for injury prevention, diagnosis and treatment. For example, it is possible that experimental methods such as applying fatigue loading until failure, or utilizing more complex loading directions/modes (e.g., superposing impingement with tensile loading of the tendon, or loading the tendon in more physiologic directions [63, 64]) may be required in cadaveric studies to produce pathology more consistent with clinical and/or imaging results (fig. 2). Furthermore, refinements of recent technological advancements such as arthroscopically insertable force probes [10, 65] for in vivo measurement of tendon forces as well as imaging methods for in vivo kinematic studies [9, 66] and soft tissue deformation analyses [67] will likely provide critical insight into the biomechanical environment of rotator cuff tendon and surrounding soft tissue stabilizers. Collectively, advances in our understanding of the in vivo, temporal biomechanical function of the rotator cuff has strong implications for rehabilitation protocols and guidelines for the design of tissue engineered constructs for healing and repair of RC defects.

References

1 Moosmayer S, Smith HJ, Tariq R, Larmo A: Prevalence and characteristics of asymptomatic tears of the rotator cuff: an ultrasonographic and clinical study. J Bone Joint Surg Br 2009;91:196.

2 Yamaguchi K, Ditsios K, Middleton WD, Hildebolt CF, Galatz LM, Teefey SA: The demographic and morphological features of rotator cuff disease. A comparison of asymptomatic and symptomatic shoulders. J Bone Joint Surg Am 2006;88:1699.

3 Karas V, Wang VM, Dhawan A, Cole BJ: Biomechanical factors in rotator cuff pathology. Sports Med Arthrosc 2011;19:202–206.

4 Wang VM, Wang FC, McNickle AG, Friel NA, Yanke AB, Chubinskaya S, Romeo AA, Verma NN, Cole BJ: Medial versus lateral supraspinatus tendon properties. Am J Sports Med 2010;38:2456.

5 Fallon J, Blevins F, Vogel K, Trotter J: Functional morphology of the supraspinatus tendon. J Orthop Res 2002;20:920–926.

6 Parsons IM, Apreleva M, Fu F, Woo SLY: The effect of rotator cuff tears on reaction forces at the glenohumeral joint. J Orthop Res 2002;20:439–446.

7 Roh MS, Wang VM, April EW, Pollock RG, Bigliani LU, Flatow EL: Anterior and posterior musculotendinous anatomy of the supraspinatus. J Shoulder Elbow Surg 2000;10:436–440.

8 Andarawis-Puri N, Ricchetti ET, Soslowsky LJ: Interaction between the supraspinatus and infraspinatus tendons. Am J Sports Med 2009;37:1831.

9 Bey MJ, Kline SK, Zauel R, Lock TR, Kolowich PA: Measuring dynamic in-vivo glenohumeral joint kinematics: technique and preliminary results. J Biomech 2008;41:711–714.

10 Bull AM, Reilly P, Wallace A, Amis A, Emery RJH: A novel technique to measure active tendon forces: application to the subscapularis tendon. Knee Surg Sports Traumatol Arthrosc 2005;13:145–150.

11 Yamamoto A, Takagishi K, Osawa T, Yanagawa T, Nakajima D, Shitara H, Kobayashi T: Prevalence and risk factors of a rotator cuff tear in the general population. J Shoulder Elbow Surg 2010;19:116–120.

12 Tempelhof S, Rupp S, Seil R: Age-related prevalence of rotator cuff tears in asymptomatic shoulders. J Shoulder Elbow Surg 1999;8:296–299.

13 Brasseur JL, Lucidarme O, Tardieu M, Tordeur M, Montalvan B, Parier J, Goux PL, Gires A, Grenier P: Ultrasonographic rotator-cuff changes in veteran tennis players: the effect of hand dominance and comparison with clinical findings. Eur Radiol 2004;14:857–864.

14 Connor PM, Banks DM, Tyson AB, Coumas JS, D'Alessandro DF: Magnetic resonance imaging of the asymptomatic shoulder of overhead athletes. Am J Sports Med 2003;31:724.

15 Fehringer EV, Sun J, VanOeveren LS, Keller BK, Matsen FA 3rd: Full-thickness rotator cuff tear prevalence and correlation with function and co-morbidities in patients sixty-five years and older. J Shoulder Elbow Surg 2008;17:881–885.

16 Fuchs B, Weishaupt D, Zanetti M, Hodler J, Gerber C: Fatty degeneration of the muscles of the rotator cuff: assessment by computed tomography versus magnetic resonance imaging. J Shoulder Elbow Surg 1999;8:599–605.

17 Kim HM, Teefey SA, Zelig A, Galatz LM, Keener JD, Yamaguchi K: Shoulder strength in asymptomatic individuals with intact compared with torn rotator cuffs. J Bone Joint Surg Am 2009;91:289.

18 Miniaci A, Dowdy PA, Willits KR, Vellet AD: Magnetic resonance imaging evaluation of the rotator cuff tendons in the asymptomatic shoulder. Am J Sports Med 1995;23:142.

19 Mazzocca AD, Rincon LM, O'Connor RW, Obopilwe E, Andersen M, Geaney L, Arciero RA: Intra-articular partial-thickness rotator cuff tears. Am J Sports Med 2008;36:110.

20 Bey MJ, Ramsey ML, Soslowsky LJ: Intratendinous strain fields of the supraspinatus tendon: effect of a surgically created articular-surface rotator cuff tear. J Shoulder Elbow Surg 2002;12:562–569.

21 Reilly P, Amis AA, Wallace AL, Emery RJH: Mechanical factors in the initiation and propagation of tears of the rotator cuff. Quantification of strains of the supraspinatus tendon in vitro. J Bone Joint Surg Br 2003;85:594–599.

22 Perry SM, Getz CL, Soslowsky LJ: Alterations in function after rotator cuff tears in an animal model. J Shoulder Elbow Surg 2009;18:296–304.

23 Sarver JJ, Dishowitz MI, Kim SY, Soslowsky LJ: Transient decreases in forelimb gait and ground reaction forces following rotator cuff injury and repair in a rat model. J Biomech 2010; 43:778–782.

24 Lake SP, Miller KS, Elliott DM, Soslowsky LJ: Effect of Fiber Distribution and Realignment on the Nonlinear and Inhomogeneous Mechanical Properties of Human Supraspinatus Tendon under Longitudinal Tensile Loading. J Orthop Res 2009; 27:1596–1602.

25 Millar NL, Hueber AJ, Reilly JH, Xu Y, Fazzi UG, Murrell GA, McInnes IB: Inflammation is present in early human tendinopathy. Am J Sports Med 2010;38:2085.

26 Hashimoto T, Nobuhara K, Hamada T: Pathologic evidence of degeneration as a primary cause of rotator cuff tear. Clin Orthop 2003;415:111.

27 Maffulli N, Wong J, Almekinders LC: Types and epidemiology of tendinopathy. Clin Sports Med 2003;22:675–692.

28 Matthews T, Hand G, Rees J, Athanasou N, Carr A: Pathology of the torn rotator cuff tendon: reduction in potential for repair as tear size increases. J Bone Joint Surg Br 2006;88:489.

29 Luo ZP, Hsu HC, Grabowski JJ, Morrey BF, An KN: Mechanical environment associated with rotator cuff tears. J Shoulder Elbow Surg 1998;7: 616–620.

30 Wakabayashi I, Itoi E, Sano H, Shibuya Y, Sashi R, Minagawa H, Kobayashi M: Mechanical environment of the supraspinatus tendon: a two-dimensional finite element model analysis. J Shoulder Elbow Surg 2003;12:612–617.

31 Seki N, Itoi E, Shibuya Y, Wakabayashi I, Sano H, Sashi R, Minagawa H, Yamamoto N, Abe H, Kikuchi K: Mechanical environment of the supraspinatus tendon: three-dimensional finite element model analysis. J Orthop Sci 2008;13:348–353.

32 Sano H, Wakabayashi I, Itoi E: Stress distribution in the supraspinatus tendon with partial-thickness tears: an analysis using two-dimensional finite element model. J Shoulder Elbow Surg 2006;15: 100–105.
33 Huang CY, Wang VM, Pawluk RJ, Bucchieri JS, Levine WN, Bigliani LU, Mow VC, Flatow EL: Inhomogeneous mechanical behavior of the human supraspinatus tendon under uniaxial loading. J Orthop Res 2005;23:924–930.
34 Yamakado K, Katsuo S, Mizuno K, Arakawa H, Hayashi S: Medial-row failure after arthroscopic double-row rotator cuff repair. Arthroscopy 2010;26:430–435.
35 Sward L, Hughes J, Amis A, Wallace W: The strength of surgical repairs of the rotator cuff. A biomechanical study on cadavers. J Bone Joint Surg Br 1992;74:585.
36 Cummins CA, Murrell GAC: Mode of failure for rotator cuff repair with suture anchors identified at revision surgery. J Shoulder Elbow Surg 2003;12: 128–133.
37 Sano H, Ishii H, Yeadon A, Backman DS, Brunet JA, Uhthoff HK: Degeneration at the insertion weakens the tensile strength of the supraspinatus tendon: a comparative mechanical and histologic study of the bone-tendon complex. J Orthop Res 1997;15: 719–726.
38 Fukuda H, Hamada K, Nakajima T, Tomonaga A: Pathology and pathogenesis of the intratendinous tearing of the rotator cuff viewed from en bloc histologic sections. Clin Orthop 1994;304:60.
39 Itoi E, Berglund LJ, Grabowski JJ, Schultz FM, Growney ES, Morrey BF, An KN: Tensile properties of the supraspinatus tendon. J Orthop Res 1995;13: 578–584.
40 Neer CS: Anterior acromioplasty for the chronic impingement syndrome in the shoulder: a preliminary report. J Bone Joint Surg Am 1972;54:41–50.
41 Neer C, Poppen N: Supraspinatus outlet. Orthop Trans 1987;11:234.
42 Bigliani LU, Ticker JB, Flatow EL, Soslowsky LJ, Mow VC: The relationship of acromial architecture to rotator cuff disease. Clin Sports Med 1991;10:823–838.
43 Petersson CJ, Gentz CF: Ruptures of the supraspinatus tendon the significance of distally pointing acromioclavicular osteophytes. Clin Orthop 1983;174: 143.
44 Cuomo F, Kummer FJ, Zuckerman JD, Lyon T, Blair B, Olsen T: The influence of acromioclavicular joint morphology on rotator cuff tears. J Shoulder Elbow Surg 1998;7:555–559.
45 Seitz AL, Michener LA: Ultrasonographic measures of subacromial space in patients with rotator cuff disease: a systematic review. J Clin Ultrasound 2011;39:146–154.
46 Epstein R, Schweitzer M, Frieman B, Fenlin J, Mitchell D: Hooked acromion: prevalence on MR images of painful shoulders. Radiology 1993;187: 479.
47 Ogawa K, Yoshida A, Inokuchi W, Naniwa T: Acromial spur: relationship to aging and morphologic changes in the rotator cuff. J Shoulder Elbow Surg 2005;14:591–598.
48 Edelson J, Luchs J: Aspects of coracoacromial ligament anatomy of interest of the arthroscopic surgeon. Arthroscopy 1995;11:715–719.
49 Toivonen DA, Tuite MJ, Orwin JF: Acromial structure and tears of the rotator cuff. J Shoulder Elbow Surg 1995;4:376–383.
50 Vaz S, Soyer J, Pries P, Clarac JP: Subacromial impingement: Influence of coracoacromial arch geometry on shoulder function. Joint Bone Spine 2000;67:305–309.
51 Yamamoto N, Muraki T, Sperling JW, Steinmann SP, Itoi E, Cofield RH, An KN: Contact between the coracoacromial arch and the rotator cuff tendons in nonpathologic situations: a cadaveric study. J Shoulder Elbow Surg 2010;19:681–687.
52 Denard PJ, Bahney TJ, Kirby SB, Orfaly RM: Contact pressure and glenohumeral translation following subacromial decompression: how much is enough? Orthopedics 2010;33:805.
53 Soslowsky LJ, Thomopoulos S, Tun S, Flanagan CL, Keefer CC, Mastaw J, Carpenter JE: Neer Award 1999. Overuse activity injures the supraspinatus tendon in an animal model: a histologic and biomechanical study. J Shoulder Elbow Surg 2000;9:79–84.
54 Schneeberger AG, Nyffeler RW, Gerber C: Structural changes of the rotator cuff caused by experimental subacromial impingement in the rat. J Shoulder Elbow Surg 1998;7:375–380.
55 Soslowsky LJ, Thomopoulos S, Esmail A, Flanagan CL, Iannotti JP, Williamson I, JD, Carpenter JE: Rotator cuff tendinosis in an animal model: role of extrinsic and overuse factors. Ann Biomed Eng 2002;30:1057–1063.
56 Sher JS, Uribe JW, Posada A, Murphy BJ, Zlatkin MB: Abnormal findings on magnetic resonance images of asymptomatic shoulders. J Bone Joint Surg Am 1995;77:10–15.
57 Neer CS, Craig EV, Fukuda H: Cuff-tear arthropathy. J Bone Joint Surg Am 1983;65:1232–1244.
58 Kumagai J, Sarkar K, Uhthoff H: The collagen types in the attachment zone of rotator cuff tendons in the elderly: an immunohistochemical study. J Rheumatol 1994;21:2096.

59 Moosmayer S, Tariq R, Stiris MG, Smith HJ: MRI of symptomatic and asymptomatic full-thickness rotator cuff tears: a comparison of findings in 100 subjects. Acta Orthop 2010;81:361–366.
60 Mall NA, Kim HM, Keener JD, Steger-May K, Teefey SA, Middleton WD, Stobbs G, Yamaguchi K: Symptomatic progression of asymptomatic rotator cuff tears: a prospective study of clinical and sonographic variables. J Bone Joint Surg Am 2010;92: 2623–2633.
61 Kelly BT, Williams RJ, Cordasco FA, Backus SI, Otis JC, Weiland DE, Altchek DW, Craig EV, Wickiewicz TL, Warren RF: Differential patterns of muscle activation in patients with symptomatic and asymptomatic rotator cuff tears. J Shoulder Elbow Surg 2005;14:165–171.
62 Yamaguchi K, Sher JS, Andersen WK, Garretson R, Uribe JW, Hechtman K, Neviaser RJ: Glenohumeral motion in patients with rotator cuff tears: a comparison of asymptomatic and symptomatic shoulders. J Shoulder Elbow Surg 2000;9:6–11.
63 Ahmad CS, Kleweno C, Jacir AM, Bell JE, Gardner TR, Levine WN, Bigliani LU: Biomechanical performance of rotator cuff repairs with humeral rotation. Am J Sports Med 2008;36:888–892.
64 Park MC, Jun BJ, Park CJ, Ahmad CS, El Attrache NS, Lee TQ: The biomechanical effects of dynamic external rotation on rotator cuff repair compared to testing with the humerus fixed. Am J Sports Med 2007;35:1931–1939.
65 Reilly P, Bull AM, Amis A, Wallace A, Emery RJ: Arthroscopically insertable force probes in the rotator cuff in vivo. Arthroscopy 2003;19:E8.
66 Boyer PJ, Massimini DF, Gill TJ, Papannagari R, Stewart SL, Warner JP, Li G: In vivo articular cartilage contact at the glenohumeral joint: preliminary report. J Orthop Sci 2008;13:359–365.
67 Bey M, Kline S, Baker A, McCarron J, Iannotti J, Derwin K: Estimation of dynamic, in vivo soft-tissue deformation: experimental technique and application in a canine model of tendon injury and repair. J Orthop Res 2011;29:822–827.

Vasili Karas
Rush University Medical Center
1611 W. Harrison Street, Suite 300, Chicago, IL 60612 (USA)
Tel. +1 312 432 2380
E-Mail vasili.karas@gmail.com

Maffulli N (ed): Rotator Cuff Tear. Med Sport Sci. Basel, Karger, 2012, vol 57, pp 27–40

The Scapula in Rotator Cuff Disease

W. Ben Kibler

Shoulder Center of Kentucky, Lexington, Ky., USA

Abstract

The scapula serves as the platform or base for the muscles of the rotator cuff. Rotator cuff function and dysfunction is therefore directly related to the functional state of the scapula. When the scapula is well stabilized, optimal positioning in both static and dynamic tasks allows the rotator cuff to function at an optimal level. However, scapular dysfunction produces an unstable base which in turn negatively affects the rotator cuff's biomechanical contributions to arm motion. Scapular alterations may be causative in rotator cuff dysfunction or may be the result of rotator cuff injury and increase the dysfunction. Possible causative mechanisms such as compromised anatomy (i.e. injury), muscle tightness, and scapular muscle weakness can contribute to the apparent dysfunction. Whether it is a cause or an effect, scapular dyskinesis is frequently identified in rotator cuff disease. Careful examination for presence of scapular dyskinesis and each of the causative mechanisms should be done as part of the comprehensive evaluation of patients with rotator cuff disease. Correction of the alterations following a logically progressed closed to open chain scapular-based program should be included as part of the overall treatment plan.

The scapula is closely related to many aspects of rotator cuff function and dysfunction. All of the rotator cuff muscles have their origin on the scapula. The static position and dynamic motion of the scapula markedly influence rotator cuff activity. This means that the muscles' capability for exerting maximal force at their insertion on the humerus is related to the stability of the scapula as a base for muscle contraction. Also, the position of the scapula in relationship to the humerus can affect the structural integrity and muscle contractility of the cuff. Excessive angulation of the humerus in relation to the acromion or the glenoid can result in external or internal impingement, and excessive angulation can decrease the cuff's ability to maintain glenohumeral (GH) concavity/compression.

Given all of these important relationships, it is not surprising to frequently find alterations in scapular kinematics associated with many aspects of the spectrum of rotator cuff disease, from impingement to tendinopathy to tear. Studies have found altered scapular kinematics, collectively termed scapular dyskinesis in 49–100% of rotator cuff patients [1–3]. Identification of the presence or absence of the alterations, and rehabilitation towards normal kinematics, should be an integral part of the treatment of rotator cuff disease.

The Scapula in Rotator Cuff Dysfunction and Disease

Many studies have evaluated scapular kinematics in subjects with rotator cuff weakness [4, 5], rotator cuff tendinopathy or impingement [6–9], and rotator cuff tear [2–4]. Alterations in scapular kinematics have been found in most studies.

In patients with clinical symptoms and/or imaging demonstrating rotator cuff impingement or rotator cuff tendinopathy, the studies have almost uniformly identified kinematic alterations consistent with scapular dyskinesis [7–11]. The exact nature of the alterations is not consistent, with varying combinations of changes in upward rotation (most showing a decrease), posterior tilt (most showing a decrease), and internal/external rotation (no change or increased internal rotation). All patients with demonstrated rotator cuff tears showed increased upward rotation of some magnitude, with most also showing decreased posterior tilt [3, 4]. Also, in a large prospective study of patients with MRI-proven full-thickness rotator cuff tears, scapular dyskinesis was identified as a major factor associated with lower functional scores [12].

The exact relationship of scapular dyskinesis and the spectrum of rotator cuff disease is not clear – is the dyskinesis a cause, an effect, or a compensation? Proposals for a causative effect include suggestions that decreased upward rotation and posterior tilt may alter the size of the subacromial space and may alter rotator cuff clearance under the coraco-acromial arch which can induce mechanical abrasion and wear; that increased anterior tilt and internal rotation will produce glenoid antetilting during arm motion, predisposing the rotator cuff to internal impingement; or that increased strain within the rotator cuff tendon due to altered muscle activation patterns may increase the observed apoptotic changes within the tendon cells [10, 13–17]. Proposals that dyskinesis is an effect point to the inhibitory effect of pain on individual muscle activation and the disruption of normal activation patterns, and on the effect of pain avoidance upon kinematic patterns [18]. If the dyskinesis results as an effect of the rotator cuff disease process, the altered mechanics would be considered a negative decompensation and could be expected to exacerbate the dysfunction of the entire shoulder complex. It appears that the increased upward rotation in patients with rotator cuff tears is a compensation to attempt to increase or maximize arm elevation or positioning in the face of weakened or absent rotator cuff activation. In this situation, it could be considered a positive compensation. Whatever the relationship, scapular dyskinesis is frequently identified in rotator cuff disease and is associated with lower function scores. Therefore, it must be identified if present, and its correction should be included as part of the overall treatment plan.

Causative Mechanisms for Scapular Dyskinesis

The scapula is stabilized on the curved ellipsoid thoracic wall by the bony strut of the clavicle and coordinated integrated muscle activation patterns [19]. Alterations in all the areas can produce dyskinesis.

Excessive thoracic kyphosis or scoliosis can change scapular motion. Acquired thoracic kyphosis produces increased internal rotation of the scapula, and elevation and decreased scapular upward rotation and posterior tilt. These kinematic alterations lead to decreased maximal arm elevation in forward flexion and abduction [20, 21].

The loss of clavicular strut function can be seen as a result of clavicular fracture, non-unions, or shortened/rotated mal-unions. In the presence of an intact AC joint, scapular dyskinesis will result as the scapula follows the position of the distal clavicle fragment. Most frequently, there will be increased scapular internal rotation, increased anterior tilt, and varying degrees of interference with upward rotation. Maximal rotator cuff strength and decreased functional outcomes scores related to decreased strength have been reported in these patients [22].

The most common causative mechanisms for scapular dyskinesis involve alterations in the soft tissues. Inflexibility and stiffness of the pectoralis minor and biceps short head produce anterior tilt and protraction due to their pull on the coracoid [23]. The most common soft tissue inflexibility is glenohumeral internal rotation deficit (GIRD), which produces a 'wind-up' of the scapula on the thorax with arm internal rotation or horizontal abduction. GIRD has been frequently associated with impingement and other rotator cuff diseases [24–27].

Several studies have documented alterations in periscapular muscle activation in patients with scapular dyskinesis and rotator cuff disease. Serratus anterior activation and strength is decreased in patients with impingement and shoulder pain, contributing to the loss of posterior tilt and upward rotation seen in these patients [7, 28, 29]. In addition, alteration of force couple activation patterns is seen. The upper trapezius/lower trapezius force couple is particularly affected, with delayed onset of activation in the lower trapezius, which would alter retraction and posterior tilt [30, 31]. Finally, fatigue in the periscapular muscles will alter kinematics. It appears that the lower portion of the stabilizing force couple, the lower trapezius and serratus anterior, are most susceptible to the effects of fatigue, which produces increased upward rotation and decreased posterior tilt [32, 33].

It appears that these multiple possible causative mechanisms are rarely isolated, but that several may be present in the same patient, in addition to GH pathology. Careful examination for presence or absence of scapular dyskinesis and each of the causative mechanisms should be done as part of the comprehensive evaluation of patients with rotator cuff disease.

Evaluation of the Scapula

Scapular evaluation should be both inclusive and dynamic. Distant contributions to normal scapular function and dyskinesis should be evaluated, and dynamic evaluation of motion, muscular activation, and corrective maneuvers should be included.

Leg and trunk muscle activity is both large and important in shoulder and arm throwing, serving, and lifting activities [34]. It is also important as a major source of facilitation of scapular muscle activation [35]. Evaluation of the legs and trunk may be performed by screening certain important parameters, and following with more detailed analysis on positive items. Lumbar lordosis, pelvic tilt, and hip rotational abnormalities should be checked. A good screening examination for leg and trunk strength is the single leg stability series (Trendelenburg and single leg squat maneuvers) [36].

Thoracic and cervical posture may be evaluated by inspection and rotation. Thoracic kyphosis or scoliosis may have a direct relationship to the motion of the scapula by producing abnormal posturing or necessitating extra motion for retraction. Excessive cervical lordosis indicates posterior cervical muscle or fascia tightness or anterior clavicular fascia tightness, which can have an effect on scapular retraction and protraction.

Objective Measurement

Coracoid-based inflexibility can be assessed by palpation of the pectoralis minor and the short head of the biceps brachii at their insertion on the coracoid tip. They will usually be tender to palpation, even whether they are not symptomatic in use, can be traced to their insertions as taut bands, and will produce symptoms of soreness and stiffness when the scapulae are manually maximally retracted and the arm is slightly abducted to approximately 40–50° [23]. A rough measurement of pectoralis minor tightness may be obtained by standing the patient against the wall and measuring the distance from the wall to the anterior acromial tip. This can be done using a 'double square' device with a patient standing with his or her back against a wall (fig. 1) [37]. A bilateral measurement is taken (in inches or centimeters) to determine if there is a notable difference between the involved and non-involved shoulder.

Visual Observation

The scapular examination should largely be accomplished from the posterior aspect. The scapula should be exposed for complete visualization. The resting posture

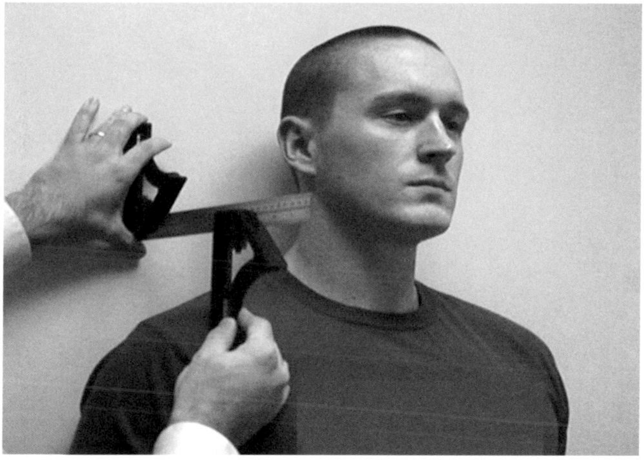

Fig. 1. Double square objective measurement for posture assessment.

should be checked for side-to-side asymmetry but especially for evidence of inferior medial or medial border prominence. If there is difficulty with determining the positions, marking the superior and inferior medial borders may help ascertain the position.

Dynamic scapular motions may be evaluated by having the patient move the arms in ascent and descent 3–5 times. This will usually bring out any weakness in the muscles and display the dyskinetic patterns. Motion in forward flexion is most likely to demonstrate medial border prominence. The addition of 3- to 5-lb weights will highlight the weakness even more [38–40]. Prominence of any part of the medial border is recorded in a 'yes' (present) or 'no' (absent) fashion. This evaluation system shows a clinical correlation of 0.64–0.84 between the clinical examination and the biomechanical findings [41].

Corrective Maneuvers

The scapular assistance test (SAT) and scapular retraction test (SRT) are corrective maneuvers that can provide information about the role of scapular dyskinesis in the total picture of dysfunction that accompanies shoulder injury and needs to be restored [5, 40, 42]. The SAT helps evaluate scapular contributions to impingement and rotator cuff strength, and the SRT evaluates contributions to rotator cuff strength. In the SAT, the examiner applies gentle pressure to assist scapular upward rotation and posterior tilt as the patient elevates the arm (fig. 2) [25]. A positive result occurs when the painful arc of impingement symptoms is relieved and the arc of motion is increased. In the SRT, the examiner grades the supraspinatus muscle

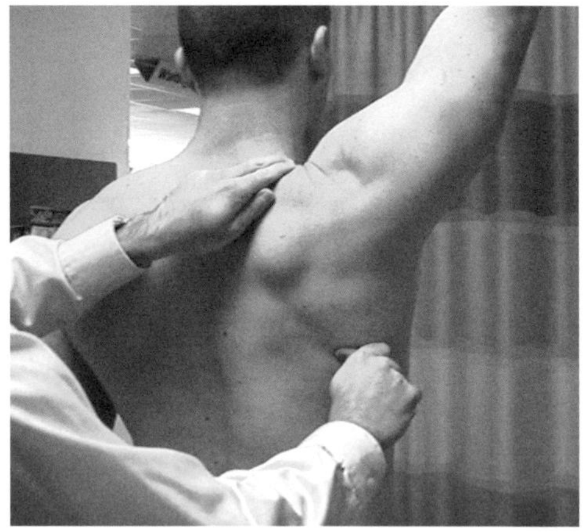

Fig. 2. Scapular assistance test.

strength following standard manual muscle testing procedures. The clinician then places and stabilizes the scapula in a retracted position (fig. 3). A positive test occurs when the demonstrated supraspinatus strength [5].

Although these tests are not capable of diagnosing a specific form of shoulder pathology, a positive SAT or SRT shows that scapular dyskinesis is directly involved in producing the symptoms and indicates the need for inclusion of early scapular rehabilitation exercises to improve scapular control.

Resting scapular position can be assessed with arms at the side. Excessive scapular internal rotation and lateral translation will be noted as prominence of the medial scapular border. A semi-dynamic assessment of scapular position using a tape measure is called the lateral scapular slide [25]. The distance between the inferior angle of the scapula and a thoracic spinous process is measured in three arm positions; at rest, hands on hip, and arms abducted to 90° and maximally internally rotated. A difference >1.5 cm suggests a loss of muscular control of the involved shoulder.

Treatment of Scapular Dyskinesis

Some patients with scapular dyskinesis have problems such as nerve injury or scapular muscle detachment which will not respond to therapy until they are repaired. Similarly, bony and/or tissue derangement issues such as acromioclavicular dislocation, fractured clavicles, labral injury, rotator cuff disease, or GH instability, may require surgical repair before the dyskinesis can be addressed. The large majority of dyskinesis cases are due to muscle weakness, inhibition, or inflexibility, and can be managed with rehabilitation.

Rehabilitation emphasis for scapular dyskinesis should start proximally and end distally [43, 44]. Initial management aims to achieve the position of optimal

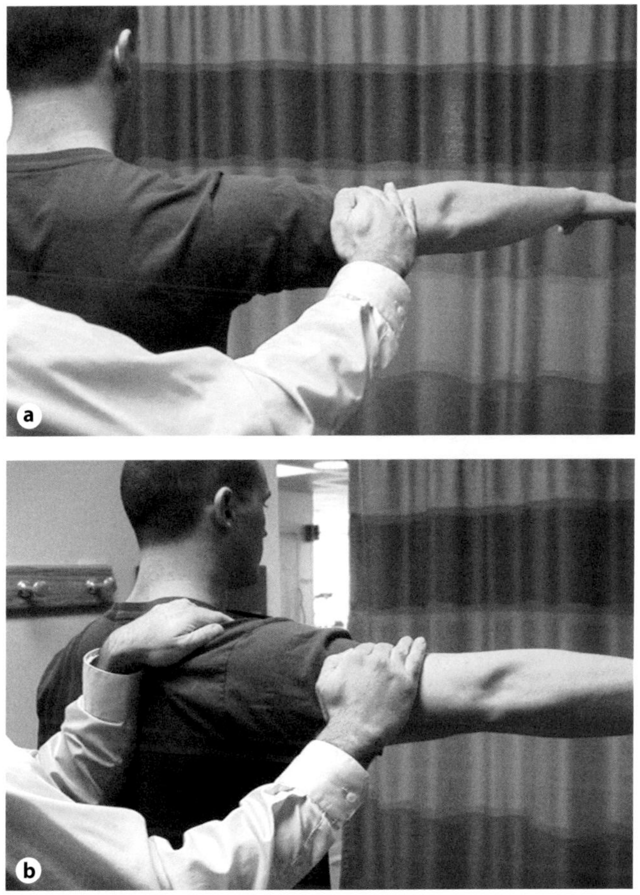

Fig. 3. Scapular retraction test.

scapular function – posterior tilt, external rotation, and upward elevation. Proximal control of core stability, which leads to control of 3D scapular motion, is achieved through an integrated rehabilitation regimen where the larger muscles of the lower extremity and trunk are utilized during the treatment of the scapula and shoulder [43]. Hip and trunk extension along with trunk rotation aid in facilitating scapular retraction. If strength or flexibility deficits are present within the proximal segments (core, pelvis, hip, etc.), they should be addressed prior to treating the scapula and/or shoulder.

Scapular dyskinesis patterns are often indicative of strength and flexibility problems in scapulothoracic and scapulohumeral muscles. Normalization of scapular range of motion is necessary before effective strengthening of the scapulothoracic muscles is possible. To normalize the scapular range of motion in rehabilitation, muscular, myofacial and/or capsular restrictions must be eliminated through manual therapeutic techniques, modalities, appropriate rest and stretching exercises. Common sites of these restrictions are the posterior rotator cuff and GH capsule, levator scapulae,

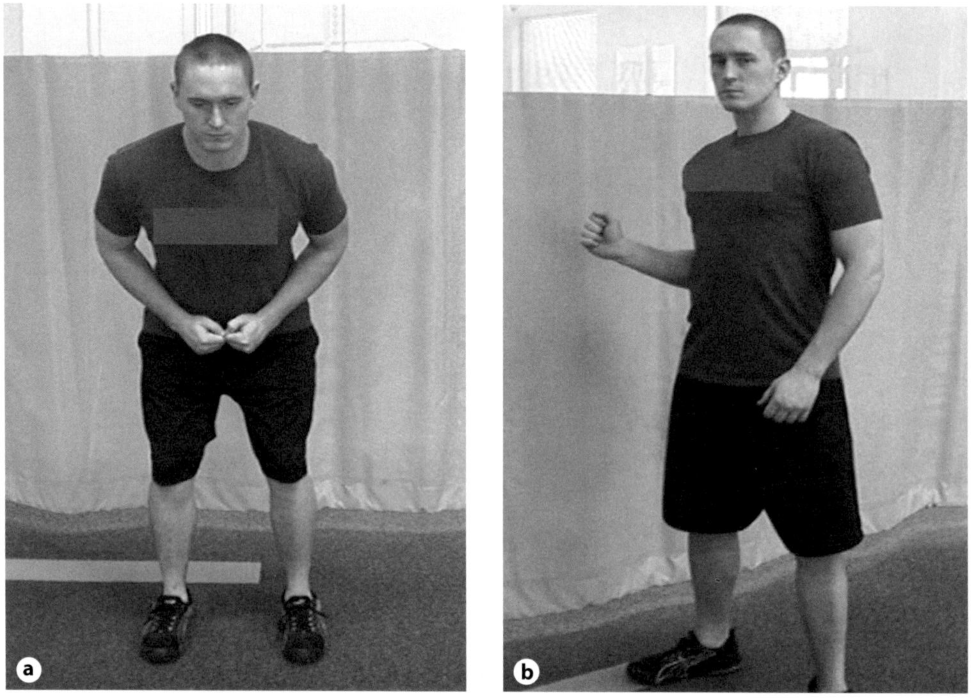

Fig. 4. Step-out exercise for early scapular motion.

upper trapezius and the coracoid-based musculature. The key to establishing this complete scapular motion is full scapular retraction, complete adduction, posterior tilt, lateral rotation and upward rotation. With no soft tissue restrictions limiting retraction, exercise can then strengthen this motion.

The serratus anterior is most important as an external rotator of the scapula, and the lower trapezius acts as a stabilizer of the acquired scapular position. Scapular stabilization protocols should focus on re-educating these muscles to act as dynamic scapula stabilizers first via the implementation of short lever, kinetic chain-assisted exercises then progress to long lever movements [45].

Scapular motion exercises begin in diagonal movement patterns such as the 'step-out' (fig. 4) which encourages scapular retraction through trunk rotation and progressing into single-plane movements such as the 'sternal lift' (fig. 5). Appropriate isometric and isotonic exercises which recruit the serratus anterior/lower trapezius force couple can be employed, which are effective when inhibition of these muscles is contributing to scapular dyskinesis. Such exercises include the low row (fig. 6), lawnmower (fig. 7), and fencing (fig. 8) maneuvers [45].

In the final phase of scapulothoracic rehabilitation, the exercises progress to include full GH motion and integrated strengthening. Horizontal dumbbell punches challenge the rotator cuff to maintain GH congruity and the scapulothoracic musculature

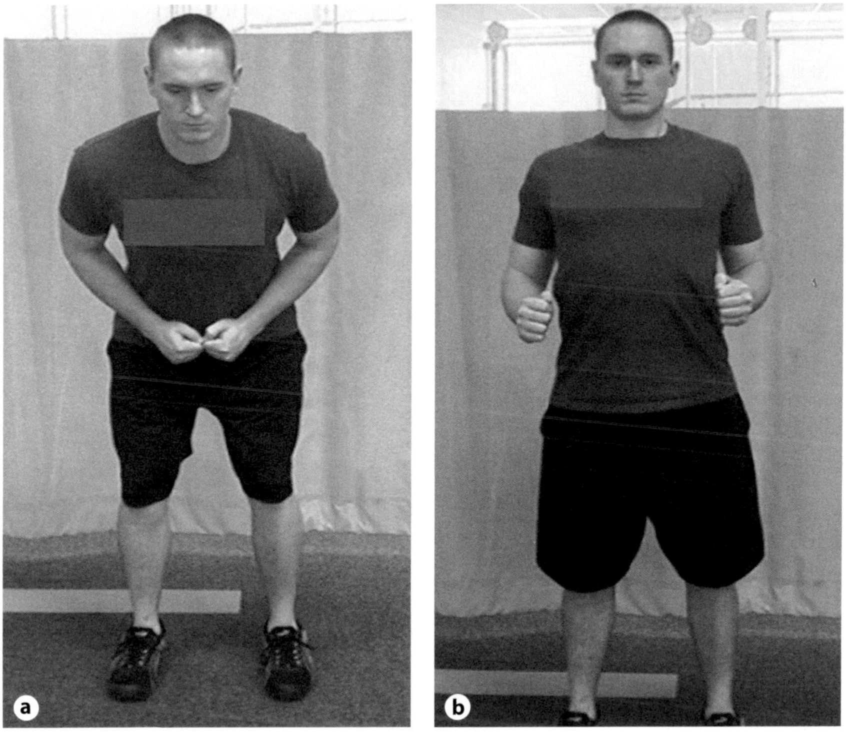

Fig. 5. Sternal lift exercise.

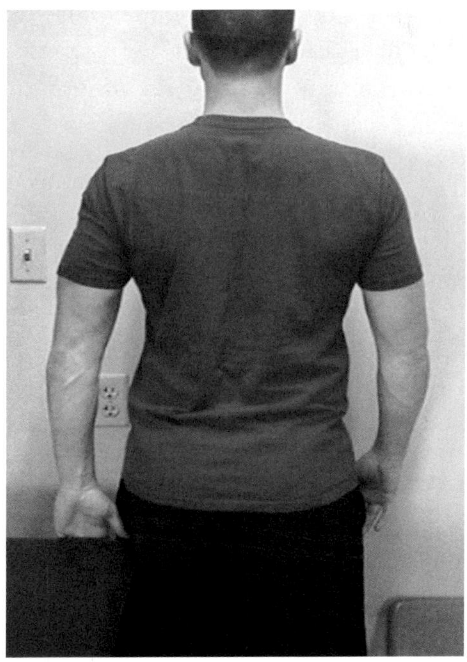

Fig. 6. Low row isometric exercise.

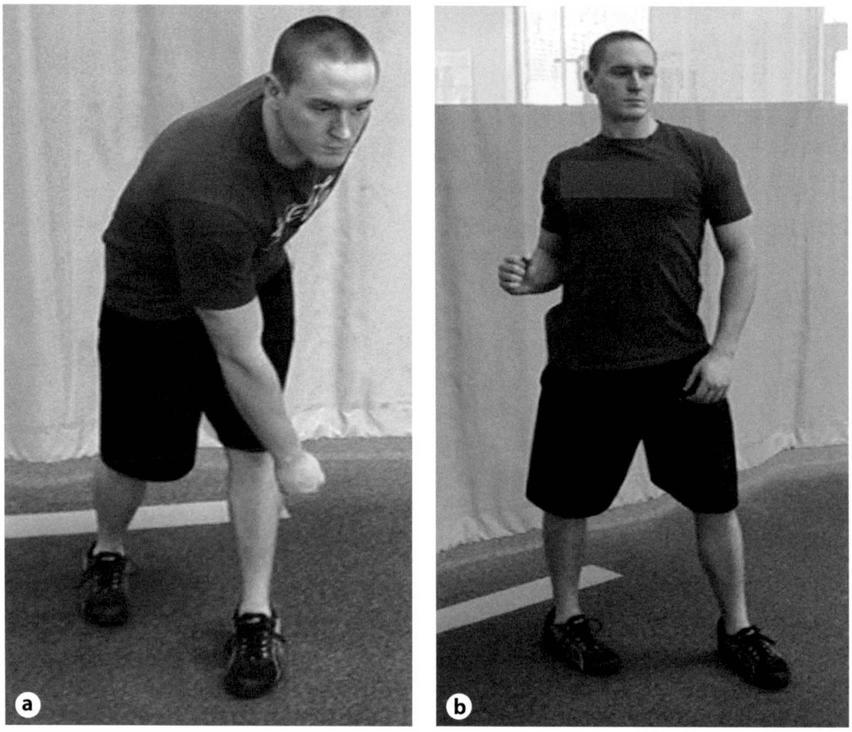

Fig. 7. Lawnmower dynamic exercise.

to stabilize the scapula with an outstretched arm. These punches, overhead presses, dumbbell 'cleans' and standing long pulls can all be done in various planes, with various amounts of leg and trunk contribution.

For scapulothoracic rehabilitation to be effective as part of rotator cuff injury, the scapula must be approached as a link within a kinetic chain. The scapula is dependent on the trunk and other proximal segments, just as the arm is dependent upon it for proper function [43, 45]. Deficits in more distant kinetic chain links may contribute to scapular dyskinesis, as well, and require evaluation and clinical attention for the rehabilitation to be complete. Thoracic spine restrictions, hip muscle tightness or weakness, low back tightness and GIRD deficit are common in patients with scapular dyskinesis and are obstacles to restoring scapular motion, strength and function.

Conclusions

Since scapular position, motion, and stability are key components of normal rotator cuff function, it is not surprising that alterations in scapular position, motion,

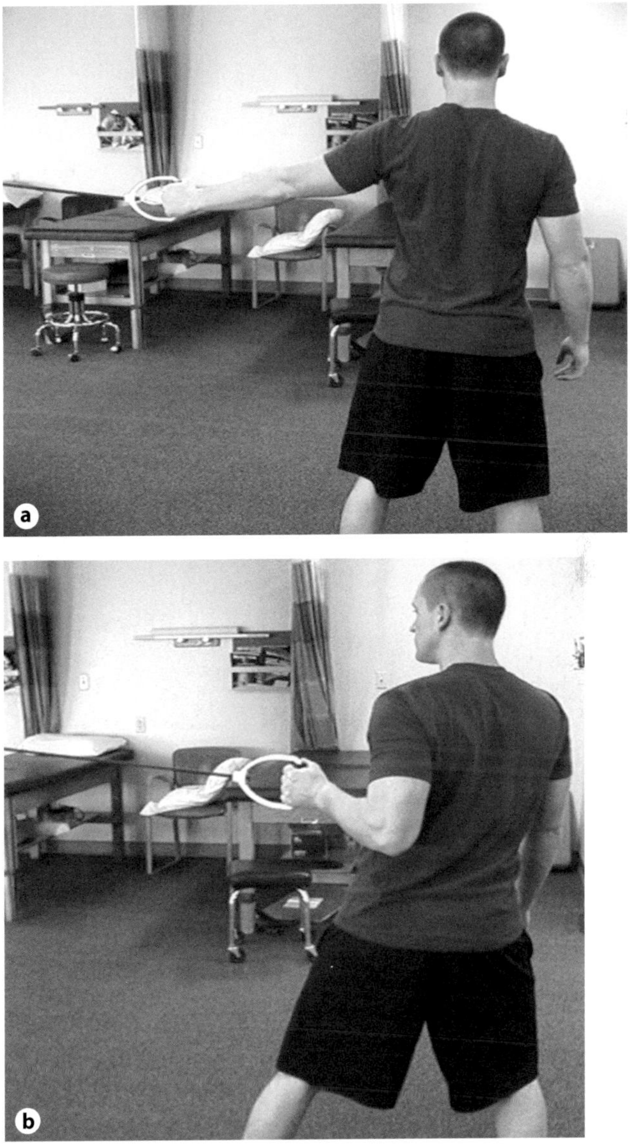

Fig. 8. Fencing dynamic exercise.

and stability collectively designated as scapular dyskinesis, should be found in association with the spectrum of rotator cuff dysfunction, from impingement through tendinopathy to tear. Dyskinesis may have causative effects to produce pathophysiology, increasing the risk of impingement or other extrinsic causes of rotator cuff disease or contributing to increased internal strain and influencing intrinsic causative factors. It may be an effect of rotator cuff disease from pain inhibition of muscle force couples. It may be a compensation for rotator cuff disease, to avoid pain-producing positions or motions, or to attempt to improve compromised motions. Probably, dyskinesis plays roles in all three circumstances depending on different pathology.

Scapular dyskinesis, a kinematic finding, has multiple causes which can be identified through careful evaluation. The clinical evaluation process can be standardized, and correlates with the actual biomechanically determined altered motions. Interventions and treatment can be based on the deficits identified.

Independent of whatever role dyskinesis plays in causation of rotator cuff disease or the causative factors of dyskinesis, scapular dyskinesis has been shown to be important in two functional problems of rotator cuff disease. Dyskinesis results in decreased capability to generate maximal rotator cuff strength, and it is associated with lower functional outcomes measurement scores.

References

1 Warner JP, Micheli LJ, Arslanian LE, Kennedy J, Kennedy R: Patterns of flexibility, laxity, and strength in normal shoulders and shoulders with instability and impingement. Am J Sports Med 1990;18:366–375.

2 Paletta GA, Warner JJP, Warren RF, Deutsch A, Altchek DW: Shoulder kinematics with two-plane x-ray evaluation in patients with anterior instability or rotator cuff tears. J Shoulder Elbow Surg 1997;6:516–527.

3 Deutsch A, Altchek DW, Schwartz E, Otis JC, Warren RF: Radiologic measurement of superior displacement of the humeral head in the impingement syndrome. J Shoulder Elbow Surg 1996;5:186–193.

4 Mell AG, LaScalza S, Guffey P, Carpenter JE, Hughes RE: Effect of rotator cuff pathology on shoulder rhythm. J Shoulder Elbow Surg 2005;14:S58–S64.

5 Kibler WB, Sciascia AD, Dome DC: Evaluation of apparent and absolute supraspinatus strength in patients with shoulder injury using the scapular retraction test. Am J Sports Med 2006;34:1643–1647.

6 Endo K, Ikata T, Katoh S, Takeda Y: Radiographic assessment of scapular rotational tilt in chronic shoulder impingement syndrome. J Orthop Sci 2001;6:3–10.

7 Ludewig PM, Cook TM: Alterations in shoulder kinematics and associated muscle activity in people with symptoms of shoulder impingement. Phys Ther 2000;80:276–291.

8 Lukasiewicz AC, McClure PW, Michener LA, Pratt N, Sennett BJ: Comparison of three-dimensional scapular position and orientation between subjects with and without shoulder impingement. J Orthop Sports Phys Ther 1999;29:574–586.

9 McClure P, Michener LA, Karduna AR: Shoulder function and three-dimensional scapular kinematics in people with and without shoulder impingement syndrome. Phys Ther 2006;86:1075–1090.

10 Graichen H, Stammberger T, Bonel H, et al: Three-dimensional analysis of shoulder girdle and supraspinatus motion patterns in patients with impingement syndrome. J Orthop Res 2001;19:1192–1198.

11 Su KP, Johnson MP, Gracely EJ, Karduna AR: Scapular rotation in swimmers with and without impingement syndrome: practice effects. Med Sci Sports Exer 2004;36:1117–1123.

12 Dunn W, Jones G: Factors associated with low outcomes scores in patients with full thickness rotator cuff tears. Feb 16, 2011.

13 Teece RM, Lunden JB, Lloyd AS, Kaiser AP, Cieminski CJ, Ludewig PM: Three-dimensional acromioclavicular joint motions during elevation of the arm. J Orthop Sports Phys Ther 2008;38:181–190.

14 Ludewig PM, Reynolds JF: The association of scapular kinematics and glenohumeral joint pathologies. J Orthop Sports Phys Ther 2009;39:90–104.

15 Michener LA, McClure PW, Karduna AR: Anatomical and biomechanical mechanisms of subacromial impingement syndrome. Clin Biomech 2003;18:369–379.

16 Hébert LJ, Moffet H, Dufour M, Moisan C: Acromiohumeral distance in a seated position in persons with impingement syndrome. J Mag Res Imaging 2003;18:72–79.
17 Karduna AR, Kerner PJ, Lazarus MD: Contact forces in the subacromial space: effects of scapular orientation. J Shoulder Elbow Surg 2005;14:393–399.
18 Falla D, Farina D, Graven-Nielsen T: Experimental muscle pain results in reorganization of coordination among trapezius muscle subdivisions during repetitive shoulder flexion. Exp Brain Res 2007;178: 385–393.
19 Ludewig PM, Phadke V, Braman JP, Hassett DR, Cieminski CJ, LaPrade RF: Motion of the shoulder complex during multiplanar humeral elevation. J Bone Joint Surg Am 2009;91:378–389.
20 Kebaetse M, McClure PW, Pratt N: Thoracic position effect on shoulder range of motion, strength, and three-dimensional scapular kinematics. Arch Phys Med Rehab 1999;80:945–950.
21 Endo K, Yukata K, Yasui N: Influence of age on scapulo-thoracic orientation. Clin Biomech 2004;19: 1009–1013.
22 McKee MD, Pedersen EM, Jones C, et al: Deficits following nonoperative treatment of displaced midshaft clavicular fractures. J Bone Joint Surg Am 2006;88:35–40.
23 Borstad JD, Ludewig PM: The effect of long versus short pectoralis minor resting length on scapular kinematics in healthy individuals. J Orthop Sports Phys Ther 2005;35:227–238.
24 Borich MR, Bright JM, Lorello DJ, Cieminski CJ, Buisman T, Ludewig PM: Scapular angular positioning at end range internal rotation in cases of glenohumeral internal rotation deficit. J Orthop Sports Phys Ther 2006;36:926–934.
25 Kibler WB: The role of the scapula in athletic function. Am J Sports Med 1998;26:325–337.
26 Harryman DT 2nd, Sidles JA, Clark JM, McQuade KJ, Gibb TD, Matsen FA 3rd: Translation of the humeral head on the glenoid with passive glenohumeral motion. J Bone Joint Surg Am 1990;72: 1334–1343.
27 Tyler TF, Nichaols SJ, Roy T, Gleim GW: Quantification of posterior capsular tightness and motion loss in patients with shoulder impingement. Am J Sports Med 2000;28:668–673.
28 Lin JJ, Hanten WP, Olson SL, et al: Functional activities characteristics of shoulder complex movements: exploration with a 3-D electromagnetic measurement system. J Rehabil Res Dev 2005;42: 199–210.
29 Cools AM, Witvrouw EE, DeClercq GA, Vanderstraeten GG, Cambier DC: Evaluation of isokinetic force production and associated muscle activity in the scapular rotators during a protraction-retraction movement in overhead athletes with impingement symptoms. Br J Sports Med 2004;38: 64–68.
30 Cools AM, Witvrouw EE, DeClercq GA, Danneels LA, Cambier DC: Scapular muscle recruitment pattern: trapezius muscle latency with and without impingement symptoms. Am J Sports Med 2003; 31:542–549.
31 Cools AM, Dewitte V, Lanszweert F, et al: Rehabilitation of scapular muscle balance. Am J Sports Med 2007;35:1744–1751.
32 Ebaugh DD, McClure PW, Karduna AR: Effects of shoulder muscle fatigue caused by repetitive overhead activities on scapulothoracic and glenohumeral kinematics. J Electromyogr Kinesiol 2006;16:224–235.
33 Tsai NT, McClure P, Karduna AR: Effects of muscle fatigue on three-dimensional scapular kinematics. Arch Phys Med Rehab 2003;84:1000–1005.
34 Kibler WB: Biomechanical analysis of the shoulder during tennis activities. Clin Sports Med 1995; 14:79–86.
35 Young JL, Herring SA, Press JM, Casazza BA: The influence of the spine on the shoulder in the throwing athlete. J Back Musculo Rehabil 1996;7:5–17.
36 Kibler WB, Press J, Sciascia AD: The role of core stability in athletic function. Sports Med 2006;36: 189–198.
37 Kluemper M, Uhl TL, Hazelrigg H: Effects of stretching and strengthening shoulder muscles on forward shoulder posture in competitive swimmers. J Sport Rehab 2006;15:58–70.
38 McClure PW, Tate AR, Kareha S, Irwin D, Zlupko E: A clinical method for identifying scapular dyskinesis. Part 1: Reliability. J Ath Train 2009;44: 160–164.
39 Tate AR, McClure PW, Kareha S, Irwin D, Barbe MF: A clinical method for identifying scapular dyskinesis: Part 2: Validity. J Ath Train 2009;44:165–173.
40 Kibler WB, Ludewig PM, McClure PW, Uhl TL, Sciascia AD: Scapula Summit 2009. J Orthop Sports Phys Ther 2009;39:A1–A13.
41 Uhl TL, Kibler WB, Gecewich B, Tripp BL: Evaluation of clinical assessment methods for scapular dyskinesis. Arthroscopy 2009;25:1240–1248.

42 Rabin A, Irrgang JJ, Fitzgerald GK, Eubanks A: The intertester reliability of the scapular assistance test. J Orthop Sports Phys Ther 2006;36:653–660.
43 Kibler WB, McMullen J, Uhl TL: Shoulder rehabilitation strategies, guidelines, and practice. Oper Tech Sports Med 2000;8:258–267.
44 Rubin B, Kibler WB: Fundamental principles of shoulder rehabilitation. Arthroscopy 2002;18:29–39.
45 Kibler WB, Sciascia AD, Uhl TL, Tambay N, Cunningham T: Electromyographic analysis of specific exercises for scapular control in early phases of shoulder rehabilitation. Am J Sports Med 2008;36: 1789–1798.

W. Ben Kibler, MD
Shoulder Center of Kentucky
1221 South Broadway
Lexington, KY 40504 (USA)
Tel. +1 859 258 8575, E-Mail wkibler@aol.com

Maffulli N (ed): Rotator Cuff Tear. Med Sport Sci. Basel, Karger, 2012, vol 57, pp 41–52

Instability and Rotator Cuff Tear

Giuseppe Porcellini[a] · Francesco Caranzano[b] · Fabrizio Campi[a] · Paolo Paladini[a]

[a]Operative Unit of Shoulder and Elbow Surgery, D. Cervesi Hospital, Cattolica/Rimini, and
[b]Orthopaedic and Traumatology Department, University of Turin, Mauriziano Hospital, Turin, Italy

Abstract

Prevalence of rotator cuff tears after traumatic dislocation increases with advancing age, as a consequence of the age-associated deterioration of structures and mechanical properties of the tendons of the rotator cuff. These act as effective stabilizers of the joint, compressing the humeral head in the three-dimensional concavity of the glenoid. It is impossible to establish whether a lesion of the capsulo-labrum complex or of the rotator cuff causes or follows a dislocation, regardless of whether it is anterior or posterior. A peripheral nerve or a brachial plexus injury can be associated with tendon lesion and instability, developing the 'terrible triad' of the shoulder. Both conservative and surgical management are possible, and surgeons must choose the most appropriate management modality according to the biologic age of the patients, functional demands, and type of lesion.

The incidence of shoulder dislocation before and after the age of 45 years is roughly equivalent [1], but the consequences of anterior glenohumeral dislocations in patients older than 40 years are markedly different than in the younger population: if in the young people the recurrence of the instability is the most common complication [2–7], in older patients, the primary issue is not recurrence of the dislocation, but the associated cuff tear [8, 9] that can lead to pain and functional deficits. The prevalence of rotator cuff tears after traumatic dislocation increases with advancing age [8], although the incidence of pre-existing rotator cuff tears is not well established. The different injury patterns are thought to be secondary to the changes in tissue properties that occur with aging, [10] and lead to degenerative weakening of the tendons [10–12]. Stevens [13], in 1926, and Codman [14], in 1934, first called attention to the possibility of tears of the rotator cuff accompanying anterior dislocation of the shoulder in elderly patients.

Prevalence and Incidence: Reports from the Literature

In 1986, Hawkins et al. [15] found, on the basis of clinical examination, an incidence of 90% of cuff lesions after dislocation in patients older than 40 years, while the incidence reported in ultrasonographic, arthrographic, and arthroscopic studies is lower: Reeves [16] and Itoi et al. [17] reported arthrographic studies in which the incidence of cuff lesions after dislocation was 30% in 28 patients older than 40 years, and 57% in patients older than 50 years. In a prospective ultrasonographic study, Toolanen et al. [11] found 25 cuff tears in 65 patients older than 40 years (38%), half partial and half full-thickness tears. A prospective study by Berbig et al. [18] evaluated 167 patients (average age 55 years, range 16–92) after a primary traumatic anterior shoulder dislocation with ultrasonography at a mean time of 13.3 days after the reduction, excluding patients with earlier shoulder surgery, and a control group of 93 healthy volunteers of similar age and sex distribution. In the case group, 53 patients had a full-thickness rotator cuff tear (incidence 31.7%); in patients less than 60 years, the percentage of tendon lesion was 8.2% for the case group (7 lesion on 82 patients), all fresh lesions at ultrasonography, and 0% for the control group. In patients older than 60 years, the percentage of cuff tears in the case group was 56% (46 lesions on 82 patients), with a pattern of acute lesion in 84.9% and of chronic lesion in 15.1%. In the control group, the incidence of cuff lesion was 44.4%, and all were chronic. The presence of a pre-existing asymptomatic tendon tear can be a confounding factor in such a study. To evaluate the prevalence of rotator cuff tears in the healthy population, Sher et al. [19] obtained magnetic resonance images of 96 asymptomatic shoulders: 34 patients had a cuff lesion (overall rate 34%); in patients older than 60 years, the rate of cuff tear (full- and partial thickness) was 54%. The prevalence of cuff tear was 28% in patients between 40 and 60 years, and 4% in patients younger than 40 years. Pevny et al. [20] reviewed 125 patients older than 40 years, without earlier shoulder injuries or surgery, who had sustained a traumatic first-time anterior shoulder dislocation secondary to ski trauma. Of the 52 patients with an average age of 56 years available to participate in the study, 17 had cuff lesions (32%) diagnosed by MRI, arthrogram or clinical evaluation. In a non-randomized prospective study, Simanket et al. [21] reported on a group of 65 patients evaluated after shoulder dislocation: 35 patients presented a cuff lesion (54%); the frequency increased to 100% in patients over the age of 70 years. Ribbans al. [22] reported 10 cuff lesions in 16 patients (61%) older than 40 years. Gumina and Postacchini [23] reported on 545 consecutive patients with anterior shoulder dislocations, a subgroup of 108 patients (20%) aged 60 years or more; they evaluated 95 patients from this subgroup by clinical or imaging study, reporting 58 cases (61%) of rotator cuff tears. The supraspinatus tendon is almost always involved [17], most often as an isolated rupture. Berbig et al. [18] found combined lesions of supraspinatus and subscapular and/or infraspinatus in 25% of shoulders. The involvement of the subscapularis tendon after shoulder dislocation is controversial: Neviaser and Neviaser [24] reported a study on 12 patients older than 40 years of age with recurrent instability of the shoulder, all with traumatic onset: 11 patients had recurrent anterior instability, and 1 patient had recurrent posterior dislocation. In this series, all patients with anterior instability had an isolated rupture of the subscapularis tendon and of the anterior capsule, without dislocation of the biceps tendon. In a case-control study of 314 consecutive arthroscopic procedures, Kim et al. [25] found 60 partial lesions of the subscapularis tendon, which were significantly associated with supraspinatus tears, cuff disease, and posterior-superior labrum fraying, and did not seem to be associated with glenohumeral instability. In an earlier observational study performed at our unit [26], with retrospective analysis of 150 prospectively gathered patients aged between 40 and 60 years, undergoing arthroscopy for rotator cuff lesions, shoulder instability, or both, there was no evidence of a statistically significant association between complete tears of the subscapularis and extensive rotator cuff disease and supraspinatus tears.

Biomechanics

Biomechanical studies of the shoulder have produced a more precise understanding of the individual contributions of the various ligaments, capsular regions and tendons to shoulder stability: shoulder muscles stabilize the glenohumeral joint by compressing the humeral head against the concave glenoid surface, allowing concentric rotation [27–30]. By this concavity-compression mechanism, the rotator cuff muscles act as the primary stabilizers of the glenohumeral joint especially during the mid-ranges of motion where the capsular ligamentous structures are lax [31]. Concavity compression is also important at the end ranges of motion, where muscle activity protects the capsular ligamentous structures by limiting the joint range of motion [32, 33] and by decreasing strain that, at these articular ranges, is usually increased on these structures [31, 34–39]. The effectiveness of the concavity-compression mechanism depends on characteristics of the shoulder muscle forces and the articular surfaces. Shoulder muscle forces may be defined by their magnitude and direction (line of action), and may be resolved into three components (fig. 1): compressive forces (stabilizing forces), translational superior-inferior directed forces, and anterior-posterior directed forces (destabilizing forces). Glenohumeral joint stability may be quantified by the ratio between the translational forces, in any direction, and the compressive forces [32, 40, 41]. The stability of the glenohumeral joint provided by concavity compression also depends on the effective glenoid arc, the area of the glenoid's articular surface available for humeral head compression [42], and may be quantified by the balance stability angle, the angle between the centre of the glenoid, and the end of the effective glenoid arc in any direction [41, 43]. The rotator cuff muscle forces are ideally aligned for effective

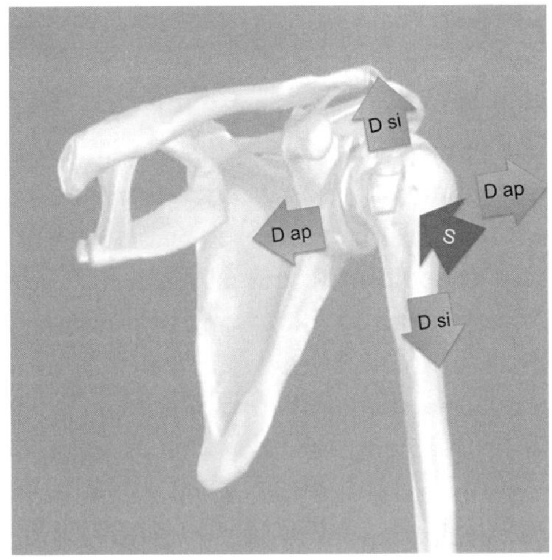

Fig. 1. Forces acting on the glenohumeral joint: stabilizing forces (S = compressive forces; black arrow) and destabilizing forces ($D_{I\text{-}S}$ = translational superior-inferior directed forces, $D_{A\text{-}P}$ = anterior-posterior directed forces; clear arrows).

compression of the glenohumeral joint at all shoulder positions [42]. Several biomechanical studies were performed to better understand and quantify the activity of cuff muscles on the stability of the joint: simulated rotator cuff activity increases the compressive forces at the glenohumeral joint and decreases the amount of humeral head translation that occurs in response to external loading; a 50% decrease in the rotator cuff muscle forces resulted in nearly a 50% increase in anterior displacement of the humeral head in response to external loading at all glenohumeral joint positions [37]. With the glenohumeral joint in its anatomic position, each rotator cuff muscle significantly contributed to anterior joint stability, and the contribution of each muscle was not significantly different from the others [44]. However, with the glenohumeral joint in end-range positions, the subscapularis was a less effective stabilizer of the glenohumeral joint than the other rotator cuff muscles, and the activity of the biceps brachii may also contribute to glenohumeral joint stability [45]. In a cadaveric model, Labriola al. [46] quantified the stability provided by active muscle forces in both mid-range and end-range glenohumeral joint positions. Compared with mid-range positions, the resultant joint force at end-range positions was directed more anteriorly, indicating that its contribution to glenohumeral joint stability was diminished. In end-range positions, simulated increase in rotator cuff muscle forces tended to improve stability, whereas increase in deltoid or pectoralis major muscle forces tended to further decrease stability. These investigations underline the importance of the action of the cuff tendons on the stability of the shoulder, but other studies were performed to quantify the shoulder instability following a tendon tear. This evaluation, performed through a muscle defect model is biased by the damage of the underlying superior capsule when the tendon defect is produced – a fact that in itself may alter stability. Therefore, a rotator cuff lesion was produced without damaging the underlying capsule in 80 cadaver shoulders to test the hypothesis that a rotator cuff lesion may limit the extent of capsular damage necessary for a dislocation to occur [47]. The supra- and infraspinatus, or the subscapularis, or all three tendons were carefully detached from their insertion. A sequential cutting protocol of four zones of the capsular ligamentous complex was implemented detaching them from the glenoid or the humerus. Stability was tested before and after each resection step; the humeral head dislocates easily with less extensive capsulo-ligamentous lesions when rotator cuff lesions are present [47]. Passive stabilization provided by the rotator cuff is more easily disrupted when associated with ligamentous lesions on the humeral side than with lesions on the glenoid side, as the close relationship of the cuff tendons with each other and with the capsule through the rotator cable is maintained with glenoid-sided lesions. Rotator cuff tendons contribute to passive stabilization of the glenohumeral joint. In the presence of cuff lesions, less extensive capsular ligamentous damage may result in a dislocation during the apprehension position. With an intact cuff, more damage can be tolerated before destabilization and dislocation occur.

Anterior and Posterior Mechanisms

McLaughlin [48] postulated that either the anterior or the posterior supporting structures of the shoulder can be disrupted after an anterior dislocation. In younger patients, the anterior capsular ligamentous structures most commonly fail after shoulder dislocation. However, in the older patient with pre-existing age-related weakening of the rotator cuff, it is more likely that the posterior rather than the anterior structures fail. Craig [49] popularized the 'posterior mechanism' of recurrent instability by analyzing the mechanical failure of cuff tissues after acute anterior shoulder dislocations in 3 patients over 60 years, all with recurrent instability. Many investigators report a strong association between cuff lesion and recurrent instability. However, when recurrent instability occurs in patients over 40, not only the posterior, but also the 'anterior mechanism' must be considered as an important contributing factor, when recurrent instability occurs in the absence of a significant rotator cuff tear [50]. In a retrospective review of 265 patients, Araghi et al. [51] identified 11 patients with recurrent anterior glenohumeral instability with onset after the age of 40, who had undergone operative management for shoulder stabilization; similar to this work, also in our previous study, the anterior mechanism – anterior capsulo-labrum detachment – seems to be the main cause of shoulder dislocation. Dislocations arising from failure of the posterior structures, with a full-thickness rotator cuff tear, seem, in our own series [26], to result from repeated dislocations rather than being the main cause. The rising number of dislocations is strongly associated with a greater number of posterior-superior lesions of the rotator cuff, supra- and infraspinatus, and this association was even stronger in patients who had experienced seven or more episodes of dislocations.

Terrible Triad of the Shoulder

The association between rotator cuff tears and nerve injury in patients over 40 years is frequent [11, 52–56]. However, there have been only a few reports with regard to the combination of shoulder dislocation, massive cuff tear (>5 cm), and neurological injury. Gonzalez and Lopez [57] in 1991 reported 2 patients, and Guven et al. [53] in 1994 reported 1 patient referring to this combination of injuries as the 'unhappy triad'. Groh and Rockwood [52] in 1995 reported 2 patients and coined the term 'terrible triad of the shoulder' for this injury association. Brown et al. [58] reported on 15 patients with concomitant rotator cuff tear and brachial plexus injuries treated with rotator cuff repair only, and concluded that these patients have a less favourable outcome than patients with isolated cuff repairs; Simonich and Wright [59] reported 6 patients with a recent anterior shoulder dislocation, massive rotator cuff tear and neurological injury. All underwent surgical cuff repair, with no routine nerve exploration at the time of rotator cuff repair, as most nerve injuries were neuropraxiae. Moreover, in patients older than 40, the potential for nerve recovery after reconstruction by graft is minimal; Simonich and Wright recommend to proceed to cuff repair as soon as possible to avoid retraction and atrophy during the nerve recovery, which can take 12–18 months, and suggest performing an electromyography, useful as baseline study, indicating a prognosis and helping clinically, because it is easy to miss an injury to the axillary nerve in patients with an associated massive cuff tear. Therefore, careful preoperative assessment is mandatory to predict the outcome. Patients with the terrible triad of the shoulder should be counselled that they have a greater than 50% chance to obtain a good outcome, but that optimal results after rotator cuff repair may take up to a year to develop. Pevny et al. [20] report an incidence of axillary nerve palsy of 8%, with an interesting association of rotator cuff tears in all patients with nerve injuries. They suggest that a rotator cuff tear should always be suspected when an axillary nerve or brachial plexus palsy is recognized.

Treatment

After relocation, accurate physical examination should be performed to expose possible tendon lesion. In younger patients, this is rare, although possible in high-energy or sports-related trauma [60]. Many investigators proposed treatment protocols (table 1). We usually adopt 20 days of immobilization after a first dislocation in patients up to 60, while this time is reduced to 2 weeks in the elderly, to avoid stiffness, and a subsequent rehabilitation program to strengthen the rotator cuff and scapular stabilizers and gradual recovery of complete range of motion; if, after 3 weeks of rehabilitation, the patient does not show significant improvement, MRI should be performed to evaluate the rotator cuff.

Table 1. Algorithms for the treatment of dislocation in the literature

Reference	Time of immobilization, start of physical therapy	Imaging examination
Hawkins and Mohtadi [61]	physical therapy at 1 week	arthrogram if poor improvement at 4 weeks
Sonnabend [62]	immobilization for 3 weeks	arthrogram or ultrasonography if pain and weakness were still present
Pevny et al. [20]	shorter immobilization to avoid stiffness in older patients	MRI: negative → rehabilitation program → repeat MRI at 3–4 weeks if poor improvement MRI: positive: arthroscopic or open cuff repair

Conservative Treatment

In older patients, shoulder dislocation is not a benign injury because of the high frequency of associated rotator cuff tears [20]. In general, the literature shows better results of operative treatment of combined instability-cuff lesion [8, 20, 50, 63, 64], but an accurate risk-benefit evaluation is mandatory. When the instability does not recur and the cuff lesion is well balanced, and the patient does not complain of pain and limitation in daily activity, conservative management is considered a possible option in elderly patients.

Operative Treatment

When a rotator cuff tear is present and is symptomatic, and when short-term conservative management does not result in improvement in terms of pain and function, surgery should be considered. The orthopaedic literature is replete with articles, reporting the successes and pitfalls of rotator cuff repairs and capsulo-labrum repairs as separate entities. There is scant literature discussing the operative treatment of patients with both. Pevny et al. [20] reported 84% of good results after early repair, compared with only 50% after conservative treatment, and concluded that early surgical repair of cuff tears yielded better results than conservative treatment. Bassett and Cofield [63] also reported better results after surgical cuff repair in terms of functional outcome and pain relief after acute dislocations. Loew et al. [8] underline how patients older than 60 have a high incidence of cuff tear arthropathy and tears after dislocation, and therefore, surgical treatment is appropriate. In older patients, shoulder dislocation is not a benign injury because of the high frequency of associated rotator cuff tears [20]. Lähteenmäki et al. [64] analyzed the results on 548 full-thickness tears (with an acute onset of symptoms), managed with early operative treatment. Despite severe preoperative symptoms, the results of early operative treatment are better than the results of either conservative treatment or late surgery, probably due to the good elasticity of the recently torn cuff. The distinction among an acute tear, acute symptoms of a chronic tear, or the acute extension of an existing chronic tear can be very difficult.

Operative Options

Hawkins et al. [65] recommend surgical repairs of both the capsulo-ligament complex and the rotator cuff in patients younger than 40 years. If a Bankart lesion is associated with partial cuff tears on the bursal side, involving less than 50% of the tendon, a Bankart repair only can be performed [66]. If a subscapularis tendon tear or a humeral avulsion of the glenohumeral ligament lesion is diagnosed, surgical repair should be performed [35] to avoid recurrence of instability. Voigt and Lill [67] proposed an algorithm for the surgical treatment of associated instability and tendon lesion in patients younger than 60 years; both capsulo-ligament reconstruction and cuff repair must be performed. In patients older than 60 or with low functional demands, cuff repair only is a good option to restore function and stability. In patients older than 70 years, in whom a cuff lesion preceding the dislocation is likely, if the repair is not possible, tendon transfer, inverse prosthesis or conservative management should be considered. Both open and arthroscopic repairs are possible. Walch and Boileau [68] proposed an open stabilization by coracoid transfer (Trillat procedure) associated to open cuff repair, and report a high incidence of arthritic changes. In a previous study [26], 50 patients aged 40–60 years with associated instability and rotator cuff tears were treated arthroscopically, 2 patients experienced recurrence of the instability, and underwent a Latarjet-Bristow procedure: at revision surgery, the cuff lesion was irreparable in both cases. Although there may be a wide spectrum of instability and cuff disease, young patients who necessitate surgery for both problems are rare. In high-demand athletes, the challenge involves the security of surgical fixation with the difficulty of complete restoration of motion. There are few reports about the management of these combined lesions in young athletes. Brislin et al. [69] perform a mini open cuff repair with combined suture anchors and transosseous sutures, or an arthroscopic repair in case of a small lesion, and then an open Bankart repair using non-absorbable anchors. They suggest that a stable repair of both lesions allows aggressive rehabilitation by minimizing the fixation pitfalls of arthroscopic-only techniques, and that the propensity for scarring and stiffness is lower with the mini open exposures. Goldberg et al. [60] report a small series of 6 elite rugby players with associated lesions who received a two-stage procedure. The mean duration between the first procedure (open-rotator cuff repair) and second procedure (open-shoulder stabilization) was 9.5 weeks (range 8–12). Overhead athletes may have some degree

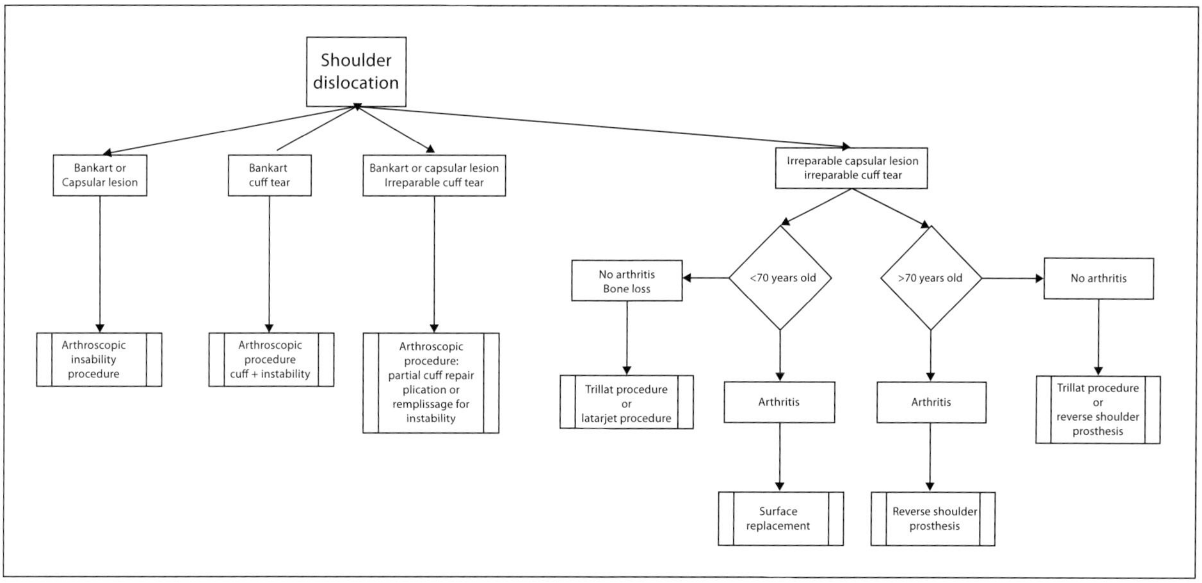

Fig. 2. Flowchart with main guidelines in case of shoulder instability.

of instability that predisposes their rotator cuffs to the microtrauma from the forceful repetitive activities of their game and training. This leads to weakening of the rotator cuff, which subsequently tears when the patient experiences an acute macrotraumatic event; athletes with shoulder instability who play contact sports should have the instability treated early, otherwise secondary changes occur, at times leading to severe rotator cuff injuries. Cole and Warner [70] considered combined rotator cuff and Bankart lesions a relative indication to perform an open repair. We recently [71] published the algorithm used in our unit for surgical management (fig. 2). The 'weakest link' is the procedure for the instability that limits aggressive rehabilitation. To avoid complications and the recurrence of instability, especially in active population, the proper surgical choice must be well evaluated, keeping in mind the most recent reports from the literature [5] about the recurrence, and identifying preoperatively such patients on the basis of sex, age, time from the first dislocation to surgery, bone loss and capsular status. Both open and arthroscopic approaches are feasible, and we suggest that the surgical option on how to manage the instability should guide and lead the final surgical choice.

Conclusions

The increase in functional demand for older individuals and the increasing age of the general population produce an increased frequency of trauma and in the necessity for a good functional result. Cuff lesions must be suspected and diagnosed promptly in older patients with a shoulder dislocation, as a long wait between the cuff rupture and surgery can jeopardize the outcome. It is not easy to establish whether a lesion of the rotator cuff causes or follows a dislocation, and both anterior and posterior mechanisms play a role in dislocation. An accurate examination after dislocation following high-energy trauma is mandatory to exclude tendon or neurological lesions, particularly in patients older than 40 years. The surgeon must consider the patient's age and functional demands, and the kind of lesion to plan the most appropriate management. Both arthroscopic and open surgeries are feasible; the operation for instability guides the surgical choice.

References

1 Rowe CR: Prognosis in dislocations of the shoulder. J Bone Joint Surg Am 1956;38:957–977.
2 Trillat A, Leclerc-Chalvet F: Luxation récidivante de l'épaule. Paris, Masson, 1973, p 126.
3 Hovelius L, Lind B, Thorling J: Primary dislocation of the shoulder: factors affecting the two-year prognosis. Clin Orthop Relat Res 1983;176:181–185.
4 Hovelius L, Eriksson G, Fredin F, et al: Recurrences after initial dislocation of the shoulder: results of a prospective study of treatment. J Bone Joint Surg Am 1983;65:343–349.
5 Hoelen MA, Burgers AM, Rozing PM: Prognosis of primary anterior shoulder dislocation in young adults. Arch Orthop Trauma Surg 1990;110:51–54.
6 Porcellini G, Campi F, Pegreffi F, et al: Predisposing factors for recurrent shoulder dislocation after arthroscopic treatment. J Bone Joint Surg Am 2009; 91:2537–2542.
7 McLaughlin MC: Trauma. Philadelphia, Saunders, 1960, pp 233–296.
8 Loew M, Thomsen M, Rickert M, Simank HG: Injury pattern in shoulder dislocation in the elderly patient (in German). Unfallchirurg 2001;104:115–118.
9 Noel B, Walch G, Tebib JG: Recurrent anterior luxation of the shoulder occurring after 40 years of age and rupture of the rotator cuff (in French). Rev Rhum Mal Osteoartic 1990;57:189–191.
10 Neviasser RJ, Neviaser TJ, Neviaser JS: Concurrent rupture of the rotator cuff and anterior dislocation of the shoulder in the older patient. J Bone Joint Surg Am 1988;70:1308–1311.
11 Toolanen G, Hildingsson C, Hedlund T, et al: Early complications after anterior dislocation of the shoulder in patients over 40 years. Acta Orthop Scand 1993;64:549–552.
12 Travlos J, Goldberg I, Boome RS: Brachial plexus lesions associated with dislocated shoulders. J Bone Joint Surg Br 1990;72:68–71.
13 Stevens JH: Dislocation of the shoulder. Ann Surg 1926;83:84–103.
14 Codman EA: The Shoulder: Rupture of the Supraspinatus Tendon and Other Lesions In or About the Subacromial Bursa. Boston, Thomas Todd Co, 1934.
15 Hawkins RJ, Bell RH, Hawkins RH, et al: Anterior dislocation of the shoulder in the older patient. Clin Orthop Relat Res 1986;206:192–195.
16 Reeves B: Acute anterior dislocation of the shoulder: clinical and experimental studies. Ann R Coil Surg Engl 1969;44:255–273.
17 ltoi E, Tabata S, Prim J: Rotator cuff tears in anterior dislocation of the shoulder. lnt Orthop 1992;19:240–244.
18 Berbig R, Weishaupt D, Prim J, Shahin O: Primary anterior shoulder dislocation and rotator cuff tears. J Shoulder Elbow Surg 1999;8:220–225.
19 Sher J, Uribe J, Posadu A, et al: Abnormal findings on magnetic resonance images of asymptomatic shoulders. J Bone Joint Surg Am 1995;77:10–15.
20 Pevny T, Hunter RE, Freeman JR: Primary traumatic anterior shoulder dislocation in patients 40 years of age and older. Arthroscopy 1998;14: 289–294.
21 Simank HG, Dauer G, Schneider S, et al: Incidence of rotator cuff tears in shoulder dislocations and results of therapy in older patients. Arch Orthop Trauma Surg 2006;126:235–240.
22 Ribbans WJ, Mitchell R, Taylor GJ: Computerised arthrotomography of primary anterior dislocation of the shoulder. J Bone Joint Surg Br 1990;72:181–185.

23 Gumina S, Postacchini R: Anterior dislocation of the shoulder in elderly patients. J Bone Joint Surg Br 1979;540–543.
24 Neviaser RJ, Neviaser N: Recurrent instability of the shoulder after age 40. J Shoulder Elbow Surg 1999;4:416–418.
25 Kim TK, Rauh PB, McFarland EG: Partial tears of the subscapularis tendon found during arthroscopic procedures on the shoulder: a statistical analysis of sixty cases. Am J Sports Med 2003;31:744–750.
26 Porcellini G, Paladini P, Campi F, et al: Shoulder instability and related rotator cuff tears: arthroscopic finding and treatment in patients aged 40 to 60 years. Arthroscopy 2006;22:270–276.
27 Howell SM, Galinat BJ, Renzi AJ, et al: Normal and abnormal mechanics of the glenohumeral joint in the horizontal plane. J Bone Joint Surg Am 1988;70:227–232.
28 Karduna AR, Williams GR, Williams JL, et al: Kinematics of the glenohumeral joint: influences of muscle forces, ligamentous constraints, and articular geometry. J Orthop Res 1996;14:986–993.
29 Kelkar R, Wang VM, Flatow EL, et al: Glenohumeral mechanics: a study of articular geometry, contact, and kinematics. J Shoulder Elbow Surg 2001;10:73–84.
30 Poppen NK, Walker PS: Normal and abnormal motion of the shoulder. J Bone Joint Surg Am 1976;58:195–201.
31 Howell SM, Kraft TA: The role of the supraspinatus and infraspinatus muscles in glenohumeral kinematics of anterior shoulder instability. Clin Orthop Relat Res 1991;263:128–134.
32 Lippett S, Vanderhoof J, Harris SL, et al: Glenohumeral stability from concavity-compression: a quantitative analysis. J Shoulder Elbow Surg 1993;2:27–34.
33 Neviaser RJ, Neviaser TJ, Neviaser JS: Anterior dislocation of the shoulder and rotator cuff rupture. Clin Orthop Relat Res 1993;291:103–106.
34 Apreleva M, Parsons IM, Pfaeffle J, et al: 3-D joint reaction forces at the glenohumeral joint during active motion. Adv Bioeng 1998;39:33–34.
35 Parsons IM, Apreleva M, Fu FH, et al: The effect of rotator cuff tears on reaction forces at the glenohumeral joint. J Orthop Res 2002;20:439–446.
36 Poppen NK, Walker PS: Forces at the glenohumeral joint in abduction. Clin Orthop Relat Res 1978;135:165–170.
37 Wuelker N, Korell M, Thren K: Dynamic glenohumeral joint stability. J Shoulder Elbow Surg 1998;7:43–52.
38 Burkhead WZ Jr, Rockwood CA Jr: Treatment of instability of the shoulder with an exercise program. J Bone Joint Surg Am 1992;74:890–896.
39 Rodosky MW, Harner CD, Fu FH: The role of the long head of the biceps muscle and superior glenoid labrum in anterior stability of the shoulder. Am J Sports Med 1994;22:121–130.
40 Lazarus MD, Sidles JA, Harryman DT, et al: Effect of a chondral-labral defect on glenoid concavity and glenohumeral stability: a cadaveric model. J Bone Joint Surg Am 1996;78:94–102.
41 Matsen FA (ed): Practical Evaluation and Management of the Shoulder. Philadelphia, Saunders, 1994, p 242.
42 Lee SB, Kim KJ, O'Driscoll SW, et al: Dynamic glenohumeral stability provided by the rotator cuff muscles in the mid-range and end-range of motion: a study in cadavera. J Bone Joint Surg Am 2000;82:849–857.
43 Rockwood CA, Matsen FA, Wirth MA, et al (eds): The Shoulder. Philadelphia, Saunders, 1998, pp 223–250.
44 Blasier RB, Guldberg MS, Rothman ED: Anterior shoulder stability: contributions of rotator cuff forces and the capsular ligaments in a cadaver model. J Shoulder Elbow Surg 1992;1:140–150.
45 Itoi E, Newman SR, Kuechle DK, et al: Dynamic anterior stabilisers of the shoulder with the arm in abduction. J Bone Joint Surg Br 1994;76:834–836.
46 Labriola JE, Lee TQ, Debski RE, et al: Stability and instability of the glenohumeral joint: the role of shoulder muscles. J Shoulder Elbow Surg 2005;14(suppl):32S–38S.
47 Pouliart N, Gagey O: Concomitant rotator cuff and capsular ligamentous lesions of the shoulder: a cadaver study. Arthroscopy 2006;22:728–735.
48 McLaughlin H: Injuries of the shoulder and arm; in McLaughlin H, Harrison L (eds): Trauma. Philadelphia, Saunders, 1959, pp 233–296.
49 Craig EV: The posterior mechanism of acute anterior shoulder dislocations. Clin Orthop Relat Res 1984;190:212–216.
50 Loehr JF, Helmig P, Søjbjerg JO, et al: Shoulder instability caused by rotator cuff lesions. An in vitro study. Clin Orthop Relat Res 1994;304:84–90.
51 Araghi A, Prasarn M, St Clair S, et al: Recurrent anterior glenohumeral instability with onset after forty years of age. Bull Hosp Joint Dis 2005;62:99–101.
52 Groh G, Rockwood C: The terrible triad: anterior dislocation of the shoulder associated with rupture of the rotator cuff and injury to the brachial plexus. J Shoulder Elbow Surg 1995;4:51–54.
53 Guven O, Akbar Z, Yalcin S, et al: Concomitant rotator cuff tear and brachial plexus injury in association with anterior shoulder dislocation: unhappy triad of the shoulder. J Orthop Trauma 1994;8:429–430.

54 Kaplan PE, Kernahan WT: Rotator cuff rupture: management with suprascapular neuropathy. Arch Phys Med Rehabil 1984;65:273–275.
55 Kay SP, Yaszemski MJ, Rockwood CA Jr: Acute tear of the rotator cuff masked by simultaneous palsy of the brachial plexus. J Bone Joint Surg Am 1988; 70:611–612.
56 Roach KE, Budiman-Mak E, Songsiridej N, et al: Development of a shoulder pain and disability index. Arthritic Care Res 1991;4:143–149.
57 Gonzalez D, Lopez R: Concurrent rotator cuff tear and brachial plexus palsy associated with anterior dislocation of the shoulder: a report of two cases. J Bone Joint Surg Am 1991;73:620–621.
58 Brown T, Newton P, Steinmann S, et al: Rotator cuff tears and associated nerve injuries. Orthopedics 2000;23:329–332.
59 Simonich SD, Wright TW: Terrible triad of the shoulder. J Shoulder Elbow Surg 2003;12:566–568.
60 Goldberg JA, Chan KY, Best JP: Surgical management of large rotator cuff tears combined with instability in elite rugby football players. Br J Sports Med 2003;37:179–181.
61 Hawkins RJ, Mohtadi NG: Controversy in anterior shoulder instability. Clin Orthop Relat Res 1991; 272:152–161.
62 Sonnabend DH: Treatment of primary anterior shoulder dislocation in patients older than 40 years of age. Clin Orthop Relat Res 1994;304:74–77.
63 Bassett RW, Cofield RH: Acute tears of the rotator cuff: the timing of surgical repair. Clin Orthop Relat Res 1983;175:18–24.
64 Lähteenmäki HE, Virolainen P, Hiltunen A, et al: Results of early operative treatment of rotator cuff tears with acute symptoms. J Shoulder Elbow Surg 2006;15:148–153.
65 Hawkins RJ, Morin WD, Bonutti PM: Surgical treatment of full-thickness rotator cuff tears in patients 40 years of age or younger. J Shoulder Elbow Surg 1999;8:259–265.
66 Habermeyer P, Lichtenberg S, Magosch P: Rotator cuff tear and shoulder instability (in German). Arthroskopie 2007;20:217–222.
67 Voigt C, Lill H: Shoulder instability and rotator cuff tear (in German). Orthopade 2009;38:70–74.
68 Walch G, Boileau P: Rotator cuff tears associated with anterior instability; in Warner JJ, Iannotti JP, Gerber C (eds): Complex and Revision Problems in Shoulder Surgery. Philadelphia, Lippincott-Raven, 1997.
69 Brislin K, Rubenstein D, Wetzler M, et al: Operative repair of anterior instability and rotator cuff tears in athlete. Oper Tech Sports Med 2002;10–2:64–68.
70 Cole BJ, Warner JJ: Arthroscopic versus open Bankart repair for traumatic anterior shoulder instability. Clin Sports Med 2000;19:19–48.
71 Porcellini G, Caranzano F, Campi F, et al: Glenohumeral instability and rotator cuff tear. Sports Med Arthrosc Rev (in press).

Giuseppe Porcellini
Operative Unit of Shoulder and Elbow Surgery
D. Cervesi Hospital, Via L.V. Beethoven 46
IT–47841 Cattolica/Rimini (Italy)
Tel. +39 0541 966 111, E-Mail gporcellini@tin.it

Maffulli N (ed): Rotator Cuff Tear. Med Sport Sci. Basel, Karger, 2012, vol 57, pp 53–64

Growth Factors and Tendon Healing

Francesco Oliva[a] · Stefano Gatti[b] · Giuseppe Porcellini[c] · Nicholas R. Forsyth[d] · Nicola Maffulli[e]

[a]Department of Orthopaedics and Traumatology, University of Rome 'Tor Vergata' School of Medicine, Rome, [b]Department of Orthopaedics and Traumatology, University of Siena School of Medicine, Siena, [c]Operative Unit of Shoulder and Elbow Surgery, 'D. Cervesi Hospital', Cattolica/Rimini, Italy; [d]The Guy Hilton Research Laboratories, Keele University Medical School, Stoke on Trent, and [e]Centre for Sports and Exercise Medicine Queen Mary University of London, Barts and The London School of Medicine and Dentistry, Mile End Hospital, London, UK

Abstract

Recent attention has focused on the biological pathways by which tendons heal leading to the identification of some growth factors (GFs) with involvement in this process. No studies have been published on the time course of the various GFs during the tendon healing process in vivo in humans. We review what is known about these GFs and their role in tendon healing.

The basic cell biology of tendons is still not fully understood, and the management of tendon injury is still challenging. Tendon injuries can be acute or chronic, and are caused by intrinsic or extrinsic factors, either alone or in combination. In acute trauma, extrinsic factors predominate. Overuse injuries and chronic tendon disorders generally have a multifactorial origin [1]. The pathologic label 'tendinosis' has been in use for more than two decades to describe collagen degeneration in tendinopathy, which is only one of the features of tendinopathy [2].

Growth factors (GFs) are synthesized and secreted by a wide variety of inflammatory cells, platelets, fibroblasts, epithelial cells, and vascular endothelial cells. In a very specific fashion, they bind to external receptors on the cell membrane, which leads to intracellular changes in DNA synthesis and expression. In this manner, GFs directly affect cellular mitogenesis and chemotaxis and are able to influence the healing cascade. Large-scale clinical trials have not been successful, possibly through inadequate delivery strategies failing to meet the physiological requirements of the tissue repair processes. These requirements are likely to comprise multiple GFs over a specific temporal pattern at an optimized ratio to meet the specific needs of the physiological process involved in tissue healing [3, 4], through processes which remain to be clarified [5].

The GF requirements of tendon cells have been investigated for over three decades. Initial experiments focussed on the actions of epidermal growth factor (EGF), insulin, and platelet-derived growth factor (PDGF) in in vitro conditions [6, 7]. Platelet-rich plasma, developed in the late 1990s [8] as a means to concentrate endogenous GFs, is now used in North America [9] and Continental Europe [10, 11].

Tendon Repair

Tendon repair can occur either intrinsically via the resident tenocytes [12] or via extrinsic mechanisms, whereby cells from the surrounding sheath or synovium invade the tissue [13]. Three biologically and temporally overlapping phases are described during tendon repair [14]. The healing process includes three phases: (1) The *inflammatory phase:* haematoma, platelet activation and invasion of cells that form a granuloma. Usually, this phase occurs 3–7 days after the injury, cells migrate from the extrinsic peritendinous tissue such as the tendon sheath, periosteum, subcutaneous tissue, and fascicles, as well as from the epitenon and endotenon [15]. (2) The *formative phase*, when cells proliferate and differentiate, continues for 8 weeks after the initial injury [16]. The migrated fibroblasts in the granuloma produce collagen (mostly collagen type III), which gradually increases its mechanical strength, so that loading can lead to elastic deformation, which allows mechanical signalling to start to influence the process. Production of collagen type I gradually takes over, and the repair callus reaches its largest size. The large transverse area compensates for tissue weakness, so that considerable traction forces can be sustained. Tenocytes become the main cell type, and collagen is continuously synthesized over the next 5 weeks. (3) Finally, in the *remodelling phase*, collagen type III is reabsorbed and replaced to produce better organization, and cross-linking increases. Finally, the callus transverse area gradually decreases as the mechanical tissue properties improve. Despite intensive remodelling over the following months, complete regeneration of the tendon is never achieved. The tissue replacing the defect remains hypercellular. The diameter of the collagen fibrils is altered, favouring thinner fibrils with reduction in the biomechanical strength of the tendon [17].

No studies have been published on the time of appearance of GF in the three different phases of the tendon healing process in humans. In a rabbit model, during healing of acute midsubstance rotator cuff tears, Kobayashi et al. [18] assessed semi-quantitatively the time expression of basic fibroblast growth factor (bFGF), insulin-like growth factor (IGF)-1, PDGF, and transforming growth factor (TGF-β) for 28 days. IGF-1 and TGF-β appear first in the blood cells in the inflammation phase; bFGF and PDGF appear later during the formative phase. TGF-β was present during

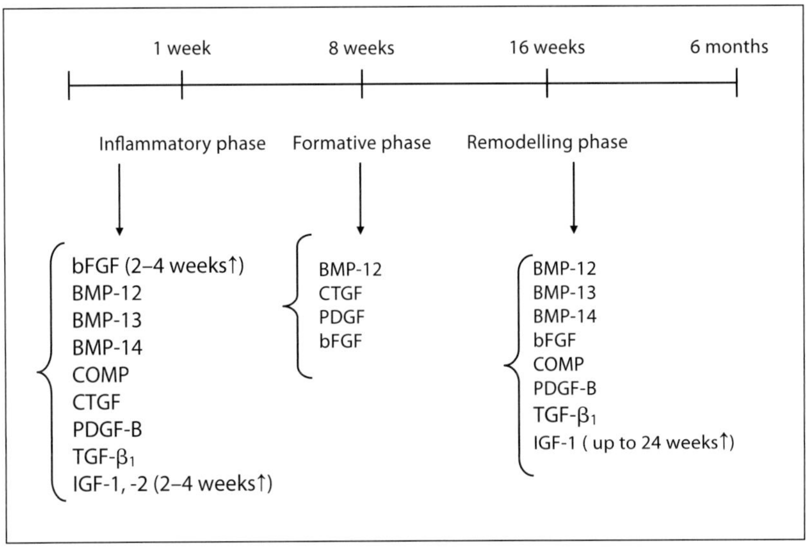

Fig. 1. The healing process of all tendons passes through three well-known stages. GFs are expressed during all these phases, promoting cell proliferation, extracellular matrix production and also participating in the final remodelling of the tendon. This figure shows the timing of some GFs studied which may in the near future be modified after new research but must be kept in mind because addition of GFs too early or late in the tendon healing process may decrease their effectiveness.

all the phases of the healing process, but the distal stump of the tear was lacking of these GFs.

Recently, Würgler-Hauri et al. [19] studied bFGF, BMP-12, BMP-13, BMP-14, cartilage oligomeric matrix protein (COMP), connective tissue growth factor (CTGF), PDGF-B, and TGF-β_1 in tendon-to-bone healing in a rat supraspinatus model for 16 weeks. Immunoassays showed an increase in the expression of all GFs at 1 week, followed by a return to control or undetectable levels by 16 weeks in both the insertion and midsubstance. Of additional note in the insertion, COMP peaked at 1 week, followed by a decrease in expression at 2 weeks. BMP-12 and CTGF were moderately expressed across all time points. Furthermore, BMP-12 and PDGF-B were moderately expressed over time in the midsubstance [19].

Growth Factors in Tendon Healing

Numerous GFs are involved in tendon repair. These include BMPs, EGF, FGF1, FGF2, IGF-1, IGF-2, PDGF-AA, PDGF-BB, PDGF-AB, TGF-β. These may be produced locally by cells in areas of injury, growth and repair, or may be delivered by blood (fig. 1).

Basic Fibroblastic Growth Factor

bFGF is a single-chain polypeptide of 146 amino acids, and is a member of the heparin-binding GF family. In humans, 22 members have been identified, all of which are structurally related signalling molecules. It is angiogenic [20] and has mitogenic effects on many mesenchymal cells such as ligament fibroblasts [21].

This GF has been shown to be involved in wound healing. Specifically, Chan et al. [22] showed that, in vitro, supplementation of bFGF increases the proliferation of rat patellar tendon fibroblasts. Chang et al. [23] showed that bFGF mRNA is upregulated in the tendon wound environment, and upregulated in tenocytes as well as in tendon sheath fibroblasts and inflammatory cells in vivo.

bFGF has also a stimulatory effect on human rotator cuff tendon cells in vitro, but suppresses collagen synthesis [24]. Kobayashi et al. [18] show an immunohistochemical peak expression of bFGF in the first week in a midsubstance injury of supraspinatus tendon in the rabbit, and it was suggested that bFGF could be used to promote the healing process of a torn rotator cuff tendon [25]. In a rabbit supraspinatus tendon bone injury, Würgler-Hauri et al. [19] supported this finding and, in addition, they detected another increase of bFGF at 8 weeks.

Bone Morphogenetic Proteins

BMPs (bone morphogenetic proteins) are a group of factors of the TGF-β superfamily that stimulate bone formation but also stimulate tendon cell mitogenesis and tendon healing. Although it is clear that BMPs stimulate tendon healing, the mechanism remains unclear [26, 27]. A combination of BMP signalling and influences of mechanical loading are likely crucial for tendon healing. This is reinforced by the BMP-14 knockout mice studies where a delayed tendon healing response and irregular type I collagen fibrils were observed [27]. However, in rat Achilles tendon injury models, BMP-13, not BMP-14, appeared to be involved in early tendon healing, BMP-14 was primarily required for the maintenance of homeostasis of mature tendons, and BMP-12 was required for both [28]. BMP-12, BMP-13 and BMP-14 have all been detected in intact human tendons by immunohistochemistry [29, 30].

Ovoid tendon cells (tenoblasts) in patellar tendons display elevated levels of both BMP-12 and BMP-13 when compared to the elongated tendon cells (tenocytes) [30]. This suggests that tenoblasts are more active in matrix remodelling and healing than tenocytes. In addition, BMP-2, BMP-7, and BMP-12 all participate in tendon-bone healing and improve formation of new bone and fibrocartilage at the healing tendon attachment site, resulting in an improved load to failure [31].

Recently, gene therapy with the BMP-12 cDNA muscle graft showed histologically better organized and homogeneous pattern of collagen fibres at all time points than the control groups [32]. Recombinant BMP-12 on a sponge carrier also stimulated rotator cuff repair in the sheep model [33]. Although BMP-14 did not appear to be directly involved in healing in the Achilles tendon model, BMP-14 gene therapy did increase tendon tensile strength in a rat model of Achilles tendon injury [34].

Insulin-Like Growth Factor

IGF is named after its hypoglycaemic effect after intravenous administration. The stimulatory effects of IGF-1 have been demonstrated in many cell types, including cartilage, bone, muscle and tendon cells [35]. During tendon healing, its role seems to stimulate the proliferation and migration of the tenoblasts during the inflammatory phase, while its increase in the remodelling phase seems to be clear [36]. In addition to the mitogenic effect, IGF-1 can also stimulate selected components of matrix synthesis, and its expression was noted in avian tenocytes [37]. Complementary to this are the observations that IGF-1 induced tenocyte migration, division, matrix expression and accelerated functional recovery from Achilles tendon injury in a rat model [38–40]. However, IGF-1 was not observed in tenocytes on day 10 following injury in a canine flexor tendon repair model, but was instead located in the surrounding inflammatory cells [41]. Similar observations were noted in studies concerning lesions of the flexor digitorum superficialis tendons of both forelimbs [42]. Similar to the canine model, IGF-1 levels had decreased by approximately 40% when compared to normal tendon at 2 weeks. Continued analysis then revealed a substantial upregulation of IGF-1, exceeding normal tendons. By 4 weeks, IGF-1 levels had increased substantially and were maintained through to 8 weeks. IGF-1 also improved aspects of healing in an equine model of collagenase-induced flexor tendinopathy [43].

The expression of the insulin-like growth factor-1-binding proteins (IGFBPs) has been studied in equine flexor tendons after acute injury and during healing over time: mRNA and protein expression for IGFBP-2, -3, and -4 was detected in normal tendon, and showed a marked increase following injury [44].

Platelet-Derived Growth Factor

PDGF was first isolated from platelets, but can be produced by many different cells, including smooth muscle cells [45]. PDGF is a basic protein of approximately 30 kDa formed by two subunits (α and β chain) that exist in three isoforms. Most studies are focussed on the homodimer PDGF-BB isoform, which has stimulatory effects on both cell division and matrix synthesis.

An investigation into the consequences of administration of PDGF-BB directly into the wound gap of rat patellar tendons showed that early supplementation (day 3 post-injury) was not beneficial to restoration of mechanical properties [46], probably from an increase in cell proliferation without matrix production. Later supplementation with PDGF-BB (on day 7 post-injury) did stimulate matrix production, with an accompanying higher peak load and pyridinoline content. PDGF-BB stimulated matrix and DNA synthesis in a dose-dependent manner in intrasynovial intermediate and proximal segments of deep flexor tendons, and extrasynovial peroneal tendons of rabbits during short-term cultures. PDGF-BB stimulated collagen synthesis and non-collagen protein synthesis in proximal intrasynovial tendon segments more than in extrasynovial peroneal tendon segments, and DNA synthesis less in proximal than in intermediate intrasynovial tendons [47].

Exogenous PDGF genes can be transferred effectively into intrasynovial tenocytes. The transfer increases significantly the expression of genes for PDGF and type I collagen [48].

PDGF holds particular promise in combination with other GFs. Tendon cells express the receptor for PDGF, but do not normally express PDGF itself [49]. When applied with IGF-1 TGF-β and bFGF, robust stimulation of tendon fibroblast migration and cell division are produced [38, 39, 50–53]. In a tissue engineering study, PDGF-BB-transduced cells stimulated adjacent rat tendon fibroblasts to increase collagen synthesis by 300% at 24 h compared to a 28% increase in IGF-1-transduced cells [54].

In a study of intrasynovial canine tendon, PDGF-BB and bFGF significantly increased flexor tendon fibroblast proliferation, collagen production and matrix synthesis when each was applied on its own. [55]. In a study on the expression of GFs in normal canine flexor tendon healing, PDGF-AA, PDGF-BB and VEGF appeared in the whole tendon section at 10 days following tendon injury [41]. Mechanical stretching of tendon fibroblasts also promoted increased concentrations of TGF-β, PDGF and bFGF, suggesting that cyclical mechanical stretching may have a positive influence on tendon and ligament healing through stimulation of cell proliferation, differentiation and matrix formation [49]. PDGF in association with hypoxia exerts a synergistic effect which increases the expression of VEGF in Achilles tendon fibroblasts [56]. In another study, PDGF gene therapy was more beneficial to tendon healing than VEGF gene therapy in an in vitro study of rat intrasynovial tendons [57].

Transforming Growth Factor-β

Originally, TGF-β was thought to be related to cellular transformation events prior to neoplastic growth. It is now clear that TGF-β has numerous physiological effects [58, 59]. The expression of TGF-β appears closely tied to the expression of a differentiated phenotype in many cell lines including the mesenchymal precursor. Tendon and ligament formation has been tied directly to factors belonging to the TGF-β superfamily [60]. Proliferation, matrix synthesis and differentiation have also been affected in tenoblasts, chondroblasts and osteoblasts [61]. Whether this is an inhibitory or stimulatory effect depends on the stage of differentiation, presence of other GFs, and assay system used [62, 63]. TGF-β is a weak stimulator of tendon cell migration and mitogenesis, but can stimulate robust expression of extracellular matrix [64]. TGF-β affects gene expression primarily through the activation of the Smad signalling pathway. The first step in the Smad pathway is the expression of TGF-β-inducible early gene (TIEG). Healing of tendons in the TIEG knockout mouse suggests the possibility of tendon healing in the absence of the Smad pathway, and the existence of TIEG-independent routes [65]. TGF-β_1 significantly increased the amount of α-smooth muscle actin (SMA) in non-vascular cells in seven human rotator cuffs, suggesting that SMA-containing cells could contribute to the retraction of the torn ends of a ruptured rotator cuff and play an important role in healing [66].

In a canine flexor tendon injury repair model, TGF-β was detected at and proximal to the repair site [41]. Complementary to these findings was the observation that, in Achilles rat tendon healing models, the failure load and stiffness of the healing tendon were increased by administration of TGF-β_1 at 2 and 4 weeks [67]. Furthermore, the application of TGF-β_1 significantly increased the tangent modulus and the tensile strength of the fibrous tissue produced in the rabbit patellar tendon after resecting the central portion, suggesting a role of TGF-β_1 in in vivo tendon regeneration [68].

TGF-β may control the switching point in the healing process from normal to pathological [69]. All three TGF-β isoforms significantly increase collagen I and III production in cultured tendon fibroblasts [70]. TGF-β_1 induced a greater degree of contraction in tendon fibroblasts cultured in collagen gels as compared with TGF-β_3 [71]. This might explain the finding that TGF-β_1 induces scar tissue formation, whereas TGF-β_3 reduces it [72]. Intraoperative administration of neutralizing antibody to TGF-β_1 improves flexor tendon excursion, but simultaneous infiltration of neutralizing antibody to TGF-β_2 nullifies this effect. Therefore, TGF-β isoforms may interact with one another to modulate collagen synthesis in healing tendons [73].

The temporal and spatial distribution of three TGF-β receptor isoforms (RI, RII, and RIII) was analysed in a rabbit zone II flexor tendon wound healing model. This demonstrated that TGF-β receptors were upregulated after injury and during repair [74]. Receptor production was concentrated in the epitenon, tendon sheath and along the repair site. Peak levels of TGF-β receptor expression were noted on day 14 and persisted until day 56.

Formation of nitric oxide is an important event in the course of tendon healing, and its inhibition results in chronic inflammation and fibrosis due to an imbalance in TGF-β expression in vivo [75]. Examining the expression of inducible nitric oxide synthase and TGF-β in macrophage infiltrates within crush-injured digital flexor tendon and synovium of rats during normal tendon healing, the levels of TGF-β are high at first, and gradually decrease after 3 weeks of injury [75].

Vascular Endothelial Growth Factors

They are important signalling proteins involved in both vasculogenesis and angiogenesis. The broad term 'VEGF' covers a number of proteins from two families that result from alternate splicing of mRNA from a single, 8 exon, VEGF gene. The most important member is VEGF-A, a glycosylated protein of 46–48 kDa composed of two disulphide-linked subunits. Other members are placenta growth factor, VEGF-B, VEGF-C and VEGF-D. The latter ones were discovered later than VEGF-A, and before their discovery VEGF-A was called just VEGF. All members of the VEGF family stimulate cellular responses by binding to tyrosine kinase receptors (the VEGFRs) on the cell surface, causing them to dimerize and become activated through trans-phosphorylation, although to different sites, times and extents [76]. Bidder et al. [77], using in situ hybridization in a canine model of tendon injury, identified cell populations within the repair site expressing message for VEGF, suggesting their potential for organizing the angiogenic response during the early postoperative phase of wound tendon healing. Recently, Pufe et al. [78] demonstrated that VEGF concentrations are negligible in healthy human adult Achilles tendons, but high in ruptured and embryonic ones.

Discussion

In vitro cell-based studies and animal models have clarified the role of single and GFs administered to enhance cell proliferation and chemotaxis [79], aid angiogenesis [80], and influence cell differentiation during wound healing [81]. Few studies have been conducted to delineate the timing of GF expression during the various phases of the healing process in tendons [19, 82]. Some authors highlight the necessity to understand the timing of administration of GFs and their dosage for designing effective GF therapy [5, 82]. It is necessary to understand the overall reactions which GFs promote in the various cells involved in tendon healing, considering not only the timing of expression of GFs, but also their up- and downregulation from the time of injury [83]. Some studies considered a single GF during biological tendon healing in relation with cell proliferation and cellularity, without considering other GFs [84]. Other studies have characterized the effect of GFs only in vitro [71], while others have characterized the timing of GF expression [85].

Recently, a randomized controlled trial assessed the efficacy and safety of platelet-rich plasma augmentation for arthroscopic repair of small and moderate RC tears compared with non-augmented repair of the RC. This study showed that surgical repair of an RC tear resulted in significant clinical and structural improvement in both groups, but augmentation of the repair with PRFM did not result in significant improved shoulder function or structural outcome when compared with arthroscopic repair without augmentation [86].

Further investigations should be conducted to advance our knowledge on the expression of GFs during healing before administration of single or multiple GFs in tendon healing trials.

The time course of GF expression is important in wound healing, and a better understanding of how, where, when and for how long such factors are expressed may help in the development of methods to manipulate their expression, accelerate healing, and reduce adhesions. The use of GFs in soft tissue problems remains, for the time being, largely experimental.

References

1 Benjamin M, Ralphs J: Functional and developmental anatomy of tendons and ligaments; in Gordon SL, Blair SJ, Fine LJ (eds): Repetitive Motion Disorders of the Upper Extremity. Rosemont/IL, American Academy of Orthopaedic Surgeons, 1995, pp 185–203.

2 Maffulli N, Khan KM, Puddu G: Overuse tendon conditions: time to change a confusing terminology. Arthroscopy 1998;14:840–843.

3 McArthur JC, Yiannoutsos C, Simpson DM, Adornato BT, Singer EJ, Hollander H, Marra C, Rubin M, Cohen BA, Tucker T, Navia BA, Schifitto G, Katzenstein D, Rask C, Zaborski L, Smith ME, Shriver S, Millar L, Clifford DB, Karalnik IJ: A phase II trial of nerve growth factor for sensory neuropathy associated with HIV infection. Neurology 2000; 54:1080–1088.

4 Nutt JG, Burchiel KJ, Comella CL, Jankovic J, Lang AE, Laws ER Jr, Lozano AM, Penn RD, Simpson RK Jr, Stacy M, Wooten GF: Randomized, double-blind trial of glial cell line-derived neurotrophic factor in PD. Neurology 2003;60:69–73.

5 Mehta V, Mass D: The use of growth factors on tendon injuries. J Hand Ther 2005;18:87–92.

6 Stein LE: Effects of serum, fibroblast growth factor, and platelet-derived growth factor on explants of rat tail tendon: a morphological study. Acta Anat (Basel) 1985;123:247–252.

7 Gauger A, Robertson C, Greenlee TK Jr, Riederer-Henderson MA: A low-serum medium for tendon cells: effects of growth factors on tendon cell growth and collagen production. In Vitro Cell Dev Biol 1985;21:291–296.

8 Marx RE, Carlson ER, Eichstaedt RM, Schimmele SR, Strauss JE, Georgeff KR: Platelet-rich plasma: growth factor enhancement for bone grafts. Oral Surg Oral Med Oral Pathol Oral Radiol Endod 1998;85:638–646.

9 Mishra A, Pavelko T: Treatment of chronic elbow tendinosis with buffered platelet-rich plasma. Am J Sports Med 2006;34:1774–1778.

10 Anitua, E, Sanchez M, Nurden AT, Zalduendo M, de la Fuente M, Orive G, Azofra J, Andia I: Autologous fibrin matrices: a potential source of biological mediators that modulate tendon cell activities. J Biomat Med Res 2006;77:285–293.

11 Sanchez M, Anitua E, Azofra J, Andia I, Padilla S, Muljika I: Comparison of surgically repaired Achilles tendon tears using platelet-rich fibrin matrices. Am J Sports Med 2007;35:245–251.

12 Gelberman RH, Manske PR, Van de Berg JS, Lesker PA, Akeson WH: Flexor tendon repair in vitro: a comparative histologic study of the rabbit, chicken, dog and monkey. J Orthop Res 1984;2:39–48.

13 Potenza AD: Tendon healing within the flexor digital sheath in the dog. J Bone Joint Surg Am 1962; 44:49–64.

14 Sharma P, Maffulli N: Biology of tendon injury: healing, modelling and remodelling. J Muscoloskelet Neuronal Interact 2006;6:181–190.

15 Reddy GK, Stehno-Bittel L, Enwemeka CS: Matrix remodeling in healing rabbit Achilles tendon. Wound Repair Regen 1999;7:518–527.

16 Maffulli N, Benazzo F: Basic sciences of tendons. Sports Med Arthrosc 2000;8:1–5.

17 Maffulli N, Moller HD, Evans CH: Tendon healing: can it be optimised? Br J Sports Med 2002;36:315–316.

18 Kobayashi M, Itoi E, Minagawa H, Miyakoshi N, Takahashi S, Tuoheti Y, Okada K, Shimada Y: Expression of growth factors in the early phase of supraspinatus tendon healing in rabbits. J Shoulder Elbow Surg 2006;15:371–377.

19 Würgler-Hauri CC, Dourte LM, Baradet TC, Williams GR, Soslowsky LJ: Temporal expression of eight growth factors in tendon-to-bone healing in a rat supraspinatus model. J Shoulder Elbow Surg 2007;16:198–203.

20 Gabra N, Khiat A, Calabres P: Detection of elevated basic fibroblast growth factor during early hours of in vitro angiogenesis using a fast ELISA immunoassay. Biochem Biophys Res Commun 1994;205: 1423–1430.
21 Lee J, Green MH, Amiel D: Synergistic effect of growth factors on cell outgrowth from explants of rabbit anterior cruciate and medial collateral ligaments. J Orthop Res 1995;13:435–441.
22 Chan BP, Chan KM, Maffulli N, Webb S, Lee KK: Effect of basic fibroblast growth factor. An in vitro study of tendon healing. Clin Orthop Relat Res 1997;342:239–247.
23 Chang J, Most D, Thunder R, Mehrara B, Longaker MT, Lineaweaver WC: Molecular studies in flexor tendon wound healing: the role of basic fibroblast growth factor gene expression. J Hand Surg Am 1998;23:1052–1058.
24 Takahasih S, Nakajima M, Kobayashi M, Wakabayashi I, Miyakoshi N, Minagawa H, et al: Effect of recombinant basic fibroblast growth factor on fibroblast-like cells from human rotator cuff tendon. Tohoku J Exp Med 2002;198:207–214.
25 Gulotta LV, Rodeo SA: Growth factors for rotator cuff repair. Clin Sports Med 2009;28:13–23.
26 Yu Y, Bliss JP, Bruce WJ, Walsh WR: Bone morphogenetic proteins and Smad expression in ovine tendon-bone healing. Arthroscopy 2007;23:205–210.
27 Chhabra A, Tsou D, Clark RT, Gaschen V, Hunziker EB, Mikic B: GDF-5 deficiency in mice delays Achilles tendon healing. J Orthop Res 2003;21:826–835.
28 Eliasson P, Fahlgren A, Aspenberg P: Mechanical load and BMP signaling during tendon repair. A role for follistatin? Clin Orthop Relat Res 2008;466: 1592–1597.
29 Fu SC, Wong YP, Chan BP, Pau HM, Cheuk YC, Lee KM, Chan KM: The roles of bone morphogenetic protein-12 in stimulating the proliferation and matrix production of human patellar tendon fibroblasts. Life Sci 2003;72:2965–2974.
30 Chuen FS, Chuk CY, Ping WY, Nar WW, Kim HL, Ming CK: Immunohistochemical characterization of cells in adult human patellar tendons. J Histochem Cytochem 2004;52:1151–1157.
31 Rodeo SA: Biologic augmentation of rotator cuff tendon repair. J Shoulder Elbow Surg 2007;16:191–197.
32 Majewski M, Betz O, Ochsner PE, Liu F, Porter RM, Evans CH: Ex vivo adenoviral transfer of bone morphogenetic protein 12 cDNA improves Achilles tendon healing in a rat model. Gene Ther 2008;15: 1139–1146.
33 Seeherman HJ, Archambault JM, Rodeo SA, Turner AS, Zekas L, D'Augusta D, Li XJ, Smith E, Wozney JM: rhBMP-12 accelerates healing of rotator cuff repairs in a sheep model. J Bone Joint Surg Am 2008;90:2206–2219.
34 Bolt P, Clerk AN, Luu HH, Kang Q, Kummer JL, Deng ZL, Olson K, Primus F, Montag AG, He TC, Haydon RC, Toolan BC: BMP-14 gene therapy increases tendon tensile strength in a rat model of Achilles tendon injury. J Bone Joint Surg Am 2007; 89:1315–1320.
35 Trippel SB, Wroblewski J, Makower A, Whelan MC, Schoenfeld D, Doctrow SR: Regulation of growth-plate chondrocytes by insulin-like growth-factor and basic fibroblast growth factor. J Bone Joint Surg Am 1993;75:177–189.
36 Molloy T, Wang Y, Murrell GA: The roles of growth factors in tendon and ligament healing. Sports Med 2003;33:381–394.
37 Tsuzaki M, Brigman BE, Yamamoto J, Lawrence WT, Simmons JG, Mohapatra NK, Lund PK, Van Wyk J, Hannafin JA, Bhargava MM, Banes AJ: IGF-I is expressed by avian flexor tendon cells. J Orthop Res 2000;8:546–556.
38 Abrahamsson SO, Lohmander S: Differential effects of insulin-like growth factor-I on matrix and DNA synthesis in various regions and types of rabbit tendons. J Orthop Res 1996;14:370–376.
39 Banes AJ, Tsuzaki M, Hu P, Brigman B, Brown T, Almekinders L, Lawrence WT, Fisher T: PDGF-BB, IGF-I and mechanical load stimulate DNA synthesis in avian tendon fibroblasts in vitro. J Biomech 1995;28:1505–1513.
40 Kurtz CA, Loebig TG, Anderson DD, DeMeo PJ, Campbell PG: Insulin-like growth factor I accelerates functional recovery from Achilles tendon injury in a rat model. Am J Sports Med 1999;27: 363–369.
41 Tsubone T, Moran SL, Amadio PC, Zhao C, An KN: Expression of growth factors in canine flexor tendon after laceration in vivo. Ann Plast Surg 2004; 53:393–397.
42 Dahlgren LA, Mohammed HO, Nixon AJ: Temporal expression of growth factors and matrix molecules in healing tendon lesions. J Orthop Res 2005;23: 84–92.
43 Dahlgren LA, Van der Meulen MC, Bertram JE, Starrak GS, Nixon AJ: Insulin-like growth factor-I improves cellular and molecular aspects of healing in a collagenase-induced model of flexor tendinitis. J Orthop Res 2002;20:910–919.
44 Dahlgren LA, Mohammed HO, Nixon AJ: Expression of insulin-like growth factor binding proteins in healing tendon lesions. J Orthop Res 2006;24:183–192.

45 Bowen-Pope DF, Ross R: Platelet-derived growth factor. Clin Endocrinol Metab 1984;13:191–205.

46 Chan BP, Fu SC, Qin L, Rolf C, Chan KM: Supplementation-time dependence of growth factors in promoting tendon healing. Clin Orthop Relat Res 2006;448:240–247.

47 Yoshikawa Y, Abrahamsson SO: Dose-related cellular effects of platelet-derived growth factor-BB differ in various types of rabbit tendons in vitro. Acta Orthop Scand 2001;72:287–292.

48 Wang XT, Liu PY, Tang JB: Tendon healing in vitro: genetic modification of tenocytes with exogenous PDGF gene and promotion of collagen gene expression. J Hand Surg Am 2004;29:884–890.

49 Skutek M, Van Griensven M, Zeichen J, Brauer N, Bosch U: Cyclic mechanical stretching modulates secretion pattern of growth factors in human tendon fibroblasts. Eur J Appl Physiol 2001;86:48–52.

50 Bynum D, Almekinders L, Benjamin M, Ralphs J, McNeilly C, Yang X, Kenamond C, Weinhold P, Tsuzaki M, Banes A: Wounding in vivo and PDGF-BB in vitro stimulate tendon surface migration and loss of connesin-43 expression. Transact Ann Mtg Orthop Res Soc 1997;22:26.

51 Banes AJ, Horesovsky G, Larson C, Tsuzaki M, Judex S, Archambault J: Mechanical load stimulates expression of novel genes in vivo and in vitro in avian flexor tendon cells. Osteoarthritis Cartilage 1999;7:141–153.

52 De Mos M, van der Windt AE, Jahr H, van Schie HT, Weinans H, Verhaar JA, van Osch GJ: Can platelet-rich plasma enhance tendon repair? A cell culture study. Am J Sports Med 2008;36: 1171–1178.

53 Eppley BL, Woodell JE, Higgins J: Platelet quantification and growth factor analysis from platelet-rich plasma: implications for wound healing. Plast Reconstr Surg 2004;114:1502–1508.

54 Uggen JC, Dines J, Uggen CW, Mason JS, Razzano P, Dines D, Grande DA: Tendon gene therapy modulates the local repair environment in the shoulder. J Am Osteopath Assoc 2005;105:20–21.

55 Thomopoulos S, Harwood FL, Silva MJ, Amiel D, Gelberman RH: Effect of several growth factors on canine flexor tendon fibroblast proliferation and collagen synthesis in vitro. J Hand Surg Am 2005; 30:441–447.

56 Petersen W, Pufe T, Zantop T, Tillmann B, Mentlein R: Hypoxia and PDGF have a synergistic effect that increases the expression of the angiogenetic peptide vascular endothelial growth factor in Achilles tendon fibroblasts. Arch Orthop Trauma Surg 2003;123: 485–488.

57 Wang XT, Liu PY, Tang JB: Tendon healing in vitro: modification of tenocytes with exogenous vascular endothelial growth factor gene increases expression of transforming growth factor-β but minimally affects expression of collagen genes. J Hand Surg Am 2005;30:222–229.

58 Sporn MB, Roberts AB: Transforming growth factor-β: recent progress and new challenges. J Cell Biol 1992;119:1017–1021.

59 Chan KM, Fu SC, Wong YP, Hui WC, Cheuk YC, Wong MW: Expression of transforming growth factor-β isoforms and their roles in tendon healing. Wound Repair Regen 2008;16:399–407.

60 Wolfman NM, Hattersley G, Cox K, Celeste AJ, Nelson R, Yamaji N, Dube JL, DiBlasio-Smith E, Nove J, Song JJ, Wozney JM, Rosen V: Ectopic induction of tendon and ligament in rats by growth and differentiation factors 5, 6, and 7, members of the TGF-β gene family. J Clin Invest 1997; 100:321–330.

61 Herpin A, Lelong C, Favrel P: Transforming growth factor-β-related proteins: an ancestral and widespread superfamily of cytokines in metazoans. Dev Comp Immunol 2004;28:461–85.

62 Fu SC, Wong YP, Cheuk YC, Lee KM, Chan KM: TGF-β_1 reverses the effects of matrix anchorage on the gene expression of decorin and procollagen type I in tendon fibroblasts. Clin Orthop Relat Res 2005; 431:226–232.

63 Anitua E, Sanchez M, Nurden AT, Zalduendo M, De la Fuente M, Azofra J, Andia I: Reciprocal actions of platelet-secreted TGF-β_1 on the production of VEGF and HGF by human tendon cells. Plast Reconstr Surg 2007;119:950–959.

64 Banes AJ, Sanderson M, Boitano S, Hu P, Brigman B, Tsuzaki M, Fischer T, Lawrence WT: Mechanical load +/– growth factors induces [Ca^{2+}]ic release, cyclin D1 expression and DNA synthesis in avian tendon cells. Proceedings of the Second World Congress of Biomechanics, Amsterdam 1994.

65 Tsubone T, Moran SL, Subramaniam M, Amadio PC, Spelsberg TC, An KN: Effect of TGF-β-inducible early gene deficiency on flexor tendon healing. J Orthop Res 2006;24:569–575.

66 Premdas J, Tang JB, Warner JP, Murray MM, Spector M: The presence of smooth muscle actin in fibroblasts in the torn human rotator cuff. J Orthop Res 2001;19:221–228.

67 Kashiwagi K, Mochizuki Y, Yasunaga Y, Ishida O, Deie M, Ochi M: Effects of transforming growth factor-β_1 on the early stages of healing of the Achilles tendon in a rat model. Scand J Plast Reconstr Surg Hand Surg 2004;38:193–197.

68 Anaguchi Y, Yasuda K, Majima T, Tohyama H, Minami A, Hayashi K: The effect of transforming growth factor-β on mechanical properties of the fibrous tissue regenerated in the patellar tendon after resecting the central portion. Clin Biomech 2005;20:959–965.
69 Blobe GC, Schiemann WP, Lodish HF: Role of transforming growth factor-β in human disease. N Engl J Med 2000;342:1350–1358.
70 Klein MB, Yalamanchi N, Pham H, Longaker MT, Chang J: Flexor tendon healing in vitro: effects of TGF-β on tendon cell collagen production. J Hand Surg Am 2002;27:615–620.
71 Campbell BH, Agarwal C, Wang JH: TGF-β_1, TGF-β_3, and PGE_2 regulate contraction of human patellar tendon fibroblasts. Biomech Model Mechanobiol 2004;2:239–245.
72 Shah M, Foreman DM, Ferguson MW: Neutralisation of TGF-β_1 and TGF-β_2 or exogenous addition of TGF-β_3 to cutaneous rat wounds reduces scarring. J Cell Sci 1995;108:985–1002.
73 Chang J, Thunder R, Most D, Longaker MT, Lineaweaver WC: Studies in flexor tendon wound healing: neutralizing antibody to TGF-β_1 increases postoperative range of motion. Plast Reconstr Surg 2000;105:148–155.
74 Ngo M, Pham H, Longaker MT, Chang J: Differential expression of transforming growth factor-β receptors in a rabbit zone II flexor tendon wound healing model. Plast Reconstr Surg 2001;108:1260–1267.
75 Darmani H, Crossan J, McLellan SD, Meek D, Adam C: Expression of nitric oxide synthase and transforming growth factor-β in crush-injured tendon and synovium. Mediators Inflamm 2004;13:299–305.
76 Ferrara N, Gerber HP: The role of vascular endothelial growth factor in angiogenesis. Acta Haematol 2002;106:148–156.
77 Bidder M, Towler DA, Gelberman RH, Boyer MI: Expression of mRNA for vascular endothelial growth factor at the repair site of healing canine flexor tendon. J Orthop Res 2000;18:247–252.
78 Pufe T, Petersen W, Tillmann B, Mentlein R: The angiogenic peptide vascular endothelial growth factor is expressed in foetal and ruptured tendons. Virchows Arch 2001;439:579–585.
79 Popova SN, Rodriguez-Sánchez B, Lidén A, Betsholtz C, Van Den Bos T, Gullberg D: The mesenchymal $\alpha_{11}\beta_1$ integrin attenuates PDGF-BB-stimulated chemotaxis of embryonic fibroblasts on collagens. Dev Biol 2004;15:427–442.
80 Zhang J, Cao R, Zhang Y, Jia T, Cao Y, Wahlberg E: Differential roles of PDGFR-α and PDGFR-β in angiogenesis and vessel stability. FASEB J 2009;23:153–163.
81 McGrath MH: Peptide growth factors and wound healing. Clin Plast Surg 1990;17:421–432.
82 Aspenberg P: Stimulation of tendon repair: mechanical loading, GDFs and platelets. A mini-review. Int Orthop 2007;31:783–789.
83 Sun HB, Li Y, Fung DT, Majeska RJ, Schaffler MB, Flatow EL: Coordinate regulation of IL-1β and MMP-13 in rat tendons following subrupture fatigue damage. Clin Orthop Relat Res 2008;466:1555–1561.
84 Aspenberg P, Virchenko O: Platelet concentrate injection improves Achilles tendon repair in rats. Acta Orthop Scand 2004;75:93–99.
85 Fu SC, Cheuk YC, Chan KM, Hung LK, Wong MW: Is cultured tendon fibroblast a good model to study tendon healing? J Orthop Res 2008;26:374–383.
86 Castricini R, Longo UG, De Benedetto M Panfoli N, Pirani P, Zini R, Maffulli N, Denaro V: Platelet-rich plasma augmentation for arthroscopic rotator cuff repair: a randomized controlled trial. Am J Sports Med 2011;39:258–265.

Francesco Oliva, MD, PhD
Department of Trauma and Orthopaedic Surgery
University of Rome 'Tor Vergata', School of Medicine
Viale Oxford 81, IT–00133 Rome (Italy)
Tel. +33 933 8567 0924, E-Mail olivafrancesco@hotmail.com

Maffulli N (ed): Rotator Cuff Tear. Med Sport Sci. Basel, Karger, 2012, vol 57, pp 65–75

Autologous Blood Products in Rotator Cuff Repair

Omer Mei-Dan[a] · Michael R. Carmont[b]

[a]Department of Orthopaedic Surgery and the Sports Injury Unit, Meir University Hospital, Kfar Saba, Israel, and [b]Princess Royal Hospital, Telford, UK

Abstract

We review the management of rotator cuff tears, the mechanism of action of autologous blood products, principally platelet-rich plasma, and the current evidence for effective use of platelet-rich plasma, particularly in relation to the shoulder and chronic rotator cuff tears, for biological augmentation of rotator cuff repair.

Background

The rotator cuff is comprised of four muscles passing between the scapula and the humeral head: the supraspinatus, infraspinatus, teres minor and subscapularis. The tendinous portion of each of these muscles blends with the capsule of the shoulder joint before inserting into a larger area on the humeral head.

During functional activity, these muscles stabilize the humeral head against the glenoid fossa and provide a strong stable base to position the hand in space. The cuff may also be subjected to contact pressures from the overlying acromial arch and these pressures may be increased by excessive unaccustomed activity, anatomical variations and abnormal positioning of the acromion. Scapular malpositioning or protraction consequently further increase these pressures as a result of relative weakness of the scapulothoracic girdle muscles.

With pathological change, tendons may becomes tendinopathic and prone to rupture and injury. Inflammation of nearby bursal tissues and attrition from the overlying bony acromial arch may exacerbate the propensity to injury and interfere with healing. The hypovascular nature of tendons means that they demonstrate a poor response to injury, and healing may thus be prolonged and often incomplete. The frequency of rotator cuff tears increases with increasing age [1]. In humans there is a tendency for healing never to occur, with the development of chronic tears. The management of these patients is challenging.

We discuss the management of rotator cuff tears, review the perceived mechanism of action of autologous blood products, principally platelet-rich plasma (PRP), and the current evidence for its effective use, particularly in relation to the shoulder and chronic rotator cuff tears.

Current Treatment

Current options for the management of rotator cuff tendon tears include both non-operative and operative modalities. Non-operative management is more than just rest and avoidance of painful activities. Aims include the prevention of predisposing factors with optimization of scapular positioning using a scapulothoracic stabilization exercise programme.

Eccentric loading exercises can be effective in the management of tendinopathy of the Achilles and patellar tendons. There has been little reported on the efficacy of these exercises for rotator cuff tendinopathy [2].

Local anaesthetic and steroid injections may reduce inflammation of bursal tissue adjacent to the rotator cuff but, in the absence of a clearly defined inflammatory background, theoretically this treatment should not be effective on the failed healing response exhibited by these lesions. Intratendinous steroid injections have been shown to increase the rate of rupture of tendons. These can be avoided by confirming extratendinous needle placement by using ultrasound guidance as the injection is being performed.

Prophylactic or preventative surgical options include endoscopic debridement of frayed ragged tendon ends to attempt to reduce tear extension [3, 4]. Impinging bony acromial prominences and acromioclavicular joint osteophytes can also be debrided to reduce attrition of the tendon.

Tears to the cuff may be repaired either as an open procedure or arthroscopically, and these repairs can be augmented by the use of autograft, xenograft and, in some instances, synthetic material [5].

PRP is a new modality in musculoskeletal medicine and orthopaedic surgery and may offer improved healing potential for both non-operative management and the augmentation of both arthroscopic and open rotator cuff surgery [6–10] (fig. 1a–c).

Action of Platelet-Rich Plasma

PRP is being increasingly used to augment healing and promote recovery. PRP has developed from the use of autologous blood injections to promote healing [11–14]. As research has progressed, scientists are increasingly aware that it is the platelets in blood

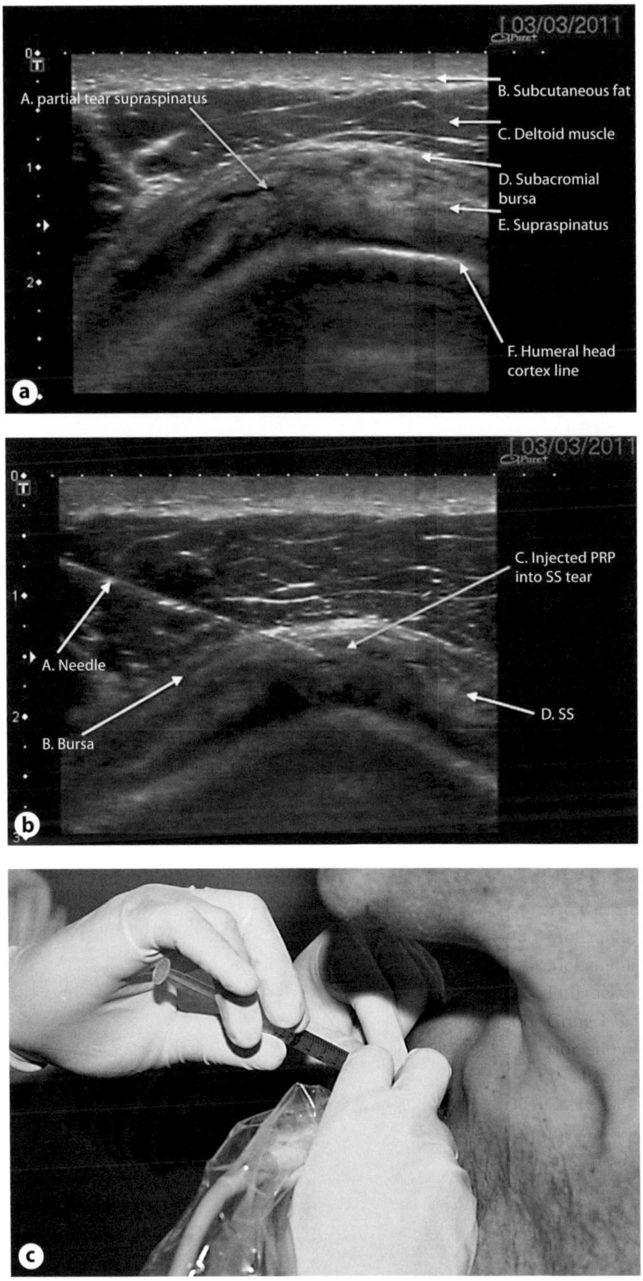

Fig. 1. **a** An axial US image of a supraspinatus partial tear (arrow A). Arrows B–F point at the anatomical landmarks of the region. The hypoechoic/black appearance of the tendons and muscles, especially in the left side periphery of the image, is the result of the anisotropic phenomena, an US artefact, and a good example why US is very operator-dependent. **b** An axial US image of a supraspinatus partial tear during its injection with PRP, seen as the white/hyperechoic area marked with arrow A. The PRP is now filling the tear within the tendon and starts to spread out into the subacromial-subdeltoid bursa along its plane, covering the supraspinatus. **c** Ultrasound-guided PRP injection.

that encourage healing rather than the white blood cells. More recently, it has been suggested that neutrophils within whole blood are actually detrimental to healing [15]. Platelets are cytoplasmic fragments of megakaryocyte leukocytes that lack nuclei but contain mitochondria, microtubules and approximately 50–80 granules per platelet. The α-granules contain many biological growth factors, which promote haemostasis, revascularization and the formation of new connective tissue in the form of extracellular matrix and fibrovascular callus [16–18]. The main growth factors are transforming growth factor-β_1 (TGF-β), platelet-derived growth factor, vascular endothelial growth factor, hepatocyte growth factor and insulin-like growth factor 1.

Preparation of Platelet-Rich Plasma

PRP and preparations rich in growth factors are obtained by the centrifugation of whole blood into its component fractions [11]. Thus, the term PRP may be applied to any fraction of autologous blood that has a higher concentration of platelets above that of normal whole blood [12, 13].

The centrifugation process allows the separation of blood into its component cells and serum. Variations in the centrifugation process alter the volume, the composition of the serum produced, and thus the concentrations of the factors. In addition, fractions may be contaminated by the presence of impurities such as leukocytes. Typically, 10% of the initial volume of autologous blood is yielded as PRP concentrate following centrifugation. Platelets in PRP needs to be at least 3–6 times higher than baseline values [19, 20]. Counter-intuitively, higher concentrations have inhibitory effects [21].

Following production, the platelets in the sample of PRP will begin secreting growth factors immediately. However, immediate administration is frequently not practical. The maximal release of growth factors occurs within the first 10 min of having produced PRP, and the majority of the factors are released after 1 h [22, 23]. Sodium citrate may be added to delay clotting and factor release. The sample can then be reactivated by the addition of calcium chloride prior to application. The administered platelets will produce additional growth factors for 7–10 days following venesection.

The coagulation of the plasma means that preparations can be applied in varying forms. The initial fluid serum can be administered by injection either percutaneously or intraoperatively for precise localized application. Alternatively, the plasma can be allowed to coagulate into a gelatinous matrix for application as a membrane over healing repair sites. Understandably, by the time of application the maximal burst of growth factors will have passed, however the healing potential of this matrix can be restored by injection of freshly activated PRP.

Different methods are available for the preparation of PRP. Since the plasma is mainly for injection or sterile application intraoperatively, it must be prepared in a

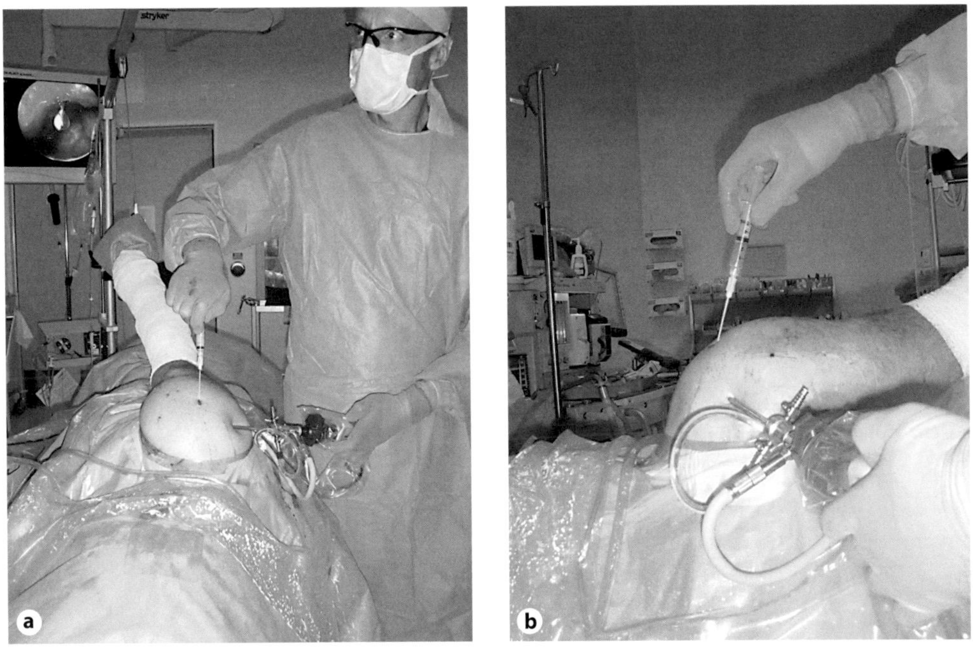

Fig. 2. a, b Arthroscopic rotator cuff repair followed by PRGF injection over the repaired tendon via the subacromial joint. When PRP is administered at arthroscopy, the injection should be performed after emptying the joint of arthroscopic fluid. Once the surgical procedure is complete, the appropriately placed needle can infiltrate the target tissues or spread around the repaired site, under dry vision, seen on the LCD behind the surgeon. After emptying the subacromial space from arthroscopic fluid, PRP is administrated under direct vision, if possible.

pure sterile manner. In some kits the plasma may be applied directly from syringes, which were used to house the blood during the centrifugation process. Cheaper financially but manually time-demanding methods involve the physical manual aspiration of high-grade PRP. This separation process may be performed in a laminar flow preparation cabinet to minimize the risk of infection, and in practice this risk is very small.

Practical Application in Shoulder Surgery

A number of additional points must be considered for the administration of PRP. For soft tissue injuries, preexisting haematomas should be aspirated before the plasma concentrate is injected to prevent dilution. Similarly, for intra-articular administration, effusions may be aspirated to optimize the concentration of plasma. Following arthroscopic procedures, the remaining irrigation fluid should be drained to prevent dilution (fig. 2a, b). Injections can be performed using a spinal needle to minimize infection (22G black). PRP matrices can be applied during open surgery.

For safety we recommend using a syringe with a nozzle with a Luer-Lok. This reduces the risk of spraying the plasma with pressurized detachment. It is obviously hazardous to spray and effectively aerosol blood products, but this also involves losing the precious plasma.

Other than the intraoperative application of PRP, additional injections may be applied during the inflammatory and proliferative stages of healing typically during the first 6 weeks following surgery.

Current Evidence of the Efficacy of Platelet-Rich Plasma

Much of the current research has been based upon tendon rupture and tendinopathy, predominantly of lower limb tendons, given the predilection of tendinopathy for these locations. In vivo, tenocytes increase in size, become elongated and are better spread following PRP application [24]. A 30% increase in tendon callus strength and stiffness of transacted rat Achilles tendons at 1 week was noted following percutaneous injections of PRP [25]. Other series report similar improvements in early healing, with increased strength of repair at 1 week post injection [26–28]. A placebo-controlled experimental trial in horses reported less inflammation and increased metabolic activity and maturation, higher strength at failure and elastic modulus in tendons treated with PRP [29].

Sanchez et al. [30] reported a decreased cross-sectional area of healed Achilles tendons at 18 months based on ultrasound findings. A recent randomized prospective study into the administration of PRP to promote healing of ruptured Achilles tendons failed to show a significant difference between treatment and control groups [31]. In this study, the repaired paratenon was distended with a large volume of PRP. This itself may compound healing of the repair by reducing the blood flow in the paratenon. Additionally the large volume of PRP used may not necessarily be therapeutic.

PRP has also been applied to the treatment of tendinopathy with predominantly case series being reported. Gaweda et al. [32] reports significantly improved outcome following the administration of PRP for patients with Achilles tendinopathy. In the management of chronic patellar tendinopathy, a single PRP injection leads to 91% improvement in symptoms in a small series of 8 athletes. Additionally, MR images revealed a noticeable reduction in tendon irregularity of the affected tendon in 80% of the patients [33].

Mishra and Pavelko [34] attempted a cohort study of the injection of PRP versus local anaesthetic for chronic elbow tendinosis. PRP administration led to a reduction of reported symptoms (60 vs. 16%), but three fifths of the control group withdrew or sought other treatments preventing definitive long-term comparisons. Similarly, a study comparing PRP and corticosteroid injection for lateral epicondylitis of the elbow showed that patients receiving PRP had reduced pain and improved function [35]. Filardo et al. [36] and Kon et al. [37] both reported prospective case series on patients with patellar tendinopathy. PRP administration led to improved Tegner and visual analogue scores [36, 37].

Comparison of the efficacy of randomized controlled studies is fraught with difficulties in interpretation and the participation of subjects. A well-designed study by De Vos at el. [38] used a single injection for treatment in a prospective randomized study of 53 patients with Achilles tendinopathy. The mean VISA-Achilles scores improved in both treatment (eccentric exercises and PRP) and control (eccentric exercises only) groups, without significant improvement in the treatment group, suggesting that the single injection of PRP did not improve outcome. The fact that a single injection was performed rather than a series of three injections means that this study may not be comparable with typical practice.

All patients are keen to recover as quickly as possible and return to normal activities. Particularly the sports community and professional athletes are keen to adopt any new technique which may give an advantage to promote performance compared to others, including during healing, recovery and rehabilitation following injury. These patients are naturally reluctant to be involved in randomized controlled studies. They are unlikely to accept receiving a placebo or the arm of a study perceived to offer inferior healing, even though this may be scientifically unfounded.

As a result, the published evidence on the use of PRP has consisted of mainly case series or cohort studies compared to published outcomes (level 4 or 5 evidence). We recently published a case report of an Olympic judoka, who had completely ruptured his elbow medial complex (both MCL and common flexor tendon origin) just 10 months before the Olympic Games. Surgery at that stage would have ruled out competition within the next 6–8 months, and he would have missed Olympic qualification. He decided upon a conservative management plan involving plasma rich in growth factors (PRGF) injections together with an accelerated rehabilitation protocol. He received two injections, at 1 and 2 weeks after the injury, and, by 6 weeks from injury, the elbow had stabilized. He went on to win a gold medal in a world cup tournament, 5.5 months following his injury [39].

The considerable interest in improved healing from competitive sportsmen has led to the International Olympic Committee producing consensus statements on PRP [40] and the World Anti-Doping Agency considering whether PRP may be considered to be performance enhancing [41].

The lack of standardization of the method of obtaining PRP leads to variation in the constituent components. Similarly, the method of administration of PRP frequently compounds comparison [42] preventing expert opinion from forming guidelines based on the current evidence [43]. PRP may be administered by injection either intraoperatively or postoperatively at predetermined stages during healing, but these have not been applied consistently during studies.

Additional Management Points

In the postoperative period, it is understandable for patients to use analgesics and anti-inflammatory (NSAIDs) medication to reduce pain. NSAIDs are inhibitors of platelet function and therefore must be avoided if PRP is used. We also recommend that patients avoid using NSAIDs for 2 days prior to PRP injections, and for 2 weeks following application.

Concern has also been raised about the concomitant use of local anaesthetics with PRP injections. The local anaesthesia alters the pH of the local tissue, and may therefore alter the efficacy of the PRP. There is no published evidence to guide us, but if necessary we recommend using only superficial infiltration with local anaesthetic.

Current Evidence for Platelet-Rich Plasma in the Shoulder

Even though PRP may be ideally suited to the treatment of degenerate tendinopathic conditions of the rotator cuff, there is a little current published evidence.

Studies have looked specifically at the growth factors found in the pathological shoulders during surgery. During rotator cuff repair, increased amounts of growth factor TGF-β were found relative to amounts found in unstable shoulders [44]. The discovery of TGF-β and vascular endothelial growth factor in the bursa of other shoulder patients [45] and osteoinductive growth factors during ovine bone and soft tissue formation [46] suggests that there may well be a role for the management of shoulder tendon pathology with PRP in the future.

There have been several articles published on human patients reporting on the outcome following surgery with the addition of PRP. Procedures reported include treatment for subacromial bursitis and impingement, open subacromial decompression and rotator cuff surgery [47–52].

Jiminez-Martin et al. [48] reported an improved pain score and reduced rehabilitation time when PRP was used in a retrospective cohort comparison when PRP was applied to traditional, mini open and arthroscopic subacromial surgery. The exogenous application of platelet leukocyte gel during open subacromial decompression was thought to contribute to faster recovery, earlier return to daily activities and less analgesic requirement [49].

Randelli et al. [50] used PRP to augment arthroscopic cuff repair in a case series of 14 patients, leading to improved pain and functional outcome without any adverse events. This research group followed up this study with a level 1 prospective randomized double-blind controlled study for augmented arthroscopic cuff repair. Patients reported significantly less pain and improved strength in external rotation and functional simple shoulder test, UCLA and Constant scores at 3 months following surgery. No difference was shown in scores between the two groups at 6, 12 and 24 months following surgery. Imaging also did not show a difference. For smaller tears (grade 1 and 2) with less retraction there was significantly higher external strength at all stages [51].

Conversely another level 1 study by Castricini et al. [52] compared the use of an autologous platelet-rich fibrin matrix for the treatment of rotator cuff tears. There was no significant difference in Constant scores in small and medium-sized tears. It is however acknowledged that other preparations of PRP may be effective and that PRP may be beneficial in large and massive rotator cuff tears.

Conclusion

As research progresses, the efficacy of autologus blood products, principally PRP and PRGF injections, is being increasingly appreciated. Whilst there is currently a lack of evidence to give firm treatment recommendations for the use of PRP in rotator cuff surgery, the absence of reported side effects means that its use is safe. The use of PRP should be considered to be experimental in all aspects of sports medicine [53]. We encourage randomized prospective studies of autologous blood products so that outcomes can be measured and firm conclusions be made.

References

1 Seida JC, LeBlanc C, Schouten JR, et al: Systematic review: non-operative and operative treatments for rotator cuff tears. Ann Intern Med 2010;15:246–255.

2 Rees JD, Wilson AM, Wolman RL: Current concepts in the management of tendon disorders. Rheumatology (Oxford) 2006;45:508–521.

3 Millstein ES, Snyder SJ: Arthroscopic evaluation and management of rotator cuff tears. Orthop Clin North Am 2003;34:507–520.

4 Beaudreuil J, Dhenain M, Coudane H, et al: Clinical practice guidelines for the surgical management of rotator cuff tears in adults. Orthop Traumatol Surg Res 2010;96:175–179.

5 Longo UG, Lamberti A, Maffulli N, et al: Tendon augmentation grafts: a systematic review. Br Med Bull 2010;94:165–188.

6 Kovacevic D, Rodeo SA: Biological augmentation of rotator cuff tendon repair. Clin Orthop Relat Res 2008;466:622–633.

7 Cheung EV, Silverio L, Sperling JW: Strategies in biologic augmentation of rotator cuff repair: a review. Clin Orthop Relat Res 2010;468:1476–1484.

8 Hall MP, Band PA, Meislin RJ, et al: Platelet-rich plasma: current concepts and application in sports medicine. J Am Acad Orthop Surg 2009;17:602–608.

9 Lopez-Vidriero E, Goudling KA, Simon DA, Sanchez M, Johnson DH: The use of platelet-rich plasma in arthroscopy and sports medicine: optimising the healing environment. Arthroscopy 2010;26:269–278.

10 Mei-Dan O, Lippi G, Sanchez M, Andia I, Maffulli N: Autologous platelet-rich plasma: a revolution in soft tissue sports injury management? Phys Sportsmed 2010;38:127–135.

11 Anitua E: Plasma rich in growth factors: preliminary results of use and preparation of sites for implants. Int J Oral Maxillofac Implants 1999;14:529–535.

12 Marx RE, Carlson ER, Eichstaedt RM, et al: Platelet-rich plasma. growth factor enhancement for bone grafts. Oral Surg Oral Med Oral Pathol Oral Radiol Endod 1998;85:638–646.

13 Andia I, Sanchez M, Maffulli N: Tendon healing and platelet-rich plasma therapies. Expert Opin Biol Ther 2010;10:1415–1426.

14 Alsousou J, Thompson M, Huley P, et al: The biology of platelet-rich plasma and its application in trauma and orthopaedic surgery. A review article. J Bone Joint Surg Br 2009;51:987.
15 Sanchez M, Anitua E, Orive G, et al: Platelet-rich therapies in the treatment of orthopaedic sports injuries. Sports Med 2009;39:345–354.
16 Harrison P, Cramer EM: Platelet α-granules. Blood Rev 1993;7:52–62.
17 Schnabel LV, Mohammed HO, Miller BJ, et al: Platelet-rich plasma enhances anabolic gene expression patterns in flexor digitorum superficialis tendons. J Orthop Res 2007;25:230–240.
18 De Mos M, Van der Windt AE, Jahr H, et al: Can platelet-rich plasma enhance tendon repair? A cell culture study. Am J Sports Med 2008;36:1171–1178.
19 Weibrich G, Hansen T, Kleis W, et al: The effect of platelet concentration in platelet-rich plasma on peri-implant bone reintegration. Bone 2004;34: 665–671.
20 Graziani F, Ivanovski S, Cei S, et al: The in vitro effect of different PRP concentrations of osteoblasts and fibroblasts. Clin Oral Implants Res 2006;17: 212–219.
21 Anitua E, Sanchez M, Nurden AT, et al: New insights into novel applications for platelet-rich fibrin therapies. Trends Biotechnol 2006;24:227–234.
22 Marx RE. Platelet-rich plasma (PRP): what is PRP and what is not PRP? Implant Dent 2001;10:225–228.
23 Marx RE. Platelet-rich plasma: evidence to support its use. J Oral Maxillofac Surg 2004;62:489–496.
24 Zhang J, Wang JH: PRP releasate promotes differentiation of tendon stem cells into active tenocytes. Am J Sports Med 2010;38:2477–2486.
25 Aspenberg P, Virchenko O: Platelet concentrate injection improves Achilles tendon repair in rats. Acta Orthop Scand 2004;75:93–99.
26 Virchenko O, Aspenberg P: How can one platelet injection after tendon injury lead to a stronger tendon after 4 weeks? Interplay between early regeneration and mechanical stimulation. Acta Orthop 2006;77:806–812.
27 Lyras DN, Kazako K, Agrogiannis IG, et al: Experimental study of tendon healing in the early phase: is IGF-1 expression influenced by platelet-rich plasma gel? Orthop Traumtol Surg Res 2010; 96:381–387.
28 Lyras DN, Kazakos K, Tryfonidis M, et al: Temporal and spatial expression of TGF-β in Achilles tendon section model after application of PRP. Foot Ankle Surg 2010;16:137–141.
29 Bosch G, Moleman M, Barnevield A, et al: The effect of PRP on neovascularisation of surgically treated equine superficial digital flexor tendon lesions. Scand J Med Sci Sports 2010.
30 Sanchez M, Anitua E, Azofra J, Andia I, Padilla S, Mujika I: Comparison of surgically repaired Achilles tendon tears using platelet-rich fibrin matrices. Am J Sports Med 2007;35:245–251.
31 Schepull T, Kvist J, Norman H, Trinks M, Berlin G, Aspenberg P: Autologous platelets have no effect on the healing of human Achilles tendon ruptures: a randomized single blind study. Am J Sports Med 2011;39:38–47.
32 Gaweda K, Tarczynska M, Krzyzanowski W: Treatment of Achilles tendinopathy with platelet-rich plasma. Int J Sports Med 2010;31:577–583.
33 Volpi P, Marinoni L, Bait C, et al: Treatment of chronic patellar tendinosis with buffered platelet-rich plasma: a preliminary study. Med Sport 2007; 60:595–603.
34 Mishra A, Pavelko T: Treatment of chronic elbow tendinosis with buffered platelet-rich plasma. Am J Sports Med 2006;34:1774–1778.
35 Peerbooms JC, Sluimer J, Bruijn DJ, et al: Positive effect of an autologous platelet concentrate in lateral epicondylitis in a double-blind randomized controlled trial: platelet-rich plasma versus corticosteroid injection with a 1-year follow-up. Am J Sports Med 2010;38:255–262.
36 Filardo G, Kon E, Della Villa S, et al: Use of platelet-rich plasma for the treatment of refractory jumper's knee. Int Orthop 2010;34:909–915.
37 Kon E, Filardo G, Delcogliano M, et al: Platelet-rich plasma: new clinical application. A pilot study for treatment of jumper's knee. Injury 2009;40:598–603.
38 De Vos RJ, Weir A, van Schie HT, Bierma-Zeinstra SM, et al: Platelet-rich plasma injection for chronic Achilles tendinopathy: a randomized controlled trial. JAMA 2010;303:144–149.
39 Mei-Dan O, Carmont MR, Kots E, et al: Early return to play following complete rupture of the medial collateral ligament of the elbow using a preparation rich in growth factors: a case report. J Shoulder Elbow Surg 2010;19:e1–e5.
40 Engebretsen L, Steffen K, Alsousou J, et al: IOC consensus paper on the use of platelet-rich plasma in sports medicine. Br J Sports Med 2010;44:1072–1081.
41 World Anti-Doping Code. International Standard 2011. Montreal, WADA, 2011.
42 Mei-Dan O, Mann G, Maffulli N: Platelet-rich plasma: any substance to it? Br J Sports Med 2010; 44:618–619.

43 Andia I, Sanchez M, Maffulli N: Platelet-rich plasma therapies for sports muscle injuries: any evidence behind clinical practice? Expert Opin Biol Ther 2011;11:509–518.
44 Sakai H, Fujita K, Sakai Y, et al: Immunolocalization of cytokines and growth factors in subacromial bursa of rotator cuff tear patients. Kobe J Med Sci 2001;47:25–34.
45 Yanagisawa K, Hamada K, Gotoh M, et al: Vascular endothelial growth factor expression in the subacromial bursa is increased in patients with impingement syndrome. J Orthop Res 2001;19:448–455.
46 Rodeo SA, Potter HG, Kawamura S, et al: Biologic augmentation of rotator cuff tendon-healing with use of a mixture of osteoinductive growth factors. J Bone Joint Surg Am 2007;89:2485–2497.
47 Maniscalco P, Gambera D, Lunati A, et al: The 'cascade' membrane: new PRP device for tendon ruptures. Description and case report on rotator cuff tendon. Acta Biomed 2008;79:223–226.
48 Jimenez-Martin A, Angulo-Gutierrez A, Gonzalez-Herranz J, et al: Surgery of subacromial syndrome with application of plasma rich in growth factors. Int J Shoulder Surg 2009;3:28–33.
49 Everts PA, Devilee RJ, Brown Mahoney C, et al: Exogenous application of platelet leucocyte gel during open subacromial decompression contributes to improved patient outcome. A prospective randomised double-blind study. Eur Surg Res 2008;40: 203–210.
50 Randelli P, Arrigoni P, Ragone V, et al: Platelet-rich plasma in arthroscopic rotator cuff repair. A prospective RCT study, 2 years' follow-up. Presented at ICSES, 2010.
51 Randelli PS, Arrigoni P, Cabitza P, et al: Autologous platelet-rich plasma for arthroscopic rotator cuff repair. A pilot study. Disabil Rehabil 2008;30:1584–1589.
52 Castricini R, Longo UG, De Benedetto M, et al: Platelet-rich plasma augmentation for arthroscopic rotator cuff repair: a randomized controlled trial. Am J Sports Med 2011;3:258–265.
53 Creaney L, Hamilton B: Growth factor delivery methods in the management of sports injuries: state of play. Br J Sports Med 2008;42:314–320.

Omer Mei-Dan
27 Prospect Terrace
Milford, Auckland 0620 (New Zealand)
Tel. +64 21 883 839
E-Mail Omer@extremegate.com

Maffulli N (ed): Rotator Cuff Tear. Med Sport Sci. Basel, Karger, 2012, vol 57, pp 76–89

Tendinopathy of the Long Head of the Biceps

Garrett M. Snyder · Scott D. Mair · Christian Lattermann

Department Orthopaedic Surgery and Sports Medicine, University of Kentucky, Lexington, Ky., USA

Abstract

Tendinopathy of the long head of the biceps is a common cause of anterior shoulder pain. As such, the anatomy and function of the tendon as well as its pathophysiology and different treatment methods have been studied extensively. The pathophysiology is a spectrum beginning with inflammation and leading to tendon degeneration. Different clinical tests and imaging modalities may all be employed to help aid in diagnosis. Conservative management is the first-line treatment, but surgical intervention may be warranted. In general, tenotomy or tenodesis is performed depending, among other things, on the age and activity level of the patient. There are several different methods for tenodesis, each with certain advantages and disadvantages. Patient factors must be considered when choosing the optimal treatment.

Biceps tendinopathy is a common cause of anterior shoulder pain. As such, its pathophysiology and treatment options have been studied extensively. Despite this research, much controversy still remains about the tendon's function in the shoulder and the best methods of treating associated pathology. This chapter will provide a brief review of the function of the long head of the biceps tendon (LHBT), as well as the pathophysiology, evaluation, and management of LHBT disorders.

Anatomy/Function

The origin of the LHBT is the supraglenoid tubercle of the scapula and the superior glenoid labrum [1]. It receives its blood supply from branches of the anterior humeral circumflex artery [1]. Both sensory and sympathetic nerve fibers have been identified in the LHBT with the highest concentration found proximally [2]. It is roughly 9 cm long and 5 cm in diameter with the proximal portion being flatter and larger [1]. It has both intra- and extra-articular components. The intra-articular portion is found

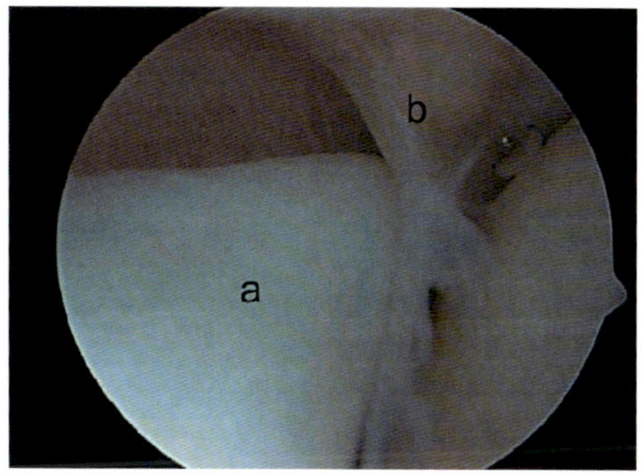

Fig. 1. Arthroscopic view of LHBT (**a**) in biceps sling (**b**).

in the rotator interval [3] and is considered extrasynovial because it is contained within an invaginated envelope of synovial membrane [4]. It becomes extra-articular once in the bicipital groove.

The bicipital groove exists between the greater and lesser tuberosities of the proximal humerus. It is teardrop shaped with its apex directed medially [5]. Secondary to the orientation of the humeral head, the LHBT makes a 30–40° turn and resides on the medial wall of the groove against the lesser tuberosity [1, 6], which makes it susceptible to irritation at this site from repetitive or overuse. It is contained within this groove by a tendoligamentous sling that consists of the subscapularis tendon, the supraspinatus tendon, the coracohumeral ligament, and the superior glenohumeral ligament [7] (fig. 1). Although the existence of a transverse humeral ligament was once thought to stabilize LHBT in its groove, recent anatomical dissection has shown that no such discrete structure exists [5]. Furthermore, the fibers of the subscapularis have been demonstrated to continue over the roof and floor of the groove [5].

The biomechanical function of the LHBT at the shoulder remains a controversial subject. It has been considered a vestigial structure [8], a humeral head depressor during abduction [9], an anterior stabilizer [10], and as a flexor and abductor of the shoulder [11]. Its primary role, however, is as a flexor and supinator of the elbow [1].

Pathophysiology

Inflammatory conditions of the LHBT lead to a continuum of progressive degeneration. Tenosynovitis/tendinitis evolving into tendinosis, delamination, pre-rupture, and finally rupture is the usual progression of events [1]. Tenosynovitis/tendinitis may cause the LHBT to initially appear hemorrhagic and if it persists, tendinosis (tendon degeneration) occurs [7]. Histologically, tendinosis is characterized by cellular infiltration, edema, fibrosis [4, 7]. Ruptured tendons have been shown to have one or more of the following: hypoxic degeneration, mucoid degeneration, tendolipomatosis, calcifying tendinopathy, and disordered arrangement of collagen fibers [12, 41].

Tendinitis of the LHBT can be divided into primary and secondary causes. Primary tendinitis is the existence of isolated tendinitis in the bicipital groove without associated shoulder pathology [4]. It is most commonly observed in young athletes and is the result of mechanical stresses on the tendon [1, 7]. Participants in sports involving repetitive overhead activities, such as throwing athletes, swimmers and volleyball players are particularly susceptible [1, 6, 7]. Secondary tendinitis occurs with associated shoulder pathology (i.e. impingement syndrome, rotator cuff disease) and is more common than primary tendinitis [4, 13]. The biceps tendon sheath is an extension of the synovial lining of the shoulder and thus is affected by inflammation of the rotator cuff [6, 7].

Mechanical causes of LHBT problems include entrapment, instability and spontaneous rupture [1]. Entrapment occurs when the intra-articular component of the LHBT becomes hypertrophied and is unable to slide into the bicipital groove. This condition is referred to as an 'hourglass biceps' [1]. Instability can manifest as either subluxation or dislocation. Partial- or full-thickness tears of the subscapularis tendon are commonly associated with LHBT subluxation and almost always associated with dislocation [7, 14]. Furthermore, rotator cuff tears may cause biceps sling incompetence which can lead to subluxation/dislocation [1]. Traumatic rupture of a normal LHBT is rare, and rupture is usually the result of chronic tendinopathy [1, 15]. Rupture usually occurs with an associated rotator cuff tear [13].

Symptoms

Symptoms of LHBT pathology are variable which can make its diagnosis elusive. The insidious onset of anterior shoulder pain localized to the bicipital groove is the most common symptom [1, 6, 7, 16]. This pain may occur at night, and may radiate into the biceps muscle and down to the radial aspect of the hand [1]. It is exacerbated by repetitive overhead activities [6]. An unstable tendon may present with a clunk during shoulder rotation, particularly with abduction [1, 6]. Rupture of the LHBT is usually noticed as an audible pop with immediate resolution of previous anterior shoulder pain [6].

Physical Examination Findings

One of the most common and reproducible findings in patients with LHBT pathology is point tenderness upon palpation of the tendon in the bicipital groove [4, 7]. The groove is directly anterior, and can be palpated easily, when the arm is internally rotated 10° [1, 6]. Two commonly used provocative tests to evaluate for LHBT

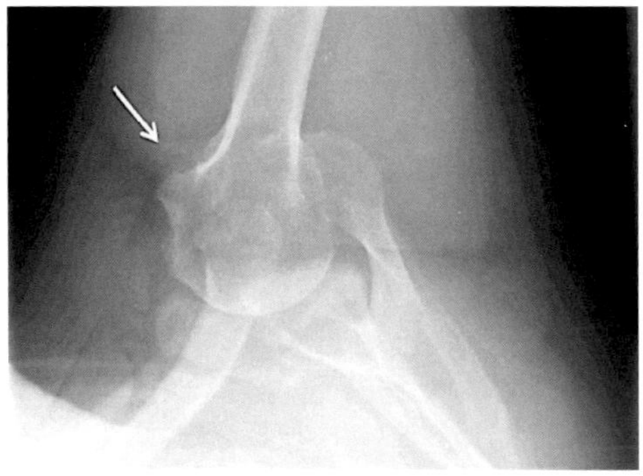

Fig. 2. Loose body (arrow) visualized in bicipital groove on a plain radiograph.

pathology are Speed's test and Yergason's test. Speed's test is positive with reproduction of bicipital groove pain with resisted forward flexion of the shoulder with the elbow fully extended, and the forearm fully supinated. A positive Yergason's test is when pain is reproduced with resisted supination of the forearm with elbow flexed at 90°. In a study by Holtby and Razmjou [17], both tests have been shown to have a low sensitivity but high specificity for detecting LHBT pathology and superior labrum anterior/posterior (SLAP) lesions. Yergason's test was found to have a sensitivity and specificity of 43 and 79% respectively. Speed's test was found to have a sensitivity and specificity of 32 and 75% respectively. Their usefulness in detecting one versus the other, however, has not been shown. An 'hourglass biceps' may limit the terminal 10–20° of arm elevation as it becomes entrapped in the bicipital groove [1]. A Popeye sign may be observed in cases of LHBT rupture. This presents as an abnormal contour of the muscle as it retracts distally.

Injections may be utilized to help differentiate LHBT pathology from other causes of shoulder pain. If the underlying cause is impingement, a subacromial injection may relieve pain [7]. Injection directly into the bicipital groove may also be done but can be difficult to perform. Ultrasound guidance may be used to improve accuracy [1].

Imaging

Plain radiographs may be useful in evaluating LHBT pathology. Calcifications or osteophytes may be seen within the bicipital groove [1] (fig. 2). The Fisk view is a described technique to visualize groove anatomy [18]. Tendinosis or a subscapularis tear may present as cystic change in the lesser tuberosity [1]. Impingement syndrome may be detected by visualization of a subacromial spur on an outlet view [6].

Ultrasound is a dynamic study that may be used to diagnose biceps rupture, subluxation or dislocation. Its usefulness, however, in detecting inflammation is unknown [7]. Furthermore, its accuracy is very operator-dependent.

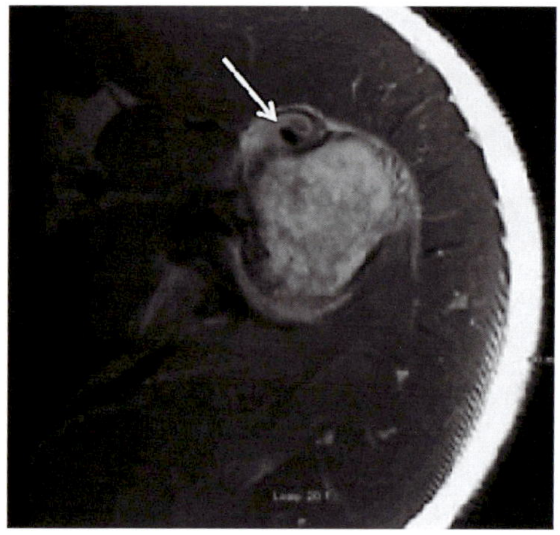

Fig. 3. Axial MR image showing fluid (arrow) surrounding LHBT.

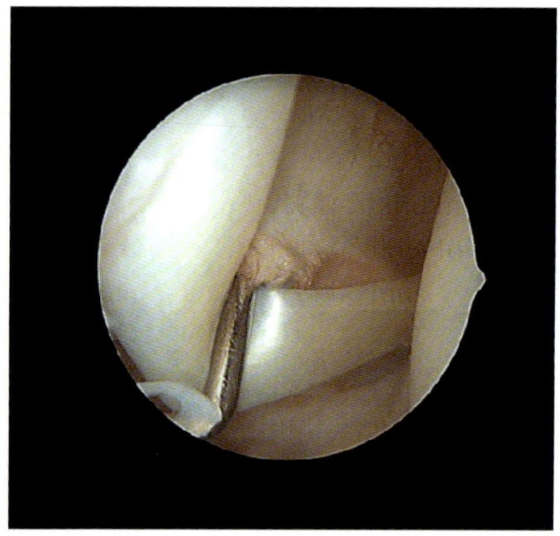

Fig. 4. Arthroscopic view of the LHBT being pulled into joint with arthroscopic probe.

Magnetic resonance imaging (MRI) is commonly used to visualize the LHBT. It also provides valuable information with respect to the surrounding structures and rotator cuff. It may be performed with or without arthrography. Increased fluid around the tendon is a sign of tendinopathy (fig. 3) and may be falsely positive with an arthrogram. Diameter change of the tendon is one of the primary criteria for diagnosing degeneration of the LHBT [19]. Signal change within the tendon is also an indication of degeneration and is best visualized on proton density-weighted fat-saturated sequences [19]. Poor correlation has been found, however, between MRI and arthroscopic findings [20].

Arthroscopic evaluation provides the definitive diagnosis of LHBT pathology [1]. The tendon should be brought into the joint so that the portion that lies in the bicipital groove may be visualized (fig. 4). An active compression test may be performed under arthroscopic visualization as described by Verma et al. [21]. The arm is forward flexed to 90° with the elbow extended, adducted 10–15°, and internally rotated. The LHBT may be observed displacing inferior and medially and may become entrapped in the joint. Correlation with clinical findings should then be used to determine treatment.

Non-Operative Management

Conservative management is usually the first-line treatment of LHBT pathology and is usually successful [6]. Activity modification and NSAID therapy are the initial interventions. Avoidance of biceps and repetitive overhead activities is helpful. Physical therapy may be utilized for implementation of modalities and iontophoresis to target inflammation. Injections, while previously mentioned for aid in diagnosis, may also prove useful for treatment. Subacromial and glenohumeral corticosteroid injections may alleviate biceps pain by addressing commonly associated shoulder inflammation [7]. The tendon sheath may also be injected within the bicipital groove. One should take care, however, not to inject the tendon itself as this may predispose to rupture [22].

Operative Management

Surgical management of LHBT pathology has been shown to be beneficial in certain scenarios and generally involves either tenotomy or tenodesis. One indication for surgery is for chronic refractory tendinitis manifested as persistent pain and with intraoperative findings of severe inflammation or hypertrophy [23, 24] (fig. 5). As previously mentioned, the biceps tendon should be pulled into the joint during arthroscopy to evaluate the part that lies in the intertubercular groove as this a common site of pathology [7]. Another indication for operative intervention is LHBT instability with or without a subscapularis tear [25] (fig. 6, 7). Arthroscopic findings of a partial tear of 25–50% are criteria that may also be used as guidelines for surgically treating the LHBT [25, 26] (fig. 8). Performing a tenotomy or tenodesis of the LHBT in the setting of an elderly person with a massive irreparable rotator cuff tear and LHBT lesion has been shown to alleviate pain and improve range of motion [27]. Symptomatic SLAP tears in patients over 50 years of age are also an indication for LHBT surgery [7, 42].

Tenotomy of the LHBT involves cutting the tendon at its proximal insertion at the superior labrum and letting the tendon retract through the groove. The patient may be placed in the lateral decubitus or beach-chair position. A standard posterior viewing portal is established and the camera is placed in the glenohumeral joint. An anterior portal is then established through the rotator interval and an arthroscopic

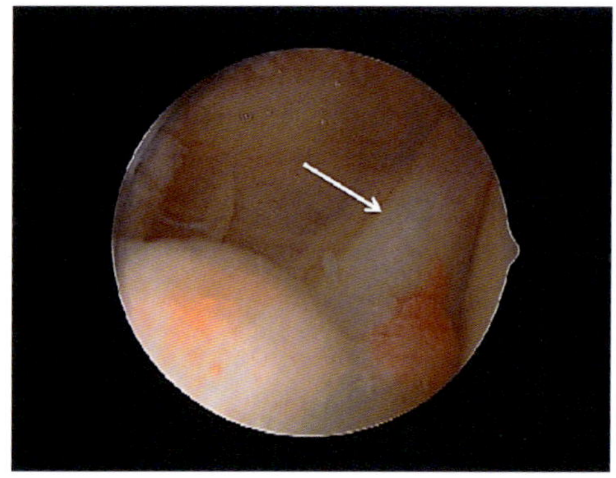

Fig. 5. Arthroscopic view of an inflamed LHBT (arrow).

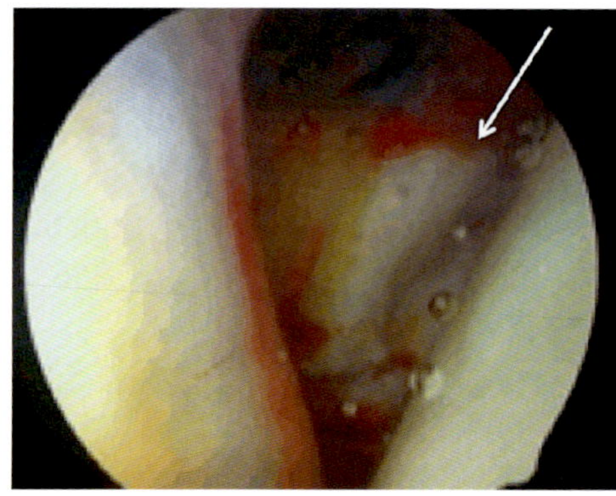

Fig. 6. Arthroscopic view of a torn subscapularis tendon (arrow).

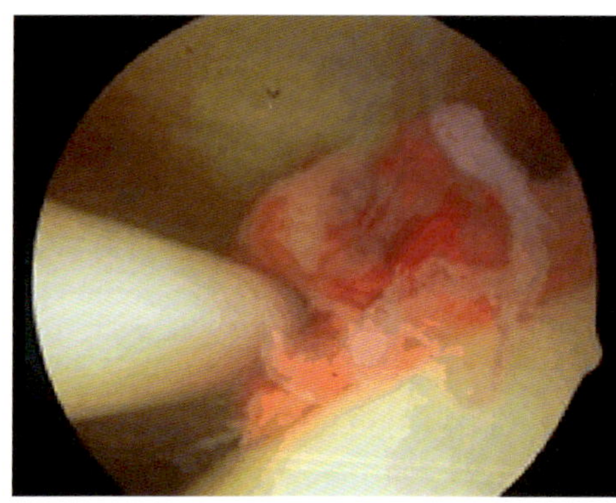

Fig. 7. Arthroscopic view of a dislocated LHBT.

basket forceps is used to cut the tendon as close as possible to the labrum (fig. 9). If, secondary to hypertrophy, the tendon does not retract, it should be debrided until it does so as this may remain a source of pain [7, 24]. This procedure has been effective in relieving pain, but patients can develop a Popeye deformity and fatigue discomfort during resisted elbow flexion [28]. A Popeye deformity occurs more frequently in

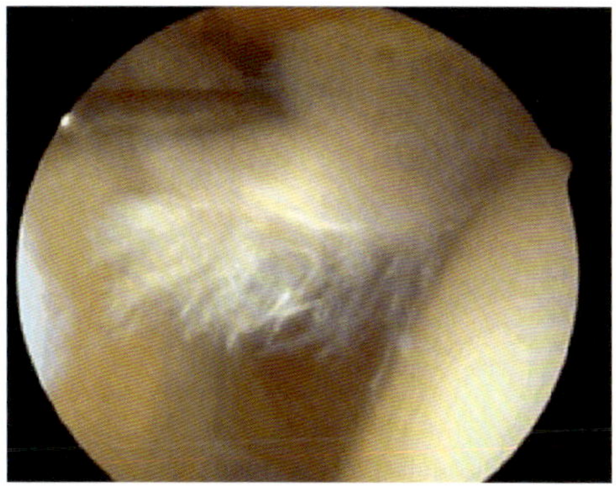

Fig. 8. Arthroscopic view of a frayed and partially torn LHBT.

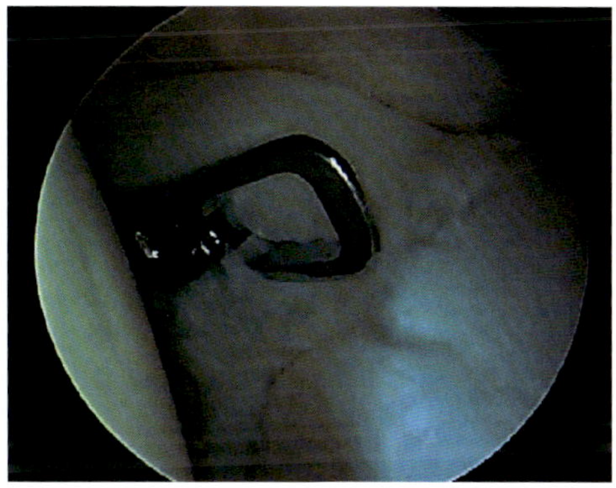

Fig. 9. Arthroscopic view of a LHBT tenotomy.

this procedure and may not be desirable in thin patients who are concerned about cosmesis [29]. Furthermore, young, heavy laborers may be affected by the muscle fatigue and cramping [28]. An advantage of a tenotomy is that there are no postoperative restrictions on activity afterward and patients quickly return to baseline activity level [29].

Tenodesis of the LHBT is preferred in young patients, laborers, and patients concerned about developing a cosmetic deformity [7]. Controversy still remains as to whether or not it is the preferred technique in athletes who present with recurrent biceps or labral pathology. There has been a wide variety of techniques for performing a tenodesis described. These techniques involve fixation either proximal to or distal to the bicipital groove. Proximal techniques are usually performed arthroscopically (table 1). The LHBT can be tenodesed into bone or soft tissue. One such soft tissue procedure is the percutaneous intra-articular transtendon (PITT) technique [30] (fig. 10). This technique has been shown to have similar fixation strength when compared with suture anchors [31]. It is a relatively easy procedure to perform and there is little associated cost since no hardware is used. Another soft tissue procedure with similar characteristics involves incorporating the LHBT into a rotator cuff repair

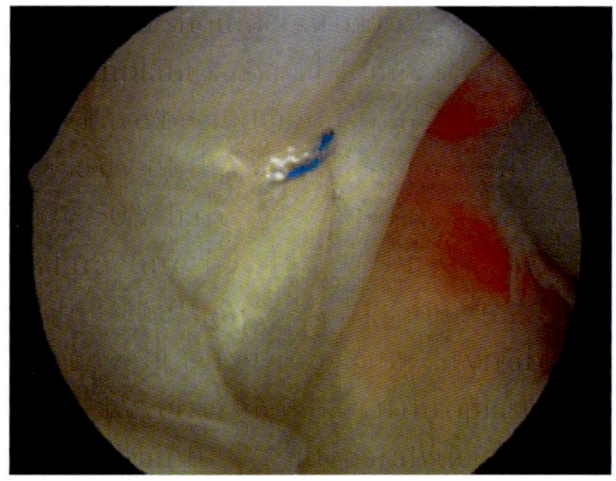

Fig. 10. Arthroscopic view of the PITT technique.

Table 1. Proximal fixation

	Soft tissue		Bone	
	PITT Roman bridge	conjoint tendon [38]	tenodesis screw [39]	suture anchors [40]
Advantages	relatively easy	restores native axis	strongest fixation	similar method to rotator cuff repair
Disadvantages	groove pain	danger to musculo-cutaneous nerve	higher cost	difficult in absence of rotator cuff tear

[43]. With any proximal fixation procedure, there is the potential for continued pain if there is pathology in the bicipital groove.

Distal procedures eliminate this potential. An open subpectoral tenodesis can be performed with rare postoperative complications [32]. With the patient in the beach-chair position, a routine arthroscopy and LHBT tenotomy as previously described is performed. A 4-cm incision is then made in the axilla over the site of the musculotendinous junction of the LHBT (fig. 11). The subcutaneous tissues are dissected bluntly and the insertion of the pectoralis major tendon is palpated. Blunt dissection is again used to palpate the LHBT on the humerus by going underneath the inferior edge of the pectoralis major tendon. The surgeon's finger is then used to pull the tendon into the wound (fig. 12). Starting 1 cm proximal to the musculotendinous junction, the tendon is whip-stitched with a #2 non-absorbable suture. The excess tendon is then cut (fig. 13). A blunt and sharp Homan retractor is then placed around the medial and lateral aspects of the humerus respectively and the periosteum is elevated exposing the bicipital groove (fig. 14). A Steinman pin is then drilled unicortically into the center of the groove. Next, a 5-mm acorn drill is passed over the Steinman pin and a unicortical hole is drilled. The Steinman pin is removed and a 2.5-mm drill is

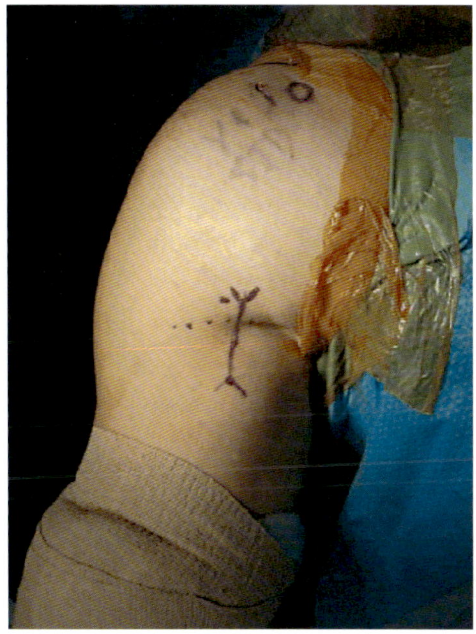

Fig. 11. Photograph of incision site for open subpectoral tenodesis.

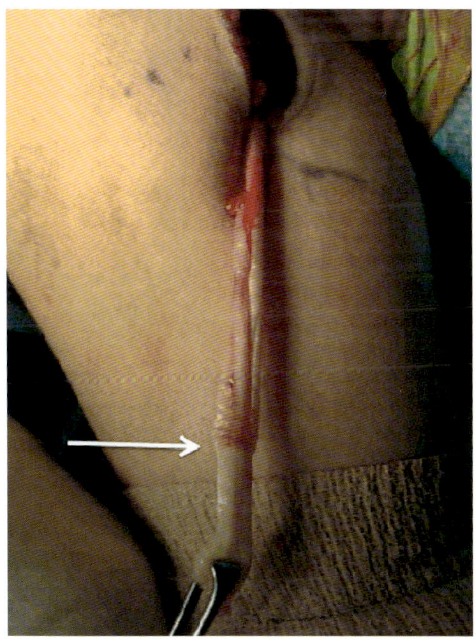

Fig. 12. Photograph of LHBT pulled through wound. Note transition zone (arrow) of extra-articular inflamed tendon and intra-articular normal tendon.

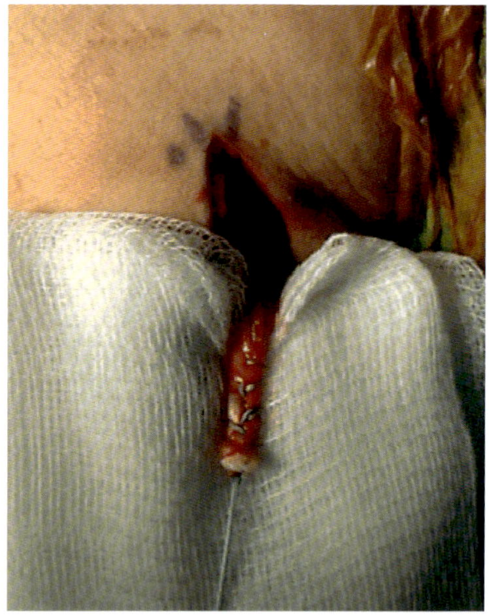

Fig. 13. Photograph of whip-stitched and cut LHBT.

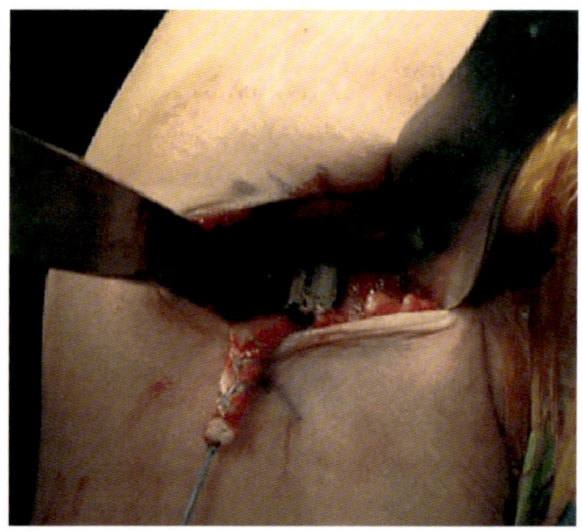

Fig. 14. Photograph of exposed bicipital groove with periosteum stripped.

used to drill two holes inferior to the 5-mm hole just medial and lateral to it aiming at the 5-mm hole (fig. 15). A suture-passer is then inserted into one of the inferior drill holes and retrieved out of the 5-mm drill hole. One limb of the previously whip-stitched tendon is then placed in the suture-passer and passed through the 5-mm hole and out one of the drill holes. These steps are repeated for the other suture limb. The tendon is then docked into the 5-mm hole and the suture limbs are tied over a bone bridge (fig. 16). This mode of fixation is known as the bone tunnel technique. Tendon fixation with an interference screw or the bone tunnel technique has been

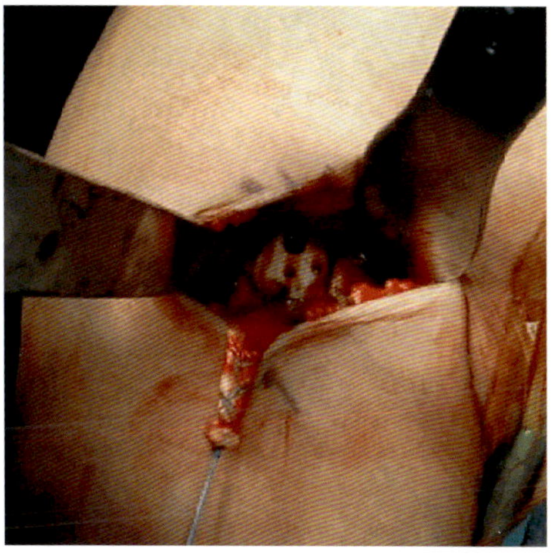

Fig. 15. Photograph of drill holes for the bone tunnel technique.

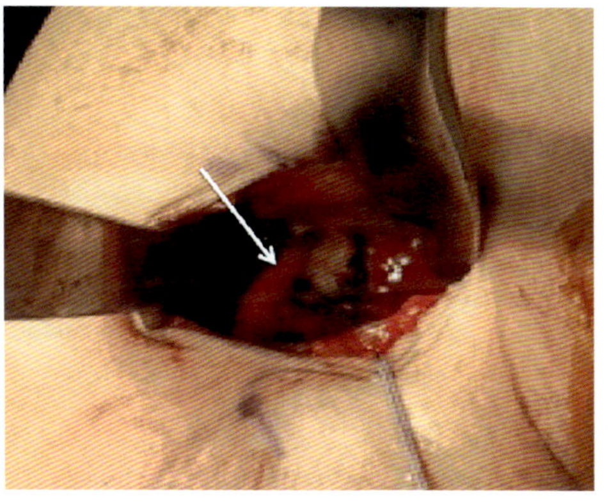

Fig. 16. Photograph of LHBT (arrow) docked into large hole with suture strands exiting below.

shown to be the strongest and second strongest modes of fixation respectively with no statistically significant difference between the two [33]. The bone tunnel technique, however, has the advantage of being cost-saving since no hardware is used.

Postoperative Rehabilitation

Rehabilitation after tenotomy can generally be aggressive. There is no immobilization, and return to activities is limited only by their symptoms [34, 35]. Heavy lifting however should be delayed in order to try and avoid a Popeye deformity [36].

Tendon-to-bone healing after a tenodesis may take up to 12 weeks with the greatest gains in strength occurring over the first 4 weeks [36, 37]. A sling is used for 4 weeks postoperatively. Pendulum exercises of the shoulder as well as passive range of motion of the elbow are allowed. Wrist and hand strengthening may be initiated early. Resisted range of motion may begin at 6 weeks postoperatively as may active elbow flexion and forearm supination [7]. Athletes may begin throwing at 3 months, can pitch at 4.5 months and can return to contact sports at 6 months out.

Conclusion

Tendinopathy is a spectrum of diseases and is a common cause of anterior shoulder pain. Different clinical tests and imaging modalities should be employed to help aid in diagnosis. Conservative management is the first-line treatment, but surgical intervention may be warranted. In general, tenotomy or tenodesis is performed depending, among other things, on the age and activity level of the patient. There are several different methods for tenodesis, each with certain advantages and disadvantages. Patient factors must be considered when choosing the optimal treatment.

References

1 Ahrens PM, Boileau P: The long head of the biceps and associated tendinopathy. J Bone Joint Surg Br 2007;89:1001–1009.

2 Alpantaki K, McLaughlin D, Karagogeos D, Hadjipavlou A, Kontakis G: Sympathetic and sensory neural elements in the tendon of the long head of the biceps. J Bone Joint Surg Am 2005;87:1580–1583.

3 Clark JM, Harryman DT: Tendons, ligaments, and capsule of the rotator cuff. Gross and microscopic anatomy. J Bone Joint Surg Am 1992;74:713–725.

4 Post M, Benca P: Primary tendinitis of the long head of the biceps. Clin Orthop Relat Res 1989;246:117–125.

5 Gleason PD, Beall DP, Sanders TG, Bond JL, Ly JQ, Holland LL, Pasque CB: The transverse humeral ligament: a separate anatomical structure or a continuation of the osseous attachment of the rotator cuff? Am J Sports Med 2006;34:72–77.

6 Patton WC, McCluskey GM III: Biceps tendinitis and subluxation. Clin Sports Med 2001;20:505–529.

7 Nho SJ, Strauss EJ, Lenart BA, Provencher MT, Mazzocca AD, Verma NN, Romeo AA: Long head of the biceps tendinopathy: diagnosis and management. J Am Acad Orthop Surg 2010;18:645–656.

8 Lippman RK: Bicipital tenosynovitis. N Y State J Med 1944:2235–2241.

9 Warner JJ, McMahon PJ: The role of the long head of the biceps brachii in superior stability of the glenohumeral joint. J Bone Joint Surg Am 1995;77:366–372.

10 Rodosky MW, Harner CD, Fu FH: The role of the long head of the biceps muscle and superior glenoid labrum in anterior stability of the shoulder. Am J Sports Med 1994 22:121–130.

11 Sakurai G, Ozaki J, Tomita Y, Nishimoto K, Tamai S: Electromyographic analysis of shoulder joint function of the biceps brachii muscle during isometric contraction. Clin Orthop Relat Res 1998;354: 123–131.

12 Kannus P, Jozsa L: Histopathological changes preceding spontaneous rupture of a tendon. A controlled study of 891 patients. J Bone Joint Surg Am 1991;73:1507–1525.

13 Neer CS II: Anterior acromioplasty for the chronic impingement syndrome in the shoulder: a preliminary report. J Bone Joint Surg Am 1972;54:41–50.

14 Walch G, Nove-Josserand L, Boileau P, Levigne C: Subluxations and dislocations of the tendon of the long head of the biceps. J Shoulder Elbow Surg 1998;7:100–108.

15 Neer CS II: Impingement lesions. Clin Orthop 1983; 173:70–77

16 Churgay CA: Diagnosis and treatment of biceps tendinitis and tendinosis. Am Fam Physician 2009; 80:470–476.

17 Holtby R, Razmjou H: Accuracy of the Speed's and Yergason's tests in detecting biceps pathology and SLAP lesions: comparison with arthroscopic findings. Arthroscopy 2004;20:231–236.

18 Fisk C: Adaptation of the technique for radiography of the bicipital groove. Radiol Technol 1965;37:47–50.
19 Buck FM, Grehn H, Hilbe M, Pfirrmann CWA, Manzanell S, Hodler J: Degeneration of the long biceps tendon: comparison of MRI with gross anatomy and histology. AJR 2009;193:1367–1375.
20 Mohtadi NG, Vellet AD, Clark ML, Hollinshead RM, Sasyniuk TM, Fick GH, Burton PJ: A prospective, double-blind comparison of magnetic resonance imaging and arthroscopy in the evaluation of patients presenting with shoulder pain. J Shoulder Elbow Surg 2004;13:258–265.
21 Verma NN, Drakos M, O'Brien SJ: The arthroscopic active compression test. Arthroscopy 2005;21: 634e1–634e4.
22 Ford LT, DeBender J: Tendon rupture after local steroid injection. South Med J 1979;72:827–830.
23 Mazzocca AD, Rios CG, Romeo AA, Arciero RA: Subpectoral biceps tenodesis with interference screw fixation. Arthroscopy 2005;21:896.
24 Boileau P, Ahrens PM, Hatzidakis AM: Entrapment of the long head of the biceps tendon: the hourglass biceps. A cause of pain and locking in the shoulder. J Shoulder Elbow Surg 2004;13:249–257.
25 Lo IKY, Burkhart SS: Arthroscopic biceps tenodesis using a bioabsorbable interference screw. Arthroscopy 2004;20:85–95.
26 Sethi N, Wright R, Yamaguchi K: Disorders of the long head of the biceps tendon. J Shoulder Elbow Surg 1999;8:644–654.
27 Boileau P, Baque F, Valerio L, Ahrens P, Chuinard C, Trojani C: Isolated arthroscopic biceps tenotomy or tenodesis improves symptoms in patients with massive irreparable rotator cuff tears. J Bone Joint Surg Am 2007;89:747–757.
28 Kelly AM, Drakos MC, Fealy S, Taylor SA, O'Brien SJ: Arthroscopic release of the long head of the biceps tendon: functional outcome and clinical results. Am J Sports Med 2005;33:208–213.
29 Frost A, Zafar MS, Maffulli N: Tenotomy versus tenodesis in the management of pathologic lesions of the tendon of the long head of the biceps brachii. Am J Sports Med 2009;37:828–833.
30 Sekiya JK, Elkousy HA, Rodosky MW: Arthroscopic biceps tenodesis using the percutaneous intra-articular transtendon technique. Arthroscopy 2003;19:1137–1141.
31 Lopez-Vidriero E, Costic RS, Fu FH, Rodosky MW: Biomechanical evaluation of two arthroscopic biceps tenodeses: double-anchor versus percutaneous intra-articular transtendon (PITT) techniques. Am J Sports Med. 2010;38:146–152.
32 Nho SJ, Reiff SN, Verma NN, Slabaugh MA, Mazzocca AD, Romeo AA: Complications associated with subpectoral biceps tenodesis: low rates of incidence following surgery. J Shoulder Elbow Surg 2010;19:764–768.
33 Ozalay M, Akpinar S, Karaeminogullari O, Balcik C, Tasci A, Tandogan RN, Gecit R: Mechanical strength of four different biceps tenodesis techniques. Arthroscopy 2005;21:992–998.
34 Hsu SH, Miller SL, Curtis AS: Long head of biceps tendon pathology: management alternatives. Clin Sports Med 2008;27:747–762.
35 Friedman DJ, Dunn JC, Higgins LD: Proximal biceps tendon: injuries and management. Sports Med Arthrosc 2008;16:162–169.
36 Ryu JHJ, Pedowitz RA: Rehabilitation of biceps tendon disorders in athletes. Clin Sports Med 2010;29:229–246.
37 Rodeo SA, Arnoczky SP, Torzilli PA, Hidaka C, Warren RF: Tendon-healing in a bone tunnel. A biomechanical and histological study in the dog. J Bone Joint Surg Am 1993;75:1795–1803.
38 Verma NN, Drakos M, O'Brien SJ: Arthroscopic transfer of the long head biceps to the conjoint tendon. Arthroscopy 2005;21:764.e1–764.e5.
39 Romeo AA, Mazzocca AD, Tauro JC: Arthroscopic biceps tenodesis. Arthroscopy 2004;20:206–213.
40 Nord KD, Smith GB, Mauck BM: Arthroscopic biceps tenodesis using suture anchors through the subclavian portal. Arthroscopy 2005;21:248–252.
41 Longo UG, Franceschi F, Ruzzini L, Rabitti C, Morini S, Maffulli N, Denaro V: Characteristics at haematoxylin and eosin staining of ruptures of the long head of the biceps tendon. Br J Sports Med 2009;43:603–607.
42 Franceschi F, Longo UG, Ruzzini L, Rizello G, Mafulli N, Denaro V: No advantages in repairing a type II superior labrum anterior and posterior lesion when associated with rotator cuff repair in patients over age 50: a randomized controlled trial. Am J Sports Med 2008;36:248–253.
43 Franceschi F, Longo UG, Ruzzini L, Rizello G, Mafulli N, Denaro V: soft tissue tenodesis of the long head of the biceps tendon associated to the Roman bridge repair. BMC Musculoskelet Disord 2008;9:78.

Christian Lattermann, MD
Center for Cartilage Repair and Restoration
Department Orthopaedic Surgery and Sports Medicine, University of Kentucky
740 South Limestone St., Kentucky Clinic K435, Lexington KY 40536 (USA)
Tel. +1 859 218 3065, E-Mail clattermann@gmail.com

Maffulli N (ed): Rotator Cuff Tear. Med Sport Sci. Basel, Karger, 2012, vol 57, pp 90–99

Conservative Treatment and Rotator Cuff Tear Progression

Umile Giuseppe Longo[a,b] · Francesco Franceschi[a,b] · Alessandra Berton[a,b] · Nicola Maffulli[c] · Vincenzo Denaro[a,b]

[a]Department of Orthopaedic and Trauma Surgery and [b]Centro Integrato di Ricerca (CIR), Campus Bio-Medico University, Rome, Italy; [c]Centre for Sports and Exercise Medicine, Queen Mary University of London, Barts and The London School of Medicine and Dentistry, Mile End Hospital, London, UK

Abstract

There is no definite consensus on the best management for patients with rotator cuff tears. No randomized controlled studies have compared the outcome of surgical versus conservative treatment. The described successful rate of conservative treatment varies widely, from 33 to 92%. Even though current evidence is not sufficient to allow definitive conclusions on conservative treatment of rotator cuff tears, non-operative management is often recommended in such patients. Prognostic factors seem to be clinical presentation, duration of symptoms and tear size. The best programme for conservative treatment is not defined. Physical therapy consists of stretching and strengthening exercises. The characteristics of exercise programmes are not standardized. In clinical practice, intra-articular injections are commonly used for treatment of shoulder pain. Systemic pharmacotherapy for patients with shoulder pain consists of non-steroidal anti-inflammatory drugs. Recently, cyclo-oxygenase-2-selective inhibitors have been introduced for management of shoulder pain. To date, few randomized controlled trials are available on conservative management of rotator cuff tears, and therefore further studies are required to clarify its role in such patients.

Rotator cuff tears are a common cause of shoulder pain and dysfunction [1–4] and the incidence ranges from 5 to 40% [5]. They are frequently encountered in primary care and in orthopaedic practice, mainly affecting the elderly population [6]. They are responsible for high direct and indirect costs in industrialized countries [7, 8]. It is essential to correctly diagnose and manage rotator cuff tear to reduce the related disability [9]. Management of rotator cuff tears can be either conservative or surgical [6, 10–17]. To date, there is not a definite consensus on the best management for patients with rotator cuff tears, and new therapeutic options are being validated, even though with contrasting results [18–21]. No randomized controlled studies have been performed to compare outcomes of surgical versus conservative treatment for rotator cuff ruptures [22–34]. Moreover, several factors limit the possibility to compare available studies. Firstly, there is a lack of uniformity in the definition of rotator cuff tendinopathy and in the assessment of results [35]. Scoring systems are different and timing of outcome variable [36]. Intervention studies are heterogeneous, and often the quality of data is poor because of inadequate methodology and inadequate sample sizes [37].

The described success rate of non-operative management varies widely, from 33 to 92% [38–40]. Satisfactory results were described in 75% of 53 patients undergoing non-operative treatment at an average follow-up longer than 7 years, particularly those with less than 6 months of pain [38]. In only 62% of 60 patients with documented rotator cuff tears at a minimum of 2 years follow-up was reported as satisfactory, with only 4% considered excellent [41]. In other settings, 70% of 136 patients at an average 1.5-year follow-up had excellent or good results [42].

Even though current evidence is not sufficient to reach clear indications for conservative management of rotator cuff tears, several authors recommend non-operative management for patients with pain without dramatic or progressive weakness [43]. On the other hand, patients with weakness, especially with sudden onset of weakness after an injury, should be investigated for an acute full-thickness tear. In this case, they would benefit from surgery [44]. Earlier surgery has been associated with better outcome, particularly in massive tears [43]. Prognostic factors are clinical presentation, duration of symptoms and tear size [42]. These aspects are correlated with each other. Symptom duration less than 1 year and tear less than 1 cm are predictors of good results with conservative treatment [29]. Rotator cuff repair could be unsuccessful when the tendon retracts beyond the glenoid rim [45–47]. Moreover, surgery could be contraindicated in the elderly population affected by co-morbidities. The elderly make up the majority of patients with rotator cuff dysfunction, with marked disabilities leading to functional decline [48].

The conservative approach consists of several interventions. They include: analgesic medication, such as non-steroidal anti-inflammatory drugs (NSAIDs), subacromial infiltration of lidocaine and corticosteroids, and physical therapy. They are commonly applied in clinical practice, but the best programme for conservative treatment is not defined by current evidence.

The aim of conservative management is to decrease shoulder pain and regain shoulder function [49]. The goals are to reduce the degree of impingement, decreasing swelling and inflammation, and to minimize risk of further injury to the rotator cuff tendons.

Physical Therapy

Physical therapy mainly consists of stretching and strengthening exercises that patients perform at home following a scheduled programme or under the supervision of a physiotherapist [50]. First of all, patients should be educated to modify activities to eliminate the offending motions, such as reaching overhead [33, 35]. An exercise programme should be tailored to the location of the tear, and aim to decrease stiffness and improve function. Such a programme would permit to maintain range of motion, prevent adhesions and decrease impingement because of posterior capsular tightness. It is important strengthening the rotator cuff, scapular stabilizers (serratus anterior, rhomboids, latissimus dorsi, and trapezius), and the deltoid. This would prevent superior humeral head migration during abduction and scapular instability predisposing to impingement syndrome. Progressively, patients will return to their daily activities.

A review of literature did not find any randomized clinical trials about exercise effectiveness in the treatment of full-thickness tears of the rotator cuff [51]. Observational studies suggest beneficial effects of physical therapy included in a treatment programme for patients with symptomatic shoulders and radiological or arthroscopic evidence of full-thickness rotator cuff tears. However, the results of case series investigations are not comparable with each other because of difference in study designs, inclusion criteria, interventions, types of exercise, outcome measurements, follow-up times, and home versus clinic-based programmes. The characteristics of an exercise programme are not standardized. Exercises can be specific or general in nature, and their duration, intensity and number of repetitions can be variable. Available evidence does not allow to define benefits closely related to physical therapy. Additionally, the physiological explanation of benefits induced by physical therapy is unclear. Hypotheses are pain modulation, coordinated movement performed by the other muscles, placebo, and reduced kinesiophobia. Influence of disease variables, such as traumatic or non-traumatic aetiology and tear size, are not known. Large (3–5 cm) and massive (>5 cm) full-thickness rotator cuff tears generally benefit from surgical intervention [52]. Nevertheless, some patients with massive tears reported functional and pain improvement with conservative treatment [53]. Pain seems to be more important for treatment choice [54–56].

Further investigations are needed to define the role of physical therapy in the management of rotator cuff tears. Indications of a specific exercise programme need to be supported by scientific evidence of efficacy.

Intra-Articular Injections

In clinical practice, several intra-articular injections are commonly used for treatment of shoulder pain. They mainly consist of subacromial injection of corticosteroids or sodium hyaluronate. These preparations have different indications but their use is not standardized [29, 31, 57, 58].

Corticosteroid injections are generally recommended in conjunction with physical therapy and oral anti-inflammatory medications. They should permit rapid pain relief allowing the patient to perform physical therapy [59]. A mixture of 3 ml of lidocaine (1%), 3 ml of bupivacaine (0.25%), and a depot corticosteroid is recommended when pain limits the patient's ability to perform exercises. Corticosteroid injections have been widely used for different causes of shoulder pain. Reported results are variable, and the literature about corticosteroid injections in patients with rotator cuff tear is limited. No significant benefits were found in patients with partial rotator cuff tear with symptoms lasting longer than 6 months who had failed physical therapy and a trial of NSAIDs [60]. Corticosteroids act on inflammation, thus acute pathology responds better to their administration. An important concern is the accuracy of delivery of the medication into the desired target. A difference in the effectiveness of the intervention performed under radiographic control has been reported in some studies [61–63]. Other authors found blind injection performed by an experienced orthopaedic surgeon as accurate as ultrasound-guided injection [64]. The effects of corticosteroids on tendon structures limit their use. They can cause collagen necrosis, weakness, and increased risk of rupture [61]. For this reason more than two injections a year, once every 6 months, are discouraged.

Patients with long-term pain may benefit from sodium hyaluronate injection. Evidence about the use of sodium hyaluronate injections in patients with shoulder pain is increasing [65–68]. Sodium hyaluronate is a normal component of synovial fluid, and contributes to preserve physiological joint friction because of its viscosity [69]. Its efficacy has been proven in a small series of patients with rotator cuff tears, with significant benefits over placebo, decreasing pain, the use of oral analgesics, and range of motion improvement [65]. As it has no side effects, it seems to be a valid treatment option. However, further studies are needed to confirm its efficacy.

Medications

Systemic drugs for patients with shoulder pain include NSAIDs [70]. Conventional NSAIDs are commonly prescribed as first-line medication. Various types of NSAIDs can be used with similar results [71]. Recently cyclo-oxygenase-2 (COX-2)-selective inhibitors have been introduced for the management of shoulder pain. Both NSAIDs and COX-2-selective inhibitors showed short-term efficacy in some controlled clinical trials [72–74]. However, both categories of drugs have side effects. Conventional NSAIDs cause adverse gastrointestinal reactions in 8–76% of patients [71]. Co-administration of proton pump inhibitors decreases the gastrointestinal risk, allowing ulcers to heal and decreasing the risk of ulcer recurrence [75, 76]. NSAIDs also have renal, haematological, dermatological, and neurological side effects [77]. There are some concerns about the cardiovascular risk of NSAIDs and COX-2 inhibitors [78–81]. Long-term therapy, lasting more than 2–3 months, was associated with increased cardiovascular effects. Selective COX-2 inhibitor showed an increase of vascular events and myocardial infarction compared to naproxen [82]. However, celecoxib, in doses around 200 mg/day, was not associated with increased cardiovascular risk [83]. Patients showed less epigastric pain than those treated with naproxen [84]. NSAIDs are recommended for short periods. They have several adverse effects and pharmacologic interactions. They interfere with diuretics, β-blockers, angiotensin-converting enzyme (ACE) inhibitors, and angiotensin type-2 receptor antagonists, influencing control of blood pressure in patients with hypertension. They can also influence bleeding in patients taking digoxin, anticoagulants and platelet inhibitors [85, 86].

Acetaminophen (paracetamol) can be an alternative for pain relief, with up to 4 g/day associated with a high safety profile. Patients with moderate to severe pain can be treated with a combination of NSAIDs or acetaminophen and a fixed dose of opioids [61]. Their safety profile varies from one to another, but they are generally contraindicated in patients with significant respiratory depression and can have a significant liability for abuse.

Possible risks and benefits of medications should be taken into account, especially in those patients who are vulnerable. As many patients with shoulder pain are elderly, these implications are relevant.

Tear Progression

The natural history and factors causing rotator cuff tears are not completely clarified [20, 21, 87–100]. Knowledge of natural history of rotator cuff tears would be useful to choose a treatment and to provide a rationale for specific interventions. It should guide timing for surgery compared with non-surgical care as it influences healing and clinical outcome [45–47, 101–106]. Moreover, characterization of factors influencing tear progression would help to identify individuals at risk and plan preventative strategies.

Several patients with asymptomatic rotator cuff tears develop symptoms with time. The progression of symptoms has been associated with significantly larger tears at baseline and a high rate of tear progression. Symptoms consist of pain and deterioration of shoulder function. Clinical scores and the active range of motion of the shoulder decreased significantly. Pain induces compensatory scapulothoracic motion during early shoulder abduction, and a more significant change of glenohumeral kinematics are most likely to occur in advanced stages of rotator cuff tears [107].

Fatty degeneration is notoriously associated with rotator cuff tears. It is irreversible and, usually, progressive [47, 102, 103, 108]. It has been proven to increase with the severity of rotator cuff tear [109]. As a tear enlarges in length or width, fatty degeneration develops. Moreover, tear progression has been demonstrated to correlate with tear location. It increases when a tear involves the more anterior aspect of the supraspinatus tendon [110]. Other factors have been studied to better characterize fatty infiltration. Age, number of tendons torn and time interval between the onset of rotator cuff symptoms and diagnosis are correlated with this phenomenon. It develops with increasing age. The presence of more than one tear is associated with earlier and faster fatty infiltration. Greater supraspinatus fatty infiltration was observed with longer delay between symptom onset and the diagnosis of rotator cuff tear [109]. These findings have clinical implications. As fatty degeneration induces poor clinical outcome [45–47, 101, 102, 104, 108, 111–117], rotator cuff repair should be performed before it develops. Elderly patients with multiple tendon tears should be treated as soon as possible.

Conclusion

There is no definite consensus on the best management of patients with rotator cuff tears. Physical therapy and injections represent the main conservative options for such patients. Further randomized controlled studies are needed to compare the outcome of surgical versus conservative treatment and to clarify the most effective regime of conservative management.

References

1 Maffulli N, Longo UG, Gougoulias N, Loppini M, Denaro V: Long-term health outcomes of youth sports injuries. Br J Sports Med 2010;44:21–25.
2 Maffulli N, Longo UG, Gougoulias N, Caine D, Denaro V: Sport injuries: a review of outcomes. Br Med Bull 2011;97:47–80.
3 Maffulli N, Longo UG, Spiezia F, Denaro V: Sports injuries in young athletes: long-term outcome and prevention strategies. Phys Sportsmed 2010;38:29–34.
4 Maffulli N, Longo UG, Spiezia F, Denaro V: Aetiology and prevention of injuries in elite young athletes. Med Sport Sci 2011;56:187–200.
5 DePalma A, Callery G, Bennett G: Variational anatomy in degenerative lesions of the shoulder joint. Instr Course Lect 1949,6:255–281.
6 Franceschi F, Longo UG, Ruzzini L, Rizzello G, Maffulli N, Denaro V: No advantages in repairing a type II superior labrum anterior and posterior lesion when associated with rotator cuff repair in patients over age 50: a randomized controlled trial. Am J Sports Med 2008;36:247–253.
7 Meislin RJ, Sperling JW, Stitik TP: Persistent shoulder pain: epidemiology, pathophysiology, and diagnosis. Am J Orthop (Belle Mead NJ) 2005;34:5–9.
8 Hegmann K, Moore J: Common neuromusculoskeletal disorders; in King PM (ed): Sourcebook of Occupational Rehabilitation. New York, Plenum Press, 1998, pp 30–32.
9 Maffulli N, Longo UG, Berton A, Loppini M, Denaro V: Biological factors in rotator cuff tears. Sports Med Arthrosc 2011 (in press).
10 Franceschi F, Longo UG, Ruzzini L, Rizzello G, Denaro V: Arthroscopic management of calcific tendinitis of the subscapularis tendon. Knee Surg Sports Traumatol Arthrosc 2007;15:1482–1485.
11 Franceschi F, Ruzzini L, Longo UG, Martina FM, Zobel BB, Maffulli N, Denaro V: Equivalent clinical results of arthroscopic single-row and double-row suture anchor repair for rotator cuff tears: a randomized controlled trial. Am J Sports Med 2007;35:1254–1260.
12 Franceschi F, Longo UG, Ruzzini L, Rizzello G, Maffulli N, Denaro V: The Roman bridge: a 'double pulley – suture bridges' technique for rotator cuff repair. BMC Musculoskelet Disord 2007;8:123.
13 Franceschi F, Longo UG, Ruzzini L, Papalia R, Rizzello G, Denaro V: To detach the long head of the biceps tendon after tenodesis or not: outcome analysis at the 4-year follow-up of two different techniques. Int Orthop 2007;31:537–545.l
14 Franceschi F, Longo UG, Ruzzini L, Rizzello G, Maffulli N, Denaro V: Arthroscopic salvage of failed arthroscopic Bankart repair: a prospective study with a minimum follow-up of 4 years. Am J Sports Med 2008;36:1330–1336.

15 Franceschi F, Longo UG, Ruzzini L, Morini S, Battistoni F, Dicuonzo G, Maffulli N, Denaro V: Circulating substance P levels and shoulder joint contracture after arthroscopic repair of the rotator cuff. Br J Sports Med 2008;42:742–745.
16 Franceschi F, Longo UG, Ruzzini L, Rizzello G, Maffulli N, Denaro V: Soft tissue tenodesis of the long head of the biceps tendon associated to the Roman bridge repair. BMC Musculoskelet Disord 2008;9:78.
17 Longo UG, Franceschi F, Spiezia F, Marinozzi A, Maffulli N, Denaro V: The low-profile Roman bridge technique for knotless double-row repair of the rotator cuff. Arch Orthop Trauma Surg 2011;131:357–361.
18 Castricini R, Longo UG, De Benedetto M, Panfoli N, Pirani P, Zini R, Maffulli N, Denaro V: Platelet-rich plasma augmentation for arthroscopic rotator cuff repair: a randomized controlled trial. Am J Sports Med 2011;39:258–265.
19 Forriol F, Longo UG, Concejo C, Ripalda P, Maffulli N, Denaro V: Platelet-rich plasma, rhOP-1 (rhBMP-7) and frozen rib allograft for the reconstruction of bony mandibular defects in sheep. A pilot experimental study. Injury 2009;40(suppl 3):S44–S49.
20 Longo UG, Lamberti A, Maffulli N, Denaro V: Tendon augmentation grafts: a systematic review. Br Med Bull 2010;94:165–188.
21 Longo UG, Lamberti A, Maffulli N, Denaro V: Tissue engineered biological augmentation for tendon healing: a systematic review. Br Med Bull 2011 (in press).
22 Ames PR, Longo UG, Denaro V, Maffulli N: Achilles tendon problems: not just an orthopaedic issue. Disabil Rehabil 2008;30:1646–1650.
23 Knobloch K, Schreibmueller L, Longo UG, Vogt PM: Eccentric exercises for the management of tendinopathy of the main body of the Achilles tendon with or without an airheel brace. A randomized controlled trial. B: Effects of compliance. Disabil Rehabil 2008;30:1692–1696.
24 Knobloch K, Schreibmueller L, Longo UG, Vogt PM: Eccentric exercises for the management of tendinopathy of the main body of the Achilles tendon with or without the airheel brace. A randomized controlled trial. A: Effects on pain and microcirculation. Disabil Rehabil 2008;30:1685–1691.
25 Longo UG, Ronga M, Maffulli N: Achilles tendinopathy. Sports Med Arthrosc 2009;17:112–126.
26 Longo UG, Ronga M, Maffulli N: Acute ruptures of the Achilles tendon. Sports Med Arthrosc 2009;17: 127–138.
27 Longo UG, Rittweger J, Garau G, Radonic B, Gutwasser C, Gilliver SF, Kusy K, Zieliński J, Felsenberg D, Maffulli N: No influence of age, gender, weight, height, and impact profile in Achilles tendinopathy in masters track and field athletes. Am J Sports Med 2009;37:1400–1405.
28 Longo UG, Rittweger J, Garau G, Radonic B, Gutwasser C, Gilliver SF, Kusy K, Zieliński J, Felsenberg D, Maffulli N: Patellar tendinopathy in master track and field athletes: influence of impact profile, weight, height, age and gender. Knee Surg Sports Traumatol Arthrosc 2011;19:508–512.
29 Maffulli N, Longo UG: Conservative management for tendinopathy: is there enough scientific evidence? Rheumatology (Oxford) 2008;47:390–391.
30 Maffulli N, Walley G, Sayana MK, Longo UG, Denaro V: Eccentric calf muscle training in athletic patients with Achilles tendinopathy. Disabil Rehabil 2008;30:1677–1684.
31 Maffulli N, Longo UG: How do eccentric exercises work in tendinopathy? Rheumatology (Oxford) 2008;47:1444–1445.
32 Maffulli N, Longo UG, Gougoulias N, Denaro V: Ipsilateral free semitendinosus tendon graft transfer for reconstruction of chronic tears of the Achilles tendon. BMC Musculoskelet Disord 2008;9:100.
33 Maffulli N, Longo UG, Loppini M, Denaro V: Current treatment options for tendinopathy. Expert Opin Pharmacother 2010;11:2177–2186.
34 Maffulli N, Longo UG, Denaro V: Novel approaches for the management of tendinopathy. J Bone Joint Surg Am 2010;92:2604–2613.
35 Maffulli N, Longo UG, Franceschi F, Rabitti C, Denaro V: Movin and bonar scores assess the same characteristics of tendon histology. Clin Orthop Relat Res 2008;466:1605–1611.
36 Longo UG, Vasta S, Maffulli N, Denaro V: Scoring systems for the functional assessment of patients with rotator cuff pathology. Sports Med Arthrosc 2011 (in press).
37 Ejnisman B, Andreoli CV, Soares BG, Fallopa F, Peccin MS, Abdalla RJ, Cohen M: Interventions for tears of the rotator cuff in adults. Cochrane Database Syst Rev 2004:CD002758.
38 Bokor DJ, Hawkins RJ, Huckell GH, Angelo RL, Schickendantz MS: Results of nonoperative management of full-thickness tears of the rotator cuff. Clin Orthop Relat Res 1993:103–110.
39 Breazeale NM, Craig EV: Partial-thickness rotator cuff tears. Pathogenesis and treatment. Orthop Clin North Am 1997;28:145–155.
40 Blair B, Rokito AS, Cuomo F, Jarolem K, Zuckerman JD: Efficacy of injections of corticosteroids for subacromial impingement syndrome. J Bone Joint Surg Am 1996;78:1685–1689.

41 Wirth MA, Basamania C, Rockwood CA Jr: Nonoperative management of full-thickness tears of the rotator cuff. Orthop Clin North Am 1997;28: 59–67.
42 Bartolozzi A, Andreychik D, Ahmad S: Determinants of outcome in the treatment of rotator cuff disease. Clin Orthop Relat Res 1994:90–97.
43 Ellman H, Hanker G, Bayer M: Repair of the rotator cuff. End-result study of factors influencing reconstruction. J Bone Joint Surg Am 1986;68:1136–1144.
44 Khan WS, Longo UG, Ahrens PM, Denaro V, Maffulli N: A systematic review of the reverse shoulder replacement in rotator cuff arthropathy, rotator cuff tears and rheumatoid arthritis. Sports Med Arthrosc 2011 (in press).
45 Harryman DT 2nd, Mack LA, Wang KY, Jackins SE, Richardson ML, Matsen FA 3rd: Repairs of the rotator cuff. Correlation of functional results with integrity of the cuff. J Bone Joint Surg Am 1991;73: 982–989.
46 Gazielly DF, Gleyze P, Montagnon C: Functional and anatomical results after rotator cuff repair. Clin Orthop Relat Res 1994:43–53.
47 Gerber C, Fuchs B, Hodler J: The results of repair of massive tears of the rotator cuff. J Bone Joint Surg Am 2000;82:505–515.
48 Lin JC, Weintraub N, Aragaki DR: Nonsurgical treatment for rotator cuff injury in the elderly. J Am Med Dir Assoc 2008;9:626–632.
49 Soslowsky LJ, Carpenter JE, Bucchieri JS, Flatow EL: Biomechanics of the rotator cuff. Orthop Clin North Am 1997;28:17–30.
50 Michener LA, Walsworth MK, Burnet EN: Effectiveness of rehabilitation for patients with subacromial impingement syndrome: a systematic review. J Hand Ther 2004;17:152–164.
51 Ainsworth R, Lewis JS: Exercise therapy for the conservative management of full-thickness tears of the rotator cuff: a systematic review. Br J Sports Med 2007;41:200–210.
52 Hawkins RH, Dunlop R: Nonoperative treatment of rotator cuff tears. Clin Orthop Relat Res 1995;321: 178–188.
53 Piccoli A, Hasson S: Conservative management of a large rotator cuff tear to increase functional abilities: a case report. Physiother Theory Pract 2004; 20:2001–2008.
54 Milgrom C, Schaffler M, Gilbert S, van Holsbeeck M: Rotator-cuff changes in asymptomatic adults. The effect of age, hand dominance and gender. J Bone Joint Surg Br 1995;77:296–298.
55 Sher JS, Uribe JW, Posada A, Murphy BJ, Zlatkin MB: Abnormal findings on magnetic resonance images of asymptomatic shoulders. J Bone Joint Surg Am 1995;77:10–15.
56 Frost P, Andersen JH, Lundorf E: Is supraspinatus pathology as defined by magnetic resonance imaging associated with clinical sign of shoulder impingement? J Shoulder Elbow Surg 1999;8:565–568.
57 Maffulli N, Testa V, Capasso G, Oliva F, Panni AS, Longo UG, King JB: Surgery for chronic Achilles tendinopathy produces worse results in women. Disabil Rehabil 2008;30:1714–1720.
58 Maffulli N, Longo UG, Maffulli GD, Rabitti C, Khanna A, Denaro V: Marked pathological changes proximal and distal to the site of rupture in acute Achilles tendon ruptures. Knee Surg Sports Traumatol Arthrosc 2011;19:680–687.
59 Siegel LB, Cohen NJ, Gall EP: Adhesive capsulitis: a sticky issue. Am Fam Physician 1999;59:1843–1852.
60 Carette S, Moffet H, Tardif J, Bessette L, Morin F, Fremont P, Bykerk V, Thorne C, Bell M, Bensen W, Blanchette C: Intra-articular corticosteroids, supervised physiotherapy, or a combination of the two in the treatment of adhesive capsulitis of the shoulder: a placebo-controlled trial. Arthritis Rheum 2003;48: 829–838.
61 Akgun K, Birtane M, Akarirmak U: Is local subacromial corticosteroid injection beneficial in subacromial impingement syndrome? Clin Rheumatol 2004;23:496–500.
62 Chen MJ, Lew HL, Hsu TC, Tsai WC, Lin WC, Tang SF, Lee YC, Hsu RC, Chen CP: Ultrasound-guided shoulder injections in the treatment of subacromial bursitis. Am J Phys Med Rehabil 2006;85:31–35.
63 Henkus HE, Cobben LP, Coerkamp EG, Nelissen RG, van Arkel ER: The accuracy of subacromial injections: a prospective randomized magnetic resonance imaging study. Arthroscopy 2006;22:277–282.
64 Rutten MJ, Maresch BJ, Jager GJ, de Waal Malefijt MC: Injection of the subacromial-subdeltoid bursa: blind or ultrasound-guided? Acta Orthop 2007;78: 254–257.
65 Shibata Y, Midorikawa K, Emoto G, Naito M: Clinical evaluation of sodium hyaluronate for the treatment of patients with rotator cuff tear. J Shoulder Elbow Surg 2001;10:209–216.
66 Itokazu M, Matsunaga T: Clinical evaluation of high-molecular-weight sodium hyaluronate for the treatment of patients with periarthritis of the shoulder. Clin Ther 1995;17:946–955.
67 Rovetta G, Monteforte P: Intra-articular injection of sodium hyaluronate plus steroid versus steroid in adhesive capsulitis of the shoulder. Int J Tissue React 1998;20:125–130.

68 Leardini G, Perbellini A, Franceschini M, Mattara L: Intra-articular injections of hyaluronic acid in the treatment of painful shoulder. Clin Ther 1988; 10:521–526.

69 Wang CT, Lin J, Chang CJ, Lin YT, Hou SM: Therapeutic effects of hyaluronic acid on osteoarthritis of the knee. A meta-analysis of randomized controlled trials. J Bone Joint Surg Am 2004;86: 538–545.

70 Andrews JR: Diagnosis and treatment of chronic painful shoulder: review of nonsurgical interventions. Arthroscopy 2005;21:333–347.

71 Van der Windt DA, van der Heijden GJ, Scholten RJ, Koes BW, Bouter LM: The efficacy of non-steroidal anti-inflammatory drugs for shoulder complaints. A systematic review. J Clin Epidemiol 1995;48:691–704.

72 Petri M, Hufman SL, Waser G, Cui H, Snabes MC, Verburg KM: Celecoxib effectively treats patients with acute shoulder tendinitis/bursitis. J Rheumatol 2004;31:1614–1620.

73 Heller B, Tarricone R: Oxaprozin versus diclofenac in NSAID-refractory periarthritis pain of the shoulder. Curr Med Res Opin 2004;20:1279–1290.

74 White RH, Paull DM, Fleming KW: Rotator cuff tendinitis: comparison of subacromial injection of a long-acting corticosteroid versus oral indomethacin therapy. J Rheumatol 1986;13:608–613.

75 Henry D, Lim LL, Garcia Rodriguez LA, Perez Gutthann S, Carson JL, Griffin M, Savage R, Logan R, Moride Y, Hawkey C, Hill S, Fries JT: Variability in risk of gastrointestinal complications with individual non-steroidal anti-inflammatory drugs: results of a collaborative meta-analysis. BMJ 1996; 312:1563–1566.

76 Forman JP, Stampfer MJ, Curhan GC: Non-narcotic analgesic dose and risk of incident hypertension in us women. Hypertension 2005;46:500–507.

77 Peterson GM: Selecting nonprescription analgesics. Am J Thers 2005;12:67–79.

78 Akarca US: Gastrointestinal effects of selective and non-selective non-steroidal anti-inflammatory drugs. Curr Pharm Des 2005;11:1779–1793.

79 Bolten WW: Problem of the atherothrombotic potential of non-steroidal anti-inflammatory drugs. Ann Rheum Dis 2006;65:7–13.

80 Ray WA, MacDonald TM, Solomon DH, Graham DJ, Avorn J: Cox-2 selective non-steroidal anti-inflammatory drugs and cardiovascular disease. Pharmacoepidemiol Drug Saf 2003;12:67–70.

81 Graham DJ, Campen D, Hui R, Spence M, Cheetham C, Levy G, Shoor S, Ray WA: Risk of acute myocardial infarction and sudden cardiac death in patients treated with cyclo-oxygenase 2-selective and non-selective non-steroidal anti-inflammatory drugs: nested case-control study. Lancet 2005;365:475–481.

82 Kearney PM, Baigent C, Godwin J, Halls H, Emberson JR, Patrono C: Do selective cyclo-oxygenase-2 inhibitors and traditional non-steroidal anti-inflammatory drugs increase the risk of atherothrombosis? Meta-analysis of randomised trials. BMJ 2006;332:1302–1308.

83 McGettigan P, Henry D: Cardiovascular risk and inhibition of cyclooxygenase: a systematic review of the observational studies of selective and nonselective inhibitors of cyclooxygenase 2. JAMA 2006;296: 1633–1644.

84 Bertin P, Behier JM, Noel E, Leroux JL: Celecoxib is as efficacious as naproxen in the management of acute shoulder pain. J Int Med Res 2003;31:102–112.

85 Stollberger C, Finsterer J: Nonsteroidal anti-inflammatory drugs in patients with cardio- or cerebrovascular disorders. Z Kardiol 2003;92:721–729.

86 Savage R: Cyclo-oxygenase-2 inhibitors: when should they be used in the elderly? Drugs Aging 2005;22:185–200.

87 Khanna A, Friel M, Gougoulias N, Longo UG, Maffulli N: Prevention of adhesions in surgery of the flexor tendons of the hand: what is the evidence? Br Med Bull 2009;90:85–109.

88 Lippi G, Longo UG, Maffulli N: Genetics and sports. Br Med Bull 2010;93:27–47.

89 Longo UG, Franceschi F, Ruzzini L, Rabitti C, Morini S, Maffulli N, Forriol F, Denaro V: Light microscopic histology of supraspinatus tendon ruptures. Knee Surg Sports Traumatol Arthrosc 2007; 15:1390–1394.

90 Longo UG, Franceschi F, Ruzzini L, Rabitti C, Morini S, Maffulli N, Denaro V: Histopathology of the supraspinatus tendon in rotator cuff tears. Am J Sports Med 2008;36:533–538.

91 Longo UG, Oliva F, Denaro V, Maffulli N: Oxygen species and overuse tendinopathy in athletes. Disabil Rehabil 2008;30:1563–1571.

92 Longo UG, Franceschi F, Ruzzini L, Rabitti C, Morini S, Maffulli N, Denaro V: Characteristics at haematoxylin and eosin staining of ruptures of the long head of the biceps tendon. Br J Sports Med 2009;43:603–607.

93 Longo UG, Franceschi F, Ruzzini L, Spiezia F, Maffulli N, Denaro V: Higher fasting plasma glucose levels within the normoglycaemic range and rotator cuff tears. Br J Sports Med 2009;43:284–287.

94 Longo UG, Franceschi F, Spiezia F, Forriol F, Maffulli N, Denaro V: Triglycerides and total serum cholesterol in rotator cuff tears: do they matter? Br J Sports Med 2010;44:948–951.

95 Longo UG, Forriol F, Campi S, Maffulli N, Denaro V: Animal models for translational research on shoulder pathologies: from bench to bedside. Sports Med Arthrosc 2011 (in press).
96 Longo UG, Berton A, Alexander S, Maffulli N, Wallace AL, Denaro V: Biological resurfacing for early osteoarthritis of the shoulder. Sports Med Arthrosc 2011 (in press).
97 Longo UG, Berton A, Khan WS, Maffulli N, Denaro V: Histopathology of rotator cuff tears. Sports Med Arthrosc 2011 (in press).
98 Longo UG, Lamberti A, Khan WS, Maffulli N, Denaro V: Synthetic augmentation for massive rotator cuff tears. Sports Med Arthrosc 2011 (in press).
99 Denaro V, Ruzzini L, Longo UG, Franceschi F, De Paola B, Cittadini A, Maffulli N, Sgambato A: Effect of dihydrotestosterone on cultured human tenocytes from intact supraspinatus tendon. Knee Surg Sports Traumatol Arthrosc 2010;18:971–976.
100 Denaro V, Ruzzini L, Barnaba SA, Longo UG, Campi S, Maffulli N, Sgambato A: Effect of pulsed electromagnetic fields on human tenocyte cultures from supraspinatus and quadriceps tendons. Am J Phys Med Rehabil 2011;90:119–127.
101 DeFranco MJ, Bershadsky B, Ciccone J, Yum JK, Iannotti JP: Functional outcome of arthroscopic rotator cuff repairs: a correlation of anatomic and clinical results. J Shoulder Elbow Surg 2007;16:759–765.
102 Gladstone JN, Bishop JY, Lo IK, Flatow EL: Fatty infiltration and atrophy of the rotator cuff do not improve after rotator cuff repair and correlate with poor functional outcome. Am J Sports Med 2007;35:719–728.
103 Goutallier D, Postel JM, Bernageau J, Lavau L, Voisin MC: Fatty muscle degeneration in cuff ruptures. Pre- and postoperative evaluation by CT scan. Clin Orthop Relat Res 1994;304:78–83.
104 Mellado JM, Calmet J, Olona M, Esteve C, Camins A, Perez Del Palomar L, Gine J, Sauri A: Surgically repaired massive rotator cuff tears: MRI of tendon integrity, muscle fatty degeneration, and muscle atrophy correlated with intraoperative and clinical findings. AJR 2005;184:1456–1463.
105 Thomazeau H, Rolland Y, Lucas C, Duval JM, Langlais F: Atrophy of the supraspinatus belly. Assessment by MRI in 55 patients with rotator cuff pathology. Acta Orthop Scand 1996;67:264–268.
106 Zanetti M, Gerber C, Hodler J: Quantitative assessment of the muscles of the rotator cuff with magnetic resonance imaging. Invest Radiol 1998;33:163–170.
107 Mall NA, Kim HM, Keener JD, Steger-May K, Teefey SA, Middleton WD, Stobbs G, Yamaguchi K: Symptomatic progression of asymptomatic rotator cuff tears: a prospective study of clinical and sonographic variables. J Bone Joint Surg Am 2010;92:2623–2633.
108 Bjorkenheim JM: Structure and function of the rabbit's supraspinatus muscle after resection of its tendon. Acta Orthop Scand 1989;60:461–463.
109 Melis B, DeFranco MJ, Chuinard C, Walch G: Natural history of fatty infiltration and atrophy of the supraspinatus muscle in rotator cuff tears. Clin Orthop Relat Res 2010;468:1498–1505.
110 Kim HM, Dahiya N, Teefey SA, Keener JD, Galatz LM, Yamaguchi K: Relationship of tear size and location to fatty degeneration of the rotator cuff. J Bone Joint Surg Am 2010;92:829–839.
111 Bigliani LU, Cordasco FA, McIlveen SJ, Musso ES: Operative treatment of failed repairs of the rotator cuff. J Bone Joint Surg Am 1992;74:1505–1515.
112 Jost B, Zumstein M, Pfirrmann CW, Gerber C: Long-term outcome after structural failure of rotator cuff repairs. J Bone Joint Surg Am 2006;88:472–479.
113 Warner JJ, Higgins L, Parsons IM, Dowdy P: Diagnosis and treatment of anterosuperior rotator cuff tears. J Shoulder Elbow Surg 2001;10:37–46.
114 Longo UG, Ramamurthy C, Denaro V, Maffulli N: Minimally invasive stripping for chronic Achilles tendinopathy. Disabil Rehabil 2008;30:1709–1713.
115 Franceschi F, Marinozzi A, Papalia R, Longo UG, Gualdi G, Denaro E: Intra- and juxta-articular osteoid osteoma: a diagnostic challenge: misdiagnosis and successful treatment: a report of four cases. Arch Orthop Trauma Surg 2006;126:660–667.
116 Maffulli N, Longo UG, Ronga M, Khanna A, Denaro V: Favorable outcome of percutaneous repair of achilles tendon ruptures in the elderly. Clin Orthop Relat Res 2010;468:1039–1046.
117 Longo UG, King JB, Denaro V, Maffulli N: Double-bundle arthroscopic reconstruction of the anterior cruciate ligament: does the evidence add up? J Bone Joint Surg Br 2008;90:995–999.

Nicola Maffulli, MD, MS, PhD, FRCS(Orth)
Centre for Sports and Exercise Medicine
Barts and The London School of Medicine and Dentistry
Mile End Hospital, 275 Bancroft Road, London E1 4DG (UK)
Tel. +44 20 8223 8839, E-Mail n.maffulli@qmul.ac.uk

Maffulli N (ed): Rotator Cuff Tear. Med Sport Sci. Basel, Karger, 2012, vol 57, pp 100–113

Operative Management of Partial- and Full-Thickness Rotator Cuff Tears

Francesco Franceschi[a,b] · Rocco Papalia[a,b] · Alessio Palumbo[a,b] · Angelo Del Buono[a,b] · Nicola Maffulli[c] · Vincenzo Denaro[a,b]

[a]Department of Orthopaedic and Trauma Surgery and [b]Centro Integrato di Ricerca (CIR), Campus Bio-Medico University, Rome, Italy; [c]Centre for Sports and Exercise Medicine, Queen Mary University of London, Barts and The London School of Medicine and Dentistry, Mile End Hospital, London, UK

Abstract

Repair of rotator cuff tears (RCT) is challenging. In RC tears, a partial (PTRCTs) or full (RCTs) discontinuation of one or more of the muscles or tendons and may occur as a result of traumatic injury or degeneration over a period of years. Many factors seem to contribute to the final outcome and a considerable number of variations during the decision-making process of patients with RCTs exist. Accurate diagnosis is fundamental to guide correct management, and the tear pattern should be carefully evaluated to plan the appropriate repair. Both non-operative and operative treatments are used to relieve pain and restore movement and function of the shoulder. Different surgical options are available. The present review describes the current evidence about diagnosis and management of partial and complete rotator tears.

Rotator cuff tears (RCTs) are the most common cause of shoulder pain and disability, occurring as result of a traumatic injury in younger patients or degenerative changes in older ones [1]. The supraspinatus is most frequently torn, but more tendons may be injured [1, 2], with partial (PTRCTs) or complete (RCTs) involvement of tendon thickness. The histopathologic changes are progressive, increase over time, and are detected in 80% of subjects older than 80 [3]. Magnetic resonance imaging (MRI) and ultrasonographic (US) findings diagnostic for partial or complete tears have been reported in 4% of patients younger than 40 years, 40% of patients over 50 years [4, 5], and up to 100% of patients older than 70 [6]. The quality of life impairment produced by RCTs is comparable to congestive heart failure, diabetes, myocardial infarction, and depression, resulting in significant pain, weakness, and limited motion [7]. Conservative and surgical management regimens have been proposed [8]. Usually, after a period varying from 6 weeks to 3 months, patients unresponsive to non-operative measures are candidates to receive surgical repair. Open, mini-open, and arthroscopic techniques have been proposed, but the choice of adequate postoperative rehabilitation programs are determinant to obtain good recovery in terms of range of motion (ROM), muscle strength, and function [7–10]. The present review describes the current evidence about diagnosis and management of partial (PTRCTs) and complete (RCTs) rotator tears.

Definition and Classification

PTRCTs are a partial disruption of the tendon fibres, with no communication between subacromial and glenohumeral spaces [11]. As reported by Ellman [6] and Snyder et al. [12], when assessing partial tears, the concept of tear depth is more important than examining the tear size. According to the involved side of the tendon, Codman [13] classified PTRCTs as 'bursal side', 'intratendinous', and 'joint-side' tears. In 1972, Neer [14] defined the condition of pain, inflammation, oedema and haemorrhage as stage I, tendon fibrosis as stage II, and the fibre disruption as stage III. Successively, other authors [15, 16] have revised this classification. Considering the average thickness of supraspinatus tendon ranges from 8 to 12 mm, Ellman [6] defined as grade I a tear depth <3 mm, or involving 25% of the tendon thickness, a grade II tear measures from 3 to 6 mm or involves 50% of tendon thickness, and a grade III involves >6 mm or more than 50% of thickness. The grading system by Ellman [6] is assessed intraoperatively. Snyder et al. [12] identified a partial articular supraspinatus tendon avulsion, defined 'PASTA lesion', and proposed a new classification evaluating size and severity of the lesions. On the other hand, in full-thickness tears (RCTs), a complete disruption of the RC fibres produces a direct communication between articular and bursal sides.

At present, the classification by Cofield [2], distinguishing small (<1 cm), medium (1–3 cm), large (3–5 cm), and massive (>5 cm) tears is likely the most used. Gerber et al. [17] referred to the tendon involvement, and defined as massive RCTs when two or more tendons are damaged.

Finally, Goutallier et al. [18] investigated the fatty degeneration of the RC muscles as the factor responsible for reduced muscle function, regardless of patient age. In stage 0, there is no fatty infiltration, mild infiltration in stage 1, muscle prevalence in stage 2, prevalent fatty infiltration in stages 3 and 4. The best management of these tears is unknown. Re-tears may occur after primary repair. However, most untreated atraumatic PTRCTs tend to progress to RCTs, and restoring tendon continuity is indicated to allow tendon to bone healing, and improve strength and function.

Diagnosis

Complete history, appropriate clinical examination, and comparison between involved and contralateral side are mandatory. In addition, areas of tenderness and passive and active ROM of the shoulder should be investigated [19]. RC strength and provocative manoeuvres are tested to choose the diagnostic and management making process. Given poor diagnostic accuracy of most clinical tests [20, 21], the diagnosis of RCTs is usually supported by imaging findings. Radiographs, MRI, arthrography, computed tomography (CT) and ultrasound are commonly used. US and MRI are the most reliable and effective imaging tools in diagnosing RCTs, particularly partial thickness tears [22].

Management

RCTs do not heal spontaneously, but remain unvaried or enlarge over time. In general, decrease of inflammation, restoring ROM, and improving rotator cuff strength are primarily targeted. As a first approach, physical therapy is indicated to improve ROM and strengthen shoulder muscles, whereas anti-inflammatory drugs and cortisone injections are administered to relieve pain [23].

If conservative measures fail, surgery is recommended. At present, traditional surgical indications are young age and history of traumatic tear. Open, mini-open, and arthroscopic procedures have been proposed (table 1). In the past, open repair has been standard practice, allowing direct inspection of the tendons. However, large incisions, long recovery time and postoperative pain induced to perform mini-open repair using a single 3- to 4-cm incision. Successively, with the advent of less invasive techniques, arthroscopy has progressively become the gold standard for management of RCTs. Compared to open or min-open procedures, arthroscopy implies shorter time of hospitalization, less pain, more cosmetic incisions, preservation of the deltoid integrity, and direct inspection of the glenohumeral joint and tendon tear [3].

Treatment for PTRCTs

Non-Operative Management

The initial management of PTRCTs involving less than 50% of the tendon thickness is conservative [24]. The duration of treatment should be tailored to the patient's features, including clinical and imaging findings, status of functional impairment, and level of activity. Rest, application of cold or heat, massage, non-steroidal anti-inflammatory oral drugs (NSAIDs), modification of activities, gentle exercises are initially indicated [11]. Oral NSAIDs and intra-articular corticosteroid injections control pain and relieve symptoms [25], whereas physical therapy is indicated to avoid stiffness secondary to decreased mobility and stretch contracted capsular structures. The anterior capsular tightness is limited by external rotation stretching

Table 1. Comparison of different managements for partial- and full-thickness RCTs

Reference (first author)	Mean age years	Imaging studies	Lesion/other lesions	Conservative management	Surgical management
Conway 2001 [67]	26	MRI and X-ray	SLAP 1 lesion in 29%, SLAP 2 lesion in 29%, SLAP 3 lesion in 7%	–	Intratendinous RCT
Deutsch 2007 [64]	49	MRI and X-ray	–	–	Converted to full-thickness lesions
Budoff 1998 [59]	46	MRI	5% SLAP lesion	–	Debridement
Park 2004 [63]	52	MRI	–	FKT before surgery	Bursal- or articular-sided
Esch 1988 [60]	25/40	MRI and X-ray	Partial-/full-thickness	–	Subacromial decompression
Itoi 1992 [62]	52	Arthrography	–	NSAIDS + FKT for 6 months	Converted to full-thickness lesions + acromioplasty or coracoid ligament resection
Snyder 1991 [12]	42	Arthrograms, ultrasounds, X-ray	33% labral lesion; 6% tendinosis of biceps tendon; 3% SLAP lesion; 3% rotator interval lesion	FKT before surgery	Debridement and subacromial decompression
Cordasco 2002 [61]	48	MRI	–	–	Acromioplasty and debridement
Baysal 2005 [8]	53	MRI and X-ray	–	–	mini-open repair
Milano 2007 [38]	45	X-ray, MRI	Cuff calcification, fatty degeneration of tendon, degenerative of biceps tendon	Preoperative for 6 months	Arthroscopic rotator cuff repair with and without subacromial decompression
Fokuda 1987 [15]	54	US, arthrography, MRI, X-ray and bursography		Spontaneous repair at the torn site was never seen	Bursal-side tears; intratendinous tears; joint side tears + acromioplasty
Audenaert 2006 [7]	42	MRI	–	–	Non-resorbable transosseously fixated patch combined with subacromial decompression

Table 1. Continued

Reference (first author)	Mean age years	Imaging studies	Lesion/other lesions	Conservative management	Surgical management
Flurin 2005 [41]	58	MRI	Supra- and infraspinatos	–	Arthroscopic repair of full-thickness RCTs
Mothadi 2008 [45]	48	MRI, X-ray	–	–	Open surgical repair VS arthroscopic acromioplasty with mini-open repair
Osti 2010 [46]	38	MRI	RCTs of <3 cm	–	Arthroscopic vs. mini-open rotator
Franceschi 2007 [48]	63	MRI	–	–	Single- and double-row suture for full-thickness RCTs
Grasso 2009 [49]	57	MRI, X-ray	–	–	Single- vs. double-row arthroscopic repair for full- thickness RCTs
Resch 2000 [55]	65	MRI	Irreparable rupture of the subscapularis tendon	FKT before surgery	Transfer of the pectoralis major muscle
Weber 1997 [68]	48	Arthrography	–	–	Arthroscopic debridement and acromioplasty vs. mini-open repair for partial thickness
Burkhart 2001 [73]	–	MRI	–	–	Arthroscopic margin convergence vs. direct tendon-To-bone repair for full-thickness RCTs
Gerber 2000 [17]		MRI	Irreparable, full-thickness tears	Preoperative for 6 months	Latissimus dorsi transfer
Boileau 2005 [75]	58	CT & MRI	Only full-thickness supraspinatus tear	–	Tension-band suture technique for full-thickness RCTs
Tauro 2004 [76]	70	MRI	Subscapularis tear	–	End-to-bone and side-to-side repair + arthroscopic rotator interval release and superior capsular release for full- thickness RCTs

exercises, adduction exercises prevent impingement contractures (60–120° of abduction), internal rotation movements with the shoulder in horizontal or cross-body adduction serve to release posteriorly the capsule [25]. When pain and range of movement improve, strengthening exercises of the rotator cuff and periscapular musculature are started to restore the normal kinematic and mechanic patterns [11, 25]. These measures are indicated for management of articular-sided or intratendinous partial-thickness lesions, but less effective in managing bursal-sided tears, probably for the strict relationship with the subacromial impingement. If the subacromial impingement is diagnosed on clinical and imaging grounds [15], surgery is recommended.

Operative Management

Many surgical treatments have been suggested for managing PTRCTs. At present, there is no agreement on the best surgical option, but patient's age, residual tendon features, tissue quality, concomitant shoulder disorders, and surgeon experience have to be taken into account. Debridement, subacromial decompression (with or without debridement), and tendon repair may be accomplished. Bursal-sided tears and articular tears involving more than 50% of tendon thickness (Ellman grade III) should be repaired, whereas debridement is recommended if less than 50% of tendon thickness is torn (Ellman grades I and II) [24]. The debridement is used for removal of necrotic and fibrotic tissues, probably responsible for generating pain and symptoms. However, before performing debridement, the glenohumeral joint and subacromial space have to be examined using standard anterior and posterior portals. By using a shaver, unhealthy tissues are removed, making the tendon surface smoother and more stable. For articular-sided tears, the Snyder suture-marking technique [12] is suggested to assess the tear thickness. A monofilament suture is passed into the tendon throughout a spinal needle, before the arthroscope is introduced into the subacromial space. If an intratendinous lesion is evidenced, the involved area of the tendon should also be debrided to stimulate the residual tendon fibres to heal. If the bursa is inflamed, bursectomy is indicated. Coexisting pathologies such as labral disruptions, long head biceps tendinopathy, or chondral lesions should also be managed at the same time.

Arthroscopic Repair of PTRCTs

Arthroscopic repair is the standard management for PTRCTs, not only because it drastically reduces the rates of re-tear or progression, but also because it provides better results than debridement alone. Although the correct surgical choice depends on residual tendon tissue [6], there is to our knowledge no validated and reliable method to directly measure the thickness of the PTRCTs. Surgeons prefer to measure these tears indirectly [6, 26, 27]. Bursal-sided and articular-sided tears, after conversion to RCTs, may be repaired using a 'transtendon' technique. In this fashion, the fibres of the articular-side are pulled, and inserted to their anatomic footprint. On the other side, intratendinous tears may be repaired after apposition of the disrupted edges.

Conversion to RCTs

After conversion to RCTs, PTRCTs are usually repaired in a single-row fashion, by placing two pairs of non-absorbable sutures, passed through the tendon and then tightened with a sliding knot.

Transtendon Repair

The abundant excision of cuff tissue and following advancement of tendon margin to the footprint area may generate increased tension on the repaired construct. Lo and Burkhart [28] proposed a 'transtendon' repair, in which the lateral aspect of the tendon footprint is preserved, while the medial side is restored by placing transtendon anchors. Once acromioplasty and complete bursectomy, if necessary, have been performed, the arthroscope is introduced into the glenohumeral joint from the standard posterior portal. Transtendon anchors are placed at the medial margin of the footprint, with an inclination angle of 45°, adjacently to the lateral aspect of the acromion. Usually, two anchors are used in lesions >1.5 cm. Once sutures have been passed through the residual tendon fibres, they are tightened in the subacromial space using a sliding knot.

Intratendinous Repair

Intratendinous repair is generally indicated in overhead athletes with intratendinous partial-thickness tears to restore the tendon articular surface, repair disrupted fibres, and improve ROM. Anterior and posterior standard portals are ordinarily used, while an additional lateral portal allows working in the subacromial space. Once the glenohumeral joint has been assessed, the intratendinous defect is tested, and using a tissue grasper repaired. Both injured tendon areas can be debrided to stimulate the healing process. Two spinal needles introduced percutaneously are passed through the tendon, to realize two or more sutures arranged in a mattress system, where articular-sided fibres are attached to healthy surrounding tissues [29].

Non-Operative Treatment

Rehabilitation may improve passive ROM and strength of the shoulder, whereas administration of systemic and local medication may relieve symptoms and pain. In patients with moderate symptoms, conservative treatment can provide satisfactory shoulder function over the years, even though the histological degenerative changes continue to progress, leading to irreparable tears in some patients [30]. There is a lack of randomized clinical trials to establish proper guidelines in terms of conservative management [31].

Operative Management

The repair of RCT should be tailored to each single patient on the basis of tear size, tendon quality, retraction staging, tear pattern, and surgeon's experience. For years, surgeons have limited their attention to provide an adequate repair of the defect, without caring for the function and biomechanics of the shoulder [32]. Different forces act on the rotator cuff muscles: in the coronal plane, all forces are dynamically balanced by the deltoid activity; in the transverse plane, posterior forces are biomechanically balanced by the anterior forces produced from subscapularis tendon. In large RCTs, as the posterior forces are unbalanced, the humeral head may migrate anterior-superiorly. Therefore, surgery has to restore the dynamic balance of these forces, rather than simply repair a defect.

Surgical Techniques

All described techniques involve reinserting the tendon on the footprint, to favour bone tendon healing [33]. Based on pre- and intraoperative findings, tendons may be reinserted at the medial or lateral edge of the footprint. The first step is assessing the glenohumeral joint to rule out associated intra-articular pathologies involving cartilages, labrum, and the tendon of the long tendon biceps. SLAP type II lesions should be fixed or repaired in patients under 50 years, while biceps tenotomy/tenodesis should be performed in older ones [34]. Biceps tenotomy has been demonstrated to improve preoperative symptoms in older patients [35], whereas an associated tenodesis is preferred in younger ones for cosmetic reasons [36]. An isolated subacromial decompression is indicated in elderly, low-demand symptomatic patients, with good motion, well-balanced coronal and transverse acting forces [32], responsive to subacromial local anaesthetic injection [37]. Subacromial decompression does not improve functional results [38]. On the other hand, growth factors are released after limited acromioplasty [39]. The coracoacromial ligament should be preserved to stabilize the humeral head in massive RCTs [40].

The tear pattern should be carefully evaluated to properly plan the repair. Tendon mobility and retraction should be examined in terms of possible reduction and insertion at the footprint. Usually, small tears require a simple tendon to bone reattachment, by placing anchors at the lateral side of the footprint [41]. For larger tears extending longitudinally, a side-to-side repair often precedes the tendon to bone reattachment. A margin convergence technique is accomplished for large U- and L-shaped tears: after shifting of tendon edges, the gap is filled with 3–4 side-to-side sutures which reinsert the tendons to the tuberosity [42]. When tendon mobility is reduced, the interval slide technique allows to release the coracohumeral ligament and extend to the spine of the scapula through the infra- and supraspinatus junction/border [43]. The biomechanical cable theory, introduced for large/massive tear, aims to re-establish an acceptable function status without the tendon gap/tear being completely closed [44]. To close the vertical aspect of the lesion, side-to-side sutures have been properly performed. Side-to-side sutures are commonly made because they allow correct apposition of the tendon ends on their insertion site, and reduce tensile and stress loads at the bone-suture junction. However, tendon to bone repair should be aimed for as it promotes more physiological healing. Comparable outcomes have been reported after arthroscopic and mini-open repair [45, 46]. The transosseous repair, originally performed in open and mini-open surgery, is a common arthroscopic procedure [47]. In the last two decades, anchors have been placed in a standard single-row fashion, but the double-row configuration has allowed to cover larger footprint areas, with no significantly different clinical benefits when compared to single row [48, 49].

In cases of irreparable and retracted RCTs, tendon transfer techniques could be considered to restore functional strength [50]. Various tendon donor sites have been described (subscapularis [51] forward portion of the supraspinatus [52], latissimus dorsi, teres major, pectoralis major, deltoid, triceps, and trapezius). In general, the latissimus dorsi and teres major tendons are used for management of posterosuperior tears [53, 54] and the pectoralis major for anterosuperior tears [55]. Tendon grafts, either biological or synthetic, can also be used to bridge large tendon defects, or reinforce weak tendon repair [55, 56].

Discussion

PTRCTs

Few studies have reported on outcome after conservative treatment of PTRCTs. On the basis of histological investigations [57, 11], partial-thickness tears of the supraspinatus do not heal but may enlarge over time. Arthrographic studies showed that 80% of conservatively managed PTRCTs progressed to RCTs at 2-year follow-up [58].

Snyder et al. [12] reported 84% of good and excellent results in a study on 31 patients who underwent combined debridement and subacromial decompression (only 18/31 patients). In another study, Budoff et al. [59] noted good and excellent outcomes in 89% of 79 shoulders undergoing debridement, declining to 81% after an average follow-up of 5 years. Esch et al. [60] found no significantly different outcomes comparing patients with RCTs and PTRCTs who had received subacromial decompression. Cordasco et al. [61] reported on 162 patients with different grades of PTRCTs, undergoing arthroscopic acromioplasty and debridement. No differences were observed between patients with normal cuff and partial-thickness tears involving less than 50% of the tendon (grades 1 and 2), even though the subgroup of patients with grade 2B partial tears (bursal-sided tears affecting less than 50% of tendon thickness) had an higher failure rate.

Itoi and Tabata [62] reported 82% (31/38) of good to excellent results after open repair, with no statistically significant differences in patients who received additional acromioplasty or coracoacromial ligament resection.

Park et al. [63] compared outcomes of patients undergoing simultaneous arthroscopic repair and decompression for management of partial (bursal- or articular-sided) and RCTs at an average postoperative follow-up of 34 months. Pain, motion, and shoulder function were improved in both groups without statistical differences, with good or excellent results in 39 (93%) of 42 patients, and satisfaction in terms of pain and functional status in 40 of 42 (95%). In a study on 41 patients with partial lesions involving more than 50% of tendon thickness, Deutsch et al. [64] converted to full-thickness tears and successively repaired in a single-row fashion, observing significantly improved ASES scores and high satisfaction rate (98%) at an average follow-up of 38 months.

A high percentage of good and excellent results was also obtained after arthroscopic transtendon repair [65–67]. Weber [68] compared a group of patients who had undergone debridement and acromioplasty with another group of patients receiving a mini-open repair: better long-term results and decreased reoperation rates were observed in patients undergoing mini-open repair compared to those operated arthroscopically.

RCTs

In patients with massive RCTs, arthroscopic debridement and decompression provide satisfactory short-term outcomes [32, 69] in terms of pain relief and functional recovery, with no strength improvement [70]. At long-term follow-up, pain and function progressively deteriorated [71]. Satisfactory clinical results have been widely reported after surgical repair of RCTs [72]. In a long-term study, Burkhart et al. [73] showed good to excellent results in almost all patients (95%), regardless of the tear size. Patients with U-shaped tears, who had undergone margin convergence repair, had outcomes comparable to patients with crescent-shaped tears who had received direct tendon-to-bone repair. Recently, a transosseous technique has been investigated: 40 patients with combined supra- and infraspinatus tears were assessed at a minimum 1-year follow-up. The rate of healing and clinical outcome was investigated on MRI and clinical examination. On MRI, 83% of patients were completely healed, whilst the failure rate was significantly associated with tear size (3.5 vs. 2.8 cm) and fatty infiltration (Goutallier 1.3 vs. 0.3 cm). After transosseous-equivalent suture-bridge repair [74], postoperative MRI assessment revealed repair integrity in 22 of 25 patients (88%), mostly when tears were limited to the supraspinatus tendon (16 of 18 patients, 89%) than to supra- and infraspinatus tendons (86%).

Boileau et al. [75] found a significant association between radiographic signs of tendon healing and postoperative strength. In a multicentre study, Mohtadi et al. [45] compared two groups with full-thickness RCTs who received two different surgical procedures – mini-open surgery and open surgery. At 3 months, statistically significant better outcomes had been reported after mini-open than open repair ($p = 0.005$). At 1- and 2-year postoperative follow-up, there was no difference in outcome between the two procedures. In another study, no statistically significant difference was found comparing the two repair technique-related outcomes for management of RCTs <3 cm [46].

If tears are larger, chronic and retracted, the interval slide technique could be an alternative procedure [28, 76] as soon as tendon transfer procedures are very effective in managing massive posterosuperior RCTs [77].

Conclusion

The management of RCTs is complex and debated. Non-operative management may be useful for mild symptomatic patients with satisfactory function. If non-operative treatment fails, full-thickness tears and partial tears should be surgically repaired. Guidelines for treatment of RCTs are not established yet, given the lack of randomized clinical trials. Careful patient evaluation and surgeon's experience are critical to develop an appropriate and individualized plan of treatment.

References

1 Binder A, Parr G, Hazleman B, et al: Pulsed electromagnetic field therapy of persistent rotator cuff tendinitis. A double-blind controlled assessment. Lancet 1984;1:695–698.

2 Cofield RH: Rotator cuff disease of the shoulder. J Bone Joint Surg Am 1985;67:974–979.

3 Milgrom C, Schaffler M, Gilbert S, et al: Rotator-cuff changes in asymptomatic adults. The effect of age, hand dominance and gender. J Bone Joint Surg Br 1995;77:296–298.

4 Sher JS, Uribe JW, Posada A, et al: Abnormal findings on magnetic resonance images of asymptomatic shoulders. J Bone Joint Surg Am 1995;77: 10–15.

5 Tempelhof S, Rupp S, Seil R: Age-related prevalence of rotator cuff tears in asymptomatic shoulders. J Shoulder Elbow Surg 1999;8:296–299.
6 Ellman H: Diagnosis and treatment of incomplete rotator cuff tears. Clin Orthop Relat Res 1990:64–74.
7 Audenaert E, Van Nuffel J, Schepens A, et al: Reconstruction of massive rotator cuff lesions with a synthetic interposition graft: a prospective study of 41 patients. Knee Surg Sports Traumatol Arthrosc 2006;14:360–364.
8 Baysal D, Balyk R, Otto D, et al: Functional outcome and health-related quality of life after surgical repair of full-thickness rotator cuff tear using a mini-open technique. Am J Sports Med 2005;33:1346–1355.
9 Bennett WF: Arthroscopic repair of full-thickness supraspinatus tears (small-to-medium): a prospective study with 2- to 4-year follow-up. Arthroscopy 2003;19:249–256.
10 Bennett WF: Arthroscopic repair of massive rotator cuff tears: a prospective cohort with 2- to 4-year follow-up. Arthroscopy 2003;19:380–390.
11 Fukuda H: The management of partial-thickness tears of the rotator cuff. J Bone Joint Surg Br 2003;85:3–11.
12 Snyder SJ, Pachelli AF, Del Pizzo W, et al: Partial-thickness rotator cuff tears: results of arthroscopic treatment. Arthroscopy 1991;7:1–7.
13 Codman EA (ed): The Shoulder. Boston, Thomas Todd, 1934.
14 Neer CS 2nd: Anterior acromioplasty for the chronic impingement syndrome in the shoulder: a preliminary report. J Bone Joint Surg Am 1972;54:41–50.
15 Fukuda H, Mikasa M, Yamanaka K: Incomplete thickness rotator cuff tears diagnosed by subacromial bursography. Clin Orthop Relat Res 1987:51–58.
16 Olsewski JM, Depew AD: Arthroscopic subacromial decompression and rotator cuff debridement for stage II and stage III impingement. Arthroscopy 1994;10:61–68.
17 Gerber C, Fuchs B, Hodler J: The results of repair of massive tears of the rotator cuff. J Bone Joint Surg Am 2000;82:505–515.
18 Goutallier D, Postel JM, Bernageau J, et al: Fatty muscle degeneration in cuff ruptures. Pre- and postoperative evaluation by CT scan. Clin Orthop Relat Res 1994:78–83.
19 Burbank KM, Stevenson JH, Czarnecki GR, et al: Chronic shoulder pain. Part I. Evaluation and diagnosis. Am Fam Physician 2008;77:453–460.
20 Hughes PC, Taylor NF, Green RA: Most clinical tests cannot accurately diagnose rotator cuff pathology: a systematic review. Aust J Physiother 2008;54:159–170.
21 Bryant L, Shnier R, Bryant C, et al: A comparison of clinical estimation, ultrasonography, magnetic resonance imaging, and arthroscopy in determining the size of rotator cuff tears. J Shoulder Elbow Surg 2002;11:219–224.
22 Rutten MJ, Spaargaren GJ, van Loon T, et al: Detection of rotator cuff tears: the value of MRI following ultrasound. Eur Radiol 20:450–457.
23 Beaudreuil J, Dhenain M, Coudane H, et al: Clinical practice guidelines for the surgical management of rotator cuff tears in adults. Orthop Traumatol Surg Res 2010;96:175–179.
24 Liem D, Alci S, Dedy N, et al: Clinical and structural results of partial supraspinatus tears treated by subacromial decompression without repair. Knee Surg Sports Traumatol Arthrosc 2008;16:967–972.
25 Matava MJ, Purcell DB, Rudzki JR: Partial-thickness rotator cuff tears. Am J Sports Med 2005;33:1405–1417.
26 Dugas JR, Campbell DA, Warren RF, et al: Anatomy and dimensions of rotator cuff insertions. J Shoulder Elbow Surg 2002;11:498–503.
27 Rudzki JR, Shaffer B: New approaches to diagnosis and arthroscopic management of partial-thickness cuff tears. Clin Sports Med 2008;27:691–717.
28 Lo IK, Burkhart SS: Transtendon arthroscopic repair of partial-thickness, articular surface tears of the rotator cuff. Arthroscopy 2004;20:214–220.
29 Brockmeier SF, Dodson CC, Gamradt SC, et al: Arthroscopic intratendinous repair of the delaminated partial-thickness rotator cuff tear in overhead athletes. Arthroscopy 2008;24:961–965.
30 Zingg PO, Jost B, Sukthankar A, et al: Clinical and structural outcomes of nonoperative management of massive rotator cuff tears. J Bone Joint Surg Am 2007;89:1928–1934.
31 Ainsworth R, Lewis JS: Exercise therapy for the conservative management of full-thickness tears of the rotator cuff: a systematic review. Br J Sports Med 2007;41:200–210.
32 Burkhart SS: Arthroscopic treatment of massive rotator cuff tears. Clinical results and biomechanical rationale. Clin Orthop Relat Res 1991:45–56.
33 Boszotta H, Prunner K: Arthroscopically assisted rotator cuff repair. Arthroscopy 2004;20:620–626.
34 Franceschi F, Longo UG, Ruzzini L, et al: No advantages in repairing a type II superior labrum anterior and posterior (SLAP) lesion when associated with rotator cuff repair in patients over age 50: a randomized controlled trial. Am J Sports Med 2008;36:247–253.
35 Szabo I, Boileau P, Walch G: The proximal biceps as a pain generator and results of tenotomy. Sports Med Arthrosc 2008;16:180–186.

36 Castagna A, Conti M, Mouhsine E, et al: Arthroscopic biceps tendon tenodesis: the anchorage technical note. Knee Surg Sports Traumatol Arthrosc 2006;14:581–585.

37 Elhassan B, Endres NK, Higgins LD, et al: Massive irreparable tendon tears of the rotator cuff: salvage options. Instr Course Lect 2008;57:153–166.

38 Milano G, Grasso A, Salvatore M, et al: Arthroscopic rotator cuff repair with and without subacromial decompression: a prospective randomized study. Arthroscopy 2007;23:81–88.

39 Randelli P, Margheritini F, Cabitza P, et al: Release of growth factors after arthroscopic acromioplasty. Knee Surg Sports Traumatol Arthrosc 2009;17:98–101.

40 Gartsman GM: Arthroscopic management of rotator cuff disease. J Am Acad Orthop Surg 1998;6:259–266.

41 Flurin PH, Landreau P, Gregory T, et al: Arthroscopic repair of full-thickness cuff tears: a multicentric retrospective study of 576 cases with anatomical assessment (in French). Rev Chir Orthop Reparatrice Appar Mot 2005;91:31–42.

42 Nho SJ, Ghodadra N, Provencher MT, et al: Anatomic reduction and next-generation fixation constructs for arthroscopic repair of crescent, L-shaped, and U-shaped rotator cuff tears. Arthroscopy 2009;25:553–559.

43 Lo IK, Burkhart SS: The interval slide in continuity: a method of mobilizing the anterosuperior rotator cuff without disrupting the tear margins. Arthroscopy 2004;20:435–441.

44 Halder AM, O'Driscoll SW, Heers G, et al: Biomechanical comparison of effects of supraspinatus tendon detachments, tendon defects, and muscle retractions. J Bone Joint Surg Am 2002;84:780–785.

45 Mohtadi NG, Hollinshead RM, Sasyniuk TM, et al: A randomized clinical trial comparing open to arthroscopic acromioplasty with mini-open rotator cuff repair for full-thickness rotator cuff tears: disease-specific quality of life outcome at an average 2-year follow-up. Am J Sports Med 2008;36:1043–1051.

46 Osti L, Papalia R, Paganelli M, et al: Arthroscopic vs mini-open rotator cuff repair. A quality of life impairment study. Int Orthop 2010;34:389–394.

47 Cole BJ, ElAttrache NS, Anbari A: Arthroscopic rotator cuff repairs: an anatomic and biomechanical rationale for different suture-anchor repair configurations. Arthroscopy 2007;23:662–669.

48 Franceschi F, Ruzzini L, Longo UG, et al: Equivalent clinical results of arthroscopic single-row and double-row suture anchor repair for rotator cuff tears: a randomized controlled trial. Am J Sports Med 2007;35:1254–1260.

49 Grasso A, Milano G, Salvatore M, et al: Single-row versus double-row arthroscopic rotator cuff repair: a prospective randomized clinical study. Arthroscopy 2009;25:4–12.

50 Singh A, Jawa A, Morman M, et al: Massive rotator cuff tears: arthroscopy to arthroplasty. Instr Course Lect 59:255–267.

51 Cofield RH: Subscapular muscle transposition for repair of chronic rotator cuff tears. Surg Gynecol Obstet 1982;154:667–672.

52 Debeyre J, Patie D, Elmelik E: Repair of ruptures of the rotator cuff of the shoulder. J Bone Joint Surg Br 1965;47:36–42.

53 Gerber C, Maquieira G, Espinosa N: Latissimus dorsi transfer for the treatment of irreparable rotator cuff tears. J Bone Joint Surg Am 2006;88:113–120.

54 Warner JJ: Management of massive irreparable rotator cuff tears: the role of tendon transfer. Instr Course Lect 2001;50:63–71.

55 Resch H, Povacz P, Ritter E, et al: Transfer of the pectoralis major muscle for the treatment of irreparable rupture of the subscapularis tendon. J Bone Joint Surg Am 2000;82:372–382.

56 Wong I, Burns J, Snyder S: Arthroscopic GraftJacket repair of rotator cuff tears. J Shoulder Elbow Surg 2010;19:104–109.

57 Hamada K, Tomonaga A, Gotoh M, et al: Intrinsic healing capacity and tearing process of torn supraspinatus tendons: in situ hybridization study of α_1 (I) procollagen mRNA. J Orthop Res 1997; 15:24–32.

58 Yamanaka K, Matsumoto T: The joint side tear of the rotator cuff. A follow-up study by arthrography. Clin Orthop Relat Res 1994:68–73.

59 Budoff JE, Nirschl RP, Guidi EJ: Debridement of partial-thickness tears of the rotator cuff without acromioplasty. Long-term follow-up and review of the literature. J Bone Joint Surg Am 1998;80:733–748.

60 Esch JC, Ozerkis LR, Helgager JA, et al: Arthroscopic subacromial decompression: results according to the degree of rotator cuff tear. Arthroscopy 1988; 4:241–249.

61 Cordasco FA, Backer M, Craig EV, et al: The partial-thickness rotator cuff tear: is acromioplasty without repair sufficient? Am J Sports Med 2002;30:257–260.

62 Itoi E, Tabata S: Incomplete rotator cuff tears. Results of operative treatment. Clin Orthop Relat Res 1992:128–135.

63 Park JY, Chung KT, Yoo MJ: A serial comparison of arthroscopic repairs for partial- and full-thickness rotator cuff tears. Arthroscopy 2004;20:705–711.

64 Deutsch A: Arthroscopic repair of partial-thickness tears of the rotator cuff. J Shoulder Elbow Surg 2007;16:193–201.
65 Waibl B, Buess E: Partial-thickness articular surface supraspinatus tears: a new transtendon suture technique. Arthroscopy 2005;21:376–381.
66 Ide J, Maeda S, Takagi K: Arthroscopic transtendon repair of partial-thickness articular-side tears of the rotator cuff: anatomical and clinical study. Am J Sports Med 2005;33:1672–1679.
67 Conway JE: Arthroscopic repair of partial-thickness rotator cuff tears and SLAP lesions in professional baseball players. Orthop Clin North Am 2001; 32:443–456.
68 Weber SC: Arthroscopic debridement and acromioplasty versus mini-open repair in the management of significant partial-thickness tears of the rotator cuff. Orthop Clin North Am 1997;28:79–82.
69 Rockwood CA Jr, Williams GR Jr, Burkhead WZ Jr: Debridement of degenerative, irreparable lesions of the rotator cuff. J Bone Joint Surg Am 1995;77:857–866.
70 Gartsman GM, Blair ME Jr, Noble PC, et al: Arthroscopic subacromial decompression. An anatomical study. Am J Sports Med 1988;16:48–50.
71 Zvijac JE, Levy HJ, Lemak LJ: Arthroscopic subacromial decompression in the treatment of full-thickness rotator cuff tears: a 3- to 6-year follow-up. Arthroscopy 1994;10:518–523.
72 Wolf BR, Dunn WR, Wright RW: Indications for repair of full-thickness rotator cuff tears. Am J Sports Med 2007;35:1007–1016.
73 Burkhart SS, Danaceau SM, Pearce CE Jr: Arthroscopic rotator cuff repair: Analysis of results by tear size and by repair technique-margin convergence versus direct tendon-to-bone repair. Arthroscopy 2001;17:905–912.
74 Frank JB, ElAttrache NS, Dines JS, et al: Repair site integrity after arthroscopic transosseous-equivalent suture-bridge rotator cuff repair. Am J Sports Med 2008;36:1496–1503.
75 Boileau P, Brassart N, Watkinson DJ, et al: Arthroscopic repair of full-thickness tears of the supraspinatus: does the tendon really heal? J Bone Joint Surg Am 2005;87:1229–1240.
76 Tauro JC: Arthroscopic repair of large rotator cuff tears using the interval slide technique. Arthroscopy 2004;20:13–21.
77 Burkhart SS: Suture anchor insertion angle and the deadman theory. Arthroscopy 2009;25:1365–1366.

Franceschi Francesco
Department of Orthopaedic and Trauma Surgery
Campus Biomedico University of Rome
Via Alvaro del Portillo
00128 Rome (Italy)
f.franceschi@unicampus.it

Maffulli N (ed): Rotator Cuff Tear. Med Sport Sci. Basel, Karger, 2012, vol 57, pp 114–121

Subscapularis Tears

Umile Giuseppe Longo[a,b,c] · Alessandra Berton[a,b] · Andrea Marinozzi[a,b] · Nicola Maffulli[d] · Vincenzo Denaro[a,b]

[a]Department of Orthopaedic and Trauma Surgery and [b]Centro Integrato di Ricerca (CIR), Campus Bio-Medico University, Rome, Italy; [c]Department of Orthopaedics, Royal Free Hampstead NHS Trust, and [d]Centre for Sports and Exercise Medicine, Queen Mary University of London, Barts and The London School of Medicine and Dentistry, Mile End Hospital, London, UK

Abstract

The subscapularis muscle is the largest and strongest muscle of the rotator cuff. It plays an essential role in the stability and function of the shoulder. Tears of the subscapularis tendon are more frequent than previously estimated. The worldwide use of arthroscopy in rotator cuff surgery has allowed to recognize the true prevalence of subscapularis lesions, as it permits to visualize the articular side where partial tears are usually localized. Subscapularis tears are generally non-traumatic, arising from intrinsic degeneration, subcoracoid and/or anterosuperior impingement. Clinical presentation is usually characterized by history of pain, typically located anteriorly, and difficulty in lifting movements across the chest, or twisting inwards that hinders activities of daily life. Special tests for the diagnosis of subscapularis tears include the lift-off, belly-press, and bear-hug tests. Imaging of the subscapularis tendon may involve plain radiography, magnetic resonance and ultrasound scanning, but MRI better characterizes subscapular tears and coexistent shoulder pathology. The management of subscapularis tears is aimed at restoring the integral role of this muscle in the shoulder. Operative management is indicated for most patients because it is the only one to allow restoration of subscapularis function. Arthroscopic repair can be safely and successfully performed. It requires tendon mobilization to reach the lesser tuberosity. If this is not possible, its footprint can be medialized up to 5–7 mm. Arthroscopic results are encouraging. At intermediate follow-up, improvement in functional scores and patient satisfaction has been reported. Outcomes are comparable to that of open repair, with a very low complication rate and no major intraoperative complications.

Introduction

The subscapularis muscle is the largest and strongest muscle of the rotator cuff. It allows internal rotation of the humerus, provides anterior stability of the shoulder, and is involved in balancing force couples of the glenohumeral joint. It provides 50%

of total cuff strength [1], and it is essential for overhead sports, such as swimming, racquet sports and throwing. It has a triangular shape and fills the subscapular fossa. It passes laterally beneath the coracoid to insert with the upper two thirds as a tendinous insertion into the lesser tuberosity, and with the lower one third as a muscular attachment to the proximal humeral metaphysis [2]. The tendinous footprint is on average 2.5 cm long in a superior to inferior direction, and is essential for normal glenohumeral biomechanics and function [3]. The superolateral aspect of the subscapularis is in contact with the superior glenohumeral ligament and the coracohumeral ligament. They form a pulley that stabilizes the biceps, whose management is important during subscapularis repair.

Epidemiology

Tears of the subscapularis are more frequent than estimated by open approaches [4, 5]. Arthroscopy has allowed to establish the true prevalence of subscapularis lesions, as it permits to visualize the articular side where partial tears are usually located [6]. The prevalence is between 27 and 30% in all shoulder arthroscopies, and between 49 and 59% in arthroscopic rotator cuff surgery [2, 7–9]. Isolated subscapularis tears are uncommon, and occur in about 10% of patients with rotator cuff tears [8]. They are frequently associated with pathology of the tendon of the long head of the biceps [10–14], as biceps pulley is anatomically related with subscapularis tendon [2, 15, 16].

Pathogenesis

Subscapularis tears are generally non-traumatic, and are associated with intrinsic degeneration, subcoracoid and/or anterosuperior impingement [17, 18]. Etiologic factors involve impingement of the subscapular tendon against the coracoid during internal rotation and against the anterosuperior glenoid rim during flexion and internal rotation [19, 20]. This would explain the higher frequency of lesions on the articular side. Traumatic tears are typical of young patients because of forced hyperextension or forced external rotation with the arm either at the side or in abduction [21, 22].

Clinical Features

Clinical presentation is usually characterized by pain, typically located anteriorly, and difficulty in lifting movements across chest or twisting inwards, which interferes with the activities of daily life. Physical examination may show tenderness at the subscapular palpation, pain with anterior elevation and internal rotation, pain or decreased strength with resisted internal rotation, and increased passive external rotation in complete tears. Special tests for the diagnosis of subscapularis tears include the lift-off, belly-press, and bear-hug tests, which involve active internal rotation of the shoulder in different positions of shoulder flexion. The lift-off test [22] is performed by placing the hand of the affected arm on the back on the midlumbar spine, and asking the patient to internally rotate the arm to lift the hand posteriorly off of the back. The test is considered positive if the patients are unable to lift the arm posteriorly off the back or if they perform the lifting manoeuvre by extending the elbow or the shoulder. The evaluation of diagnostic accuracy for the lift-off test produced mixed results. Some authors [9] reported a sensitivity of 17.6% and a specificity of 100% using weakness as a criterion, while others [23–26] confirmed not only good specificity (100%, 99%), but also good sensitivity (62%, 94%) for the lift-off test using weakness and/or pain as criteria. The belly press test [27] is performed with the arm at the side and the elbow flexed to 90°, by having the patient press the palm into his or her abdomen by internally rotating the shoulder. The test is considered positive (1) if the patient shows weakness in comparison to the opposite shoulder, or (2) if the patient pushes the hand against the abdomen by elbow extension or shoulder extension, indicating inability to exert force against the abdomen by active internal rotation produced by the subscapularis. This test appears to specific for demonstrating a subscapularis muscle tendon tear when positive [9, 26], even if its specificity is lower than the lift-off test.

The bear-hug test [9] uses resisted internal rotation with the palm of the hand held on the opposite shoulder with the fingers extended while the elbow is held in maximal anterior translation anterior to the body. As for the belly press, the bear hug appears to be valuable as a specific test to demonstrate a subscapularis muscle tendon tear when positive [9, 26], even though its specificity is lower than the lift-off test.

Imaging of the subscapularis tendon involves the use of plain radiography, magnetic resonance and ultrasound scanning, but MRI better characterizes subscapular tendon tears and coexistent shoulder pathology. Radiographs can be performed in five views (anteroposterior) views in internal and external rotation, axillary view, outlet view, 30° caudal-tilt view), but are usually normal. Sometimes lesser tuberosity cysts, specific for subscapularis tears even though not very sensitive, can be detected on plain radiographs [28], and, in massive tears, proximal migration of the humerus may be demonstrated [29–36]. On MRI, complete tears can be recognized by retracted tendon margin leaving the lesser tuberosity bare, while partial tears produce high signal intensity on T2 images. Especially for partial thickness tears it is important to consider other elements for the diagnosis because it is often overlooked [37]. They involve: narrowed coracohumeral interval (5 mm in patients with subscapularis tears instead of the normal 10 mm [38]), medial subluxation of the tendon of the long head of the biceps, associated with tear of the upper tendon border, and cysts of the lesser tuberosity, as appreciated on plain radiographs

[28]. Ultrasound scanning is a good alternative to MRI, with high sensitivity and specificity with lower cost [39], even though some authors prefer MRI for its higher definition.

Management

Management of tears of the subscapularis tendon aims to restore the integral role of this muscle in the kinematics of the shoulder. It is important to recognize and treat subscapularis tendon tears because this muscle plays an essential role in the stability of glenohumeral joint and in rotator cuff function. Conservative treatment consists of physical therapy and judicious use of corticosteroid injections, and is reserved for old patients with small, non-traumatic, and minimally disabling tears. Operative treatment is indicated for most patients because it is the only modality which restores subscapularis function. Arthroscopic repair can be safely and successfully performed. It requires tendon mobilization to reach the lesser tuberosity. If this is not possible, its footprint can be medialized up to 5–7 mm. Subscapularis mobilization can be difficult because of greater tendon retraction because of chronicity of tear and because of the risk to scar against the coracoid in proximity to neurovascular structures. Moreover, it is difficult to work in the limited subcoracoid space.

First of all, a diagnostic arthroscopy is performed. A 30° arthroscope is inserted through a posterior portal to inspect the subscapularis. The bare lesser tuberosity can be diagnostic for partial tear, which are usually located at the upper articular surface. The size of the tear can be estimated comparing it to the footprint, which is 2.5 cm long [3]. For retracted tear, the 'comma sign', between the superior glenohumeral ligament and the medial head of the coracohumeral ligament, identifies the upper border of the subscapularis [40]. Once the tear has been identified, an anterosuperolateral portal, angled 5–10° to the lesser tuberosity, parallel to the subscapularis tendon, is produced to undertake the coracoplasty. The tendon of the long head of the biceps is inspected and, if required, a tenodesis is performed [11, 13, 30, 41]. Identification of the tip of the coracoid is important because it serves as landmarks to conserve orientation, avoiding inferior incision, and to secure neurovascular structures that are >2.5 cm from the tip of the coracoid [42]. An indication for coracoplasty is a coracohumeral interval <6 mm, as can be estimated comparing it to the shaver [17, 38]. Mobilization is necessary for retracted tears. Three-sided release of the subscapularis is performed. The anterior release consists in denuding the posterolateral aspect of the coracoid. The superior release consists in the removal of adhesion between coracoid neck and base and soft tissue. The posterior release consists in positioning a 15° elevator between the posterior subscapularis and the anterior glenoid neck. To restore the footprint, the lesser tuberosity is prepared to obtain a bleeding base. Only one suture anchor with a knotless repair is used in tears of the upper portion, while at least two anchors are needed for complete tears.

Postoperative Management

Postoperatively, patients need a sling for 4–6 weeks. During this period, no overhead motion is allowed, while elbow flexion, wrist exercises, and hand exercises are encouraged. External rotation to 30° is possible only for partial tears. After 6 weeks, patients start a stretching programme of passive external rotation and forward flexion. At 12 weeks, a strengthening programme using resistance bands to light weights is started.

Results

Arthroscopic results are encouraging. Preliminary results were reported in 2002 by Burkhart and Tehrany [43], who performed arthroscopic subscapularis repair in 25 patients. Subsequent reports confirmed their findings. At intermediate follow-up, functional scores improve and patient satisfaction is good or excellent. The University of California Los Angeles (UCLA) scores generally change from 10.7–16 preoperatively to 30.5–32 postoperatively, the American Shoulder and Elbow Surgeons (ASES) score improves from 40.5 to 91.2, and the relative Constant score from 58 to 96 [8, 43–48].

Outcomes are at least equivalent to those obtained with open repair, with a very low complication rate and no major intraoperative complications.

Conclusions

Arthroscopic rotator cuff repair techniques have been developed, allowing to better clarify pathologies of the subscapularis tendon. To date, there are few randomized controlled trials on the management of subscapularis tendon tears. Unfortunately the aetiology of rotator cuff tears, including subscapularis tendon, is still largely unknown [49–75].

Clearly, studies of higher levels of evidence should be conducted. Future trials should use validated functional and clinical outcomes, adequate methodology, and be sufficiently powered.

References

1 Keating JF, Waterworth P, Shaw-Dunn J, Crossan J: The relative strengths of the rotator cuff muscles. A cadaver study. J Bone Joint Surg Br 1993;75:137–140.

2 Arai R, Sugaya H, Mochizuki T, Nimura A, Moriishi J, Akita K: Subscapularis tendon tear: an anatomic and clinical investigation. Arthroscopy 2008;24:997–1004.

3 Richards DP, Burkhart SS, Tehrany AM, Wirth MA: The subscapularis footprint: an anatomic description of its insertion site. Arthroscopy 2007;23:251–254.
4 Codman E: Lesions of the supraspinatus tendon and other lesions in or about the subacromial bursa; in The Shoulder. Boston, Thomas Todd Co, 1934, pp 65–67.
5 Frankle M, Cofield R: Rotator cuff tears including the subscapularis (abstract). Fifth International Conference of Surgery of the Shoulder, Paris 1992, p 52.
6 Sakurai G, Ozaki J, Tomita Y, Kondo T, Tamai S: Incomplete tears of the subscapularis tendon associated with tears of the supraspinatus tendon: cadaveric and clinical studies. J Shoulder Elbow Surg 1998;7:510–515.
7 Bennett WF: Subscapularis, medial, and lateral head coracohumeral ligament insertion anatomy. Arthroscopic appearance and incidence of 'hidden' rotator interval lesions. Arthroscopy 2001;17:173–180.
8 Lafosse L, Jost B, Reiland Y, Audebert S, Toussaint B, Gobezie R: Structural integrity and clinical outcomes after arthroscopic repair of isolated subscapularis tears. J Bone Joint Surg Am 2007;89:1184–1193.
9 Barth JR, Burkhart SS, De Beer JF: The bear-hug test: a new and sensitive test for diagnosing a subscapularis tear. Arthroscopy 2006;22:1076–1084.
10 Franceschi F, Ruzzini L, Longo UG, Martina FM, Zobel BB, Maffulli N, Denaro V: Equivalent clinical results of arthroscopic single-row and double-row suture anchor repair for rotator cuff tears: a randomized controlled trial. Am J Sports Med 2007;35:1254–1260.
11 Franceschi F, Longo UG, Ruzzini L, Papalia R, Rizzello G, Denaro V: To detach the long head of the biceps tendon after tenodesis or not: outcome analysis at the 4-year follow-up of two different techniques. Int Orthop 2007;31:537–545.
12 Franceschi F, Longo UG, Ruzzini L, Rizzello G, Maffulli N, Denaro V: No advantages in repairing a type II superior labrum anterior and posterior lesion when associated with rotator cuff repair in patients over age 50: a randomized controlled trial. Am J Sports Med 2008;36:247–253.
13 Franceschi F, Longo UG, Ruzzini L, Rizzello G, Maffulli N, Denaro V: Soft tissue tenodesis of the long head of the biceps tendon associated to the roman bridge repair. BMC Musculoskelet Disord 2008;9:78.
14 Longo UG, Franceschi F, Ruzzini L, Rabitti C, Morini S, Maffulli N, Denaro V: Characteristics at haematoxylin and eosin staining of ruptures of the long head of the biceps tendon. Br J Sports Med 2009;43:603–607.
15 Lafosse L, Reiland Y, Baier GP, Toussaint B, Jost B: Anterior and posterior instability of the long head of the biceps tendon in rotator cuff tears: a new classification based on arthroscopic observations. Arthroscopy 2007;23:73–80.
16 Habermeyer P, Magosch P, Pritsch M, Scheibel MT, Lichtenberg S: Anterosuperior impingement of the shoulder as a result of pulley lesions: a prospective arthroscopic study. J Shoulder Elbow Surg 2004;13:5–12.
17 Lo IK, Burkhart SS: The etiology and assessment of subscapularis tendon tears: a case for subcoracoid impingement, the roller-wringer effect, and tuff lesions of the subscapularis. Arthroscopy 2003;19:1142–1150.
18 Gerber C, Sebesta A: Impingement of the deep surface of the subscapularis tendon and the reflection pulley on the anterosuperior glenoid rim: a preliminary report. J Shoulder Elbow Surg 2000;9:483–490.
19 Castricini R, Longo UG, De Benedetto M, Panfoli N, Pirani P, Zini R, Maffulli N, Denaro V: Platelet-rich plasma augmentation for arthroscopic rotator cuff repair: a randomized controlled trial. Am J Sports Med 2011;39:258–265.
20 Franceschi F, Longo UG, Ruzzini L, Rizzello G, Denaro V: Arthroscopic management of calcific tendinitis of the subscapularis tendon. Knee Surg Sports Traumatol Arthrosc 2007;15:1482–1485.
21 Neviaser RJ, Neviaser TJ: Recurrent instability of the shoulder after age 40. J Shoulder Elbow Surg 1995;4:416–418.
22 Gerber C, Krushell RJ: Isolated rupture of the tendon of the subscapularis muscle. Clinical features in 16 cases. J Bone Joint Surg Br 1991;73:389–394.
23 Itoi E, Minagawa H, Yamamoto N, Seki N, Abe H: Are pain location and physical examinations useful in locating a tear site of the rotator cuff? Am J Sports Med 2006;34:256–264.
24 Leroux JL, Thomas E, Bonnel F, Blotman F: Diagnostic value of clinical tests for shoulder impingement syndrome. Rev Rhum Engl Ed 1995;62:423–428.
25 Hertel R, Ballmer FT, Lombert SM, Gerber C: Lag signs in the diagnosis of rotator cuff rupture. J Shoulder Elbow Surg 1996;5:307–313.
26 Rigsby R, Sitler M, Kelly JD: Subscapularis tendon integrity: an examination of shoulder index tests. J Athl Train 2010;45:404–406.

27 Gerber C, Hersche O, Farron A: Isolated rupture of the subscapularis tendon. J Bone Joint Surg Am 1996;78:1015–1023.
28 Studler U, Pfirrmann CW, Jost B, Rousson V, Hodler J, Zanetti M: Abnormalities of the lesser tuberosity on radiography and MRI: association with subscapularis tendon lesions. AJR 2008;191:100–106.
29 Longo UG, Lamberti A, Maffulli N, Denaro V: Tendon augmentation grafts: a systematic review. Br Med Bull 2010;94:165–188.
30 Longo UG, Franceschi F, Spiezia F, Marinozzi A, Maffulli N, Denaro V: The low-profile Roman bridge technique for knotless double-row repair of the rotator cuff. Arch Orthop Trauma Surg 2011; 131:357–361.
31 Longo UG, Lamberti A, Maffulli N, Denaro V: Tissue engineered biological augmentation for tendon healing: a systematic review. Br Med Bull 2011;98:31–59.
32 Longo UG, Franceschi F, Spiezia F, Forriol F, Maffulli N, Denaro V: Triglycerides and total serum cholesterol in rotator cuff tears: do they matter? Br J Sports Med 2010;44:948–951.
33 Longo UG, Forriol F, Campi S, Maffulli N, Denaro V: Animal models for translational research on shoulder pathologies: from bench to bedside. Sports Med Arthrosc 2011 (in press).
34 Longo UG, Berton A, Alexander S, Maffulli N, Wallace AL, Denaro V: Biological resurfacing for early osteoarthritis of the shoulder. Sports Med Arthrosc 2011 (in press).
35 Longo UG, Vasta S, Maffulli N, Denaro V: Scoring systems for the functional assessment of patients with rotator cuff pathology. Sports Med Arthrosc 2011 (in press).
36 Longo UG, Lamberti A, Khan WS, Maffulli N, Denaro V: Synthetic augmentation for massive rotator cuff tears. Sports Med Arthrosc 2011 (in press).
37 Tung GA, Yoo DC, Levine SM, Brody JM, Green A: Subscapularis tendon tear: primary and associated signs on MRI. J Comp Assist Tomogr 2001;25:417–424.
38 Richards DP, Burkhart SS, Campbell SE: Relation between narrowed coracohumeral distance and subscapularis tears. Arthroscopy 2005;21:1223–1228.
39 Teefey SA, Hasan SA, Middleton WD, Patel M, Wright RW, Yamaguchi K: Ultrasonography of the rotator cuff. A comparison of ultrasonographic and arthroscopic findings in one hundred consecutive cases. J Bone Joint Surg Am 2000;82:498–504.
40 Lo IK, Burkhart SS: The comma sign: an arthroscopic guide to the torn subscapularis tendon. Arthroscopy 2003;19:334–337.
41 Franceschi F, Longo UG, Ruzzini L, Rizzello G, Maffulli N, Denaro V: The Roman bridge: a 'double pulley-suture bridges' technique for rotator cuff repair. BMC Musculoskelet Disord 2007;8:123.
42 Lo IK, Burkhart SS, Parten PM: Surgery about the coracoid: Neurovascular structures at risk. Arthroscopy 2004;20:591–595.
43 Burkhart SS, Tehrany AM: Arthroscopic subscapularis tendon repair: technique and preliminary results. Arthroscopy 2002;18:454–463.
44 Adams CR, Schoolfield JD, Burkhart SS: The results of arthroscopic subscapularis tendon repairs. Arthroscopy 2008;24:1381–1389.
45 Bennett WF: Arthroscopic repair of anterosuperior (supraspinatus/subscapularis) rotator cuff tears: a prospective cohort with 2- to 4-year follow-up. Classification of biceps subluxation/instability. Arthroscopy 2003;19:21–33.
46 Bennett WF: Arthroscopic repair of isolated subscapularis tears: a prospective cohort with 2- to 4-year follow-up. Arthroscopy 2003;19:131–143.
47 Ide J, Tokiyoshi A, Hirose J, Mizuta H: Arthroscopic repair of traumatic combined rotator cuff tears involving the subscapularis tendon. J Bone Joint Surg Am 2007;89:2378–2388.
48 Kim SH, Oh I, Park JS, Shin SK, Jeong WK: Intra-articular repair of an isolated partial articular-surface tear of the subscapularis tendon. Am J Sports Med 2005;33:1825–1830.
49 Lippi G, Longo UG, Maffulli N: Genetics and sports. Br Med Bull 2010;93:27–47.
50 Longo UG, Franceschi F, Ruzzini L, Rabitti C, Morini S, Maffulli N, Forriol F, Denaro V: Light microscopic histology of supraspinatus tendon ruptures. Knee Surg Sports Traumatol Arthrosc 2007;15:1390–1394.
51 Longo UG, Franceschi F, Ruzzini L, Rabitti C, Morini S, Maffulli N, Denaro V: Histopathology of the supraspinatus tendon in rotator cuff tears. Am J Sports Med 2008;36:533–538.
52 Maffulli N, Longo UG, Franceschi F, Rabitti C, Denaro V: Movin and Bonar scores assess the same characteristics of tendon histology. Clin Orthop Relat Res 2008;466:1605–1611.
53 Maffulli N, Franceschi F, Longo UG, Ruzzini L, Denaro V: Clinical evidence for suture anchor repair of rotator cuff tears does add up: some just do not want to see it. Arthroscopy 2010;26:1568–1570.
54 Maffulli N, Longo UG, Loppini M, Denaro V: Current treatment options for tendinopathy. Expert Opin Pharmacother 2010;11:2177–2186.
55 Maffulli N, Longo UG, Denaro V: Novel approaches for the management of tendinopathy. J Bone Joint Surg Am 2010;92:2604–2613.

56 Maffulli N, Longo UG, Gougoulias N, Caine D, Denaro V: Sport injuries: a review of outcomes. Br Med Bull 2011;97:47–80.
57 Maffulli N, Longo UG, Spiezia F, Denaro V: Sports injuries in young athletes: long-term outcome and prevention strategies. Phys Sportsmed 2010;38:29–34.
58 Maffulli N, Longo UG, Spiezia F, Denaro V: Aetiology and prevention of injuries in elite young athletes. Med Sport Sci 2011;56:187–200.
59 Maffulli N, Longo UG, Berton A, Loppini M, Denaro V: Biological factors in rotator cuff tears. Sports Med Arthrosc 2011 (in press).
59 Maffulli N, Longo UG, Berton A, Loppini M, Denaro V: Biological factors in rotator cuff tears. Sports Med Arthrosc 2011 (in press).
60 Longo UG, Ramamurthy C, Denaro V, Maffulli N: Minimally invasive stripping for chronic Achilles tendinopathy. Disabil Rehabil 2008;30:1709–1713.
61 Longo UG, Ronga M, Maffulli N: Achilles tendinopathy. Sports Med Arthrosc 2009;17:112–126.
62 Longo UG, Oliva F, Denaro V, Maffulli N: Oxygen species and overuse tendinopathy in athletes. Disabil Rehabil 2008;30:1563–1571.
63 Khanna A, Friel M, Gougoulias N, Longo UG, Maffulli N: Prevention of adhesions in surgery of the flexor tendons of the hand: what is the evidence? Br Med Bull 2009;90:85–109.
64 Ames PR, Longo UG, Denaro V, Maffulli N: Achilles tendon problems: not just an orthopaedic issue. Disabil Rehabil 2008;30:1646–1650.
65 Franceschi F, Marinozzi A, Papalia R, Longo UG, Gualdi G, Denaro E: Intra- and juxta-articular osteoid osteoma: a diagnostic challenge: misdiagnosis and successful treatment: a report of four cases. Arch Orthop Trauma Surg 2006;126:660–667.
66 Maffulli N, Longo UG, Gougoulias N, Denaro V: Ipsilateral free semitendinosus tendon graft transfer for reconstruction of chronic tears of the Achilles tendon. BMC Musculoskelet Disord 2008;9:100.
67 Maffulli N, Walley G, Sayana MK, Longo UG, Denaro V: Eccentric calf muscle training in athletic patients with Achilles tendinopathy. Disabil Rehabil 2008;30:1677–1684.
68 Longo UG, Rittweger J, Garau G, Radonic B, Gutwasser C, Gilliver SF, Kusy K, Zieliński J, Felsenberg D, Maffulli N: No influence of age, gender, weight, height, and impact profile in achilles tendinopathy in masters track and field athletes. Am J Sports Med 2009;37:1400–1145.
69 Longo UG, Ronga M, Maffulli N: Acute ruptures of the achilles tendon. Sports Med Arthrosc 2009;17: 127–138.
70 Maffulli N, Longo UG: Conservative management for tendinopathy: is there enough scientific evidence? Rheumatology 2008;47:390–391.
71 Maffulli N, Longo UG: How do eccentric exercises work in tendinopathy? Rheumatology 2008;47: 1444–1445.
72 Maffulli N, Longo UG, Ronga M, Khanna A, Denaro V: Favorable outcome of percutaneous repair of achilles tendon ruptures in the elderly. Clin Orthop Relat Res 2010;468:1039–1046.
73 Maffulli N, Longo UG, Gougoulias N, Loppini M, Denaro V: Long-term health outcomes of youth sports injuries. Br J Sports Med 2010;44:21–25.
74 Longo UG, Franceschi F, Ruzzini L, Spiezia F, Maffulli N, Denaro V: Higher fasting plasma glucose levels within the normoglycaemic range and rotator cuff tears. Br J Sports Med 2009;43:284–287.
75 Longo UG, King JB, Denaro V, Maffulli N: Double-bundle arthroscopic reconstruction of the anterior cruciate ligament: does the evidence add up? J Bone Joint Surg Br 2008;90:995–999.

Nicola Maffulli, MD, MS, PhD, FRCS(Orth)
Centre for Sports and Exercise Medicine
Barts and The London School of Medicine and Dentistry
Mile End Hospital, 275 Bancroft Road, London E1 4DG (UK)
Tel. + 44 20 8223 8839, E-Mail n.maffulli@qmul.ac.uk

Maffulli N (ed): Rotator Cuff Tear. Med Sport Sci. Basel, Karger, 2012, vol 57, pp 122–141

Single- and Double-Row Repair for Rotator Cuff Tears – Biology and Mechanics

Rocco Papalia[a,b] · Francesco Franceschi[a,b] · Sebastiano Vasta[a,b] · Biagio Zampogna[a,b] · Nicola Maffulli[c] · Vincenzo Denaro[a,b]

[a]Department of Orthopaedic and Trauma Surgery and [b]Centro Integrato di Ricerca (CIR), Campus Bio-Medico University, Rome, Italy; [c]Centre for Sports and Exercise Medicine, Barts and The London School of Medicine and Dentistry, Mile End Hospital, London, UK

Abstract

Objectives: We critically review the existing studies comparing the features of single- and double-row repair, and discuss suggestions about the surgical indications for the two repair techniques. **Data Sources:** All currently available studies comparing the biomechanical, clinical and the biological features of single and double row. **Main Results:** Biomechanically, the double-row repair has greater performances in terms of higher initial fixation strength, greater footprint coverage, improved contact area and pressure, decreased gap formation, and higher load to failure. Results of clinical studies demonstrate no significantly better outcomes for double-row compared to single-row repair. Better results are achieved by double-row repair for larger lesions (tear size 2.5–3.5 cm). **Conclusions:** Considering the lack of statistically significant differences between the two techniques and that the double row is a high cost and a high surgical skill-dependent technique, we suggest using the double-row technique only in strictly selected patients.

Rotator cuff disorders are the most common cause of shoulder pain and impairments in adults with a prevalence ranging from 5 to 39% [1–3]. The pathogenesis is multifactorial, and includes repetitive microtrauma, age-related degeneration, impingement and major trauma [4, 5]. Rotator cuff tears have been classified into full-thickness tears (defined as a complete interruption of the tendon fibres) and partial thickness tears (classified as articular-sided, bursal-sided and intratendinous) [1]. Since the technological advancements allowed arthroscopy to reach comparable results to open or mini-open surgery, the surgical management of the rotator cuff tears is largely based on arthroscopic repair [6]. The aim of the arthroscopic repair is to restore the anatomical footprint. A larger area of the tendon-to-bone contact would lead to a better osseous incorporation favouring the healing process and the

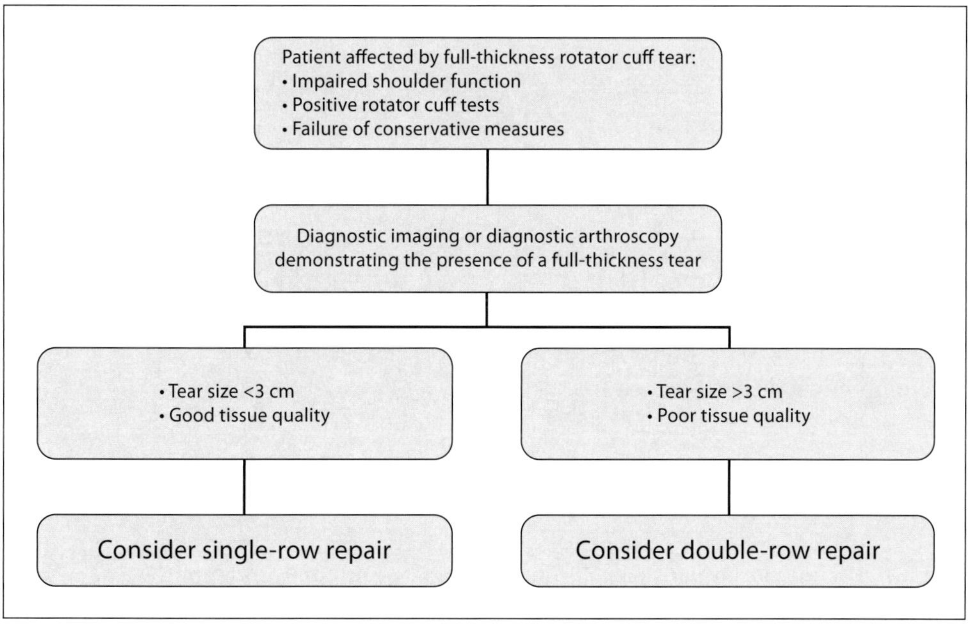

Fig. 1. Management algorithm based on current literature evidence.

recovery of the mechanical strength and function [7]. The surgical options comprehend single-row, double-row and the transosseous technique. Currently the most frequently used technique is the single-row repair, which consists of placing the suture anchors in a single row at the lateral aspect of the tendon footprint on the humeral head. The most important postoperative complication is the re-tear of the rotator cuff, leading often to a revision surgery [8–10]. Many factors have been identified as responsible for the repair failure, such as the quality of the tissues (relatively to the muscles, the tendons and the bone), neurovascular damage, preoperative size of the lesion, the failure of the suture or the knot [9, 11–14]. It has also been proposed that the single-row suture anchors do not provide an adequate tendon-to-bone contact leading to an impaired healing process [15]. This theory has induced some surgeons to develop alternative techniques. In 2003, Lo and Burkhart [16] introduced double-row rotator cuff repair. It consists of placing one row of anchors in the medial aspect of the tendon footprint and a second row more laterally. Cadaveric [17–19] and clinical [20] studies have shown the double-row technique to provide a larger coverage of the footprint restoring a closer anatomical condition. These advantages may be useful, especially during the early postoperative period when the tendon-to-bone interface is still weak and the healing process is not completed [21]. Although on the biological and biomechanical level the double-row technique was seen to be advantageous, on the clinical level it is still unclear if it is superior to the single-row suture anchor technique (fig. 1).

Description of the Surgical Techniques

Single Row [22]

Single-row anchor repair consists of placing one row of suture anchors just inside the lateral aspect of the footprint. Different suturing fashions can be used: single-row anchor-simple (SRA-s): simple stitch repair with one row of two double-loaded suture anchors; single-row anchor-mattress (SRA-m): horizontal mattress stitch repair with one line of two double-loaded suture anchors. Single-row anchor-arthroscopic Mason-Allen (SRAama): arthroscopic Mason-Allen stitch repair using one row of two double-loaded suture anchors.

Double Row [22]

Double-row anchor repair consists of placing one medial and one lateral row of suture anchors to closer approach the original rotator cuff footprint. The possible suturing fashions are: double-row anchor-simple mattress (DRA-sm): it consists of combining simple (lateral/double-loaded) and horizontal mattress stitches (medial/single-loaded) repair by two rows placing four suture anchors. Double-row anchor-arthroscopic Mason-Allen mattress (DRA-amam): arthroscopic Mason-Allen (lateral/double-loaded) and horizontal mattress stitches (medial/single-loaded) repair are combined placing two lines using a total of four suture anchors.

Transosseous Repair [23]

The transosseous repair technique consists of performing three vertical transosseous tunnels through the greater tuberosity from the articular aspect to the lateral cortex of the proximal humerus leaving a bone bridge of 8 mm between each tunnel. To reattach the injured tendons to the footprint, two horizontal mattress sutures are tied over the lateral cortex (modified McLaughlin technique).

Results

Biomechanical Studies

To investigate the features of double-row repair techniques, numerous studies have been performed, comparing the biomechanical properties of single-row to double-row repair, with different types of anchors and of suture patterns (table 1). Both animal [22, 24–31] and human [17, 18, 32–37] specimens have been used. Most biomechanical

Table 1. Biomechanical studies comparing single-row to double-row repair

Study (first author)	Specimens (involved tendon)	Technique	Testing methods	Results	Conclusions
Ahmad, 2008 [32]	18 human cadaver shoulders (supra-spinatus)	SR: 2 anchors single-loaded DR: 4 anchors, 2 medial (with mattress fashion sutures), 2 lateral (with simple fashion sutures)	Gap formation with rotational component	For the single-row repair, average gap formation per 100 cycles in the positions of neutral, internal, and external humeral rotation was 1.47±0.63, 3.11±1.55, and 2.24±0.94 mm, respectively For the double-row repair, average gap formation per 100 cycles in the positions of neutral, internal, and external humeral rotation was 1.25±0.54, 2.29±1.10, and 1.57±0.48 mm, respectively	Double-row repair has better fixation strength than single-row repairs when exposed to cyclic loading and changes in humeral rotation position
Barber, 2010 [24]	40 bovine shoulders (infra-spinatus)	Group 1: 2 triple-loaded screw suture anchors in a SR with simple stitches Group 2: 2 triple-loaded screw anchors in a SR with simple stitches over a fourth suture passed perpendicularly ('rip-stop' stitch) Group 3: DR, 2 medial and 2 lateral screw anchors with a single vertical mattress stitch passed from the medial anchors and 2 simple stitches passed from the lateral anchors Group 4: DR, 2 medial double-loaded screw anchors tied in 2 mattress stitches and 2 push-in lateral anchors capturing the medial sutures in a 'crisscross' spanning stitch Group 5: 2 medial double-loaded screw anchors tied in 2 mattress stitches and 2 push-in lateral anchors creating a 'suture-bridge' stitch	Cyclic loading displacement (5 and 10 mm), total displacement, and ultimate failure load	Group 1 was more resistant to stretching to a 5- and 10-mm gap than the DR with or without the addition of a rip-stop suture ($p < 0.05$)The addition of a rip-stop stitch made the repair more resistant to gap formation than a DR ($p < 0.05$) The crisscross DR created by 2 medial double-loaded suture anchors and 2 lateral push-in anchors stretched more than any other group ($p < 0.05$)	Triple-loaded anchors placed in a single row (group 1) are more resistant to stretching than the DR groups

Table 1. Continued

Study (first author)	Specimens (involved tendon)	Technique	Testing methods	Results	Conclusions
Baums, 2010 [25]	32 sheep shoulders (infra-spinatus)	DR: DR1: Ethibond sutures and DR2: HiFi sutures; suture technique: arthroscopic Mason-Allen stitches (lateral/double-loaded suture anchor system) and mattress stitches medial/single-loaded SR: SR1: Ethibond sutures and SR2: HiFi sutures; suture technique: arthroscopic Mason-Allen stitches	Load to failure rate and stiffness of single- vs. double-row suture techniques	SR2 showed lowest load-to-failure result with 155.7±31.1 N compared to DR1 (293.4±16.1 N) and DR2 (397.7±7.4 N) ($p < 0.001$) Stiffness was highest in DR2 (162±7.3 N/mm) and lowest in SR2 (84.4±19.9 mm) ($p < 0.001$)	High initial failure strength for DR
Baums, 2008 [22]	32 fresh-frozen sheep shoulders (infra-spinatus)	SR: 2 anchors double-loaded with Mason-Allen stitch (subgroups: SR1: Ethibond sutures (SRAE); SR2: HiFi sutures(SRAH)) DR: 4 anchors with Mason-Allen stitch (lateral/double-loaded)-horizontal mattress stitch (medial/single-loaded) (subgroups DR1: Ethibond sutures (DRAE); DR2: HiFi sutures (DRAH))	Displacement to gap formation of 5 and 10 mm at the repair site, cycles to failure, and the mode of failure	DRAE and DRAH had a lower frequency of 5- ($p = 0.135$) and 10-mm gap formation ($p = 0.135$) All DRAE and DRAH resisted 3,000 cycles while only three SRAE and one SRAH resisted 3,000 cycles ($p < 0.001$) The ultimate tensile strength in double-row specimens was significantly higher than in others ($p < 0.001$) There was no significant variation in using different suture material ($p < 0.05$)	Improvement of initial fixation strength and ultimate tensile load with double-row fixation with arthroscopic Mason-Allen/medial mattress stitches
Baums, 2009 [22]	40 fresh-frozen sheep shoulders (infra-spinatus)	SRA-s: single-row repair using simple stitches; SRA-m: single-row repair using horizontal mattress stitches; SRAama: single-row repair using arthroscopic Mason-Allen stitches. DRA-sm: double-row repair using a combination of simple and horizontal mattress stitches DRA-amam: double-row with arthroscopic Mason-Allen/horizontal mattress stitches	Evaluation of the tendon-bone interface contact pressure by pressure-sensitive film system	Contact pressure was lowest in SRA-m followed by SRA-s SRA-ama showed highest contact pressure of all single-row treatment groups ($p < 0.05$) DRA-amam presented the highest overall contact pressure ($p < 0.05$), whereas DRA-sm exerted contact pressure equal to that of SRA-ama	Contact pattern between the anchors could be increased by using the double-row technique, resulting in more footprint coverage compared to patterns utilizing the single-row techniques

Table 1. Continued

Study (first author)	Specimens (involved tendon)	Technique	Testing methods	Results	Conclusions
Zhang, 2010 [31]	10 matched pairs of fresh-frozen sheep shoulders (infra-spinatus with partial thickness tears)	DR: 2 medial anchors with horizontal mattress sutures at and 2 lateral anchors with horizontal mattress sutures. SR: transtendon single-row mattress sutures	Cycling loading and tensile testing to failure. Gap formation, stiffness, failure load and strain over the footprint area were measured	Gap formation for the transtendon SR was significantly smaller ($p < 0.05$) when compared with the DR The strain over the footprint area for the transtendon SR was significantly smaller ($p < 0.05$) when compared with the DR	Transtendon single-row fixation exhibited superior biomechanical properties when compared with double-row fixation
Kim, 2006 [17]	18 cadaveric shoulders (supra-spinatus)	DR: double-row suture anchor technique: 2 medial anchors with horizontal mattress sutures and 2 lateral anchors with simple SR: single lateral row of 2 anchors with simple sutures	Cyclic loading from 10 to 180 N for 200 cycles, tensile testing to failure and gap formation	Gap formation for the DR was significantly smaller ($p < 0.05$) when compared with SR for the first cycle (1.67±0.75 vs. 3.10±1.67 mm, respectively) and the last cycle (3.58±2.59 vs. 7.64±3.74 mm, respectively) The initial strain over the footprint area for the DR was nearly one third ($p < 0.05$) the strain of the SR	Double-row repair improved initial strength and stiffness and decreased gap formation
Lorbach, 2008 [27]	48 porcine shoulders (infra-spinatus)	SR: SR1: simple transosseous sutures, SR2: a double mattress repair or a modified Mason-Allen repair, and SR3: the Opus AutoCuff system performing an inclined mattress suture. DR: DR1: lateral row 2 double-loaded anchors with 4 simple sutu-res, 2 double-loaded anchors medial row with double mattress sutures. DR2: 2 anchors singly-loaded for medial row with 2 mattress sutures, and the ends of the sutures were crossed to fix the sutures laterally (suture bridge technique) using 2 knotless fixation devices	Cyclic load (10 to 60–200 N) to measure gap formation, ultimate load to failure and type of failure	DR1 had the highest ultimate tensile strength (398±98 N) compared to SR1 (105±21 N; $p < 0.0001$), SR Mason-Allen repair (256±73 N; $p = 0.003$) or SR double mattress repair (290±56 N; $p = 0.043$), the magnum implant (163±13 N; $p < 0.0001$), and DR2 (163±59 N; $p < 0.0001$) Lowest gap formation was found for DR1 (3.1±0.1 mm)	DR1 achieved superior results in failure load and gap formation compared to SR1 and showed similar loads and gap formation with DR2

Table 1. Continued

Study (first author)	Specimens (involved tendon)	Technique	Testing methods	Results	Conclusions
Ma, 2006 [18]	10 pairs of fresh-frozen human supra-spinatus tendons	SR: 3 different stitch configurations: two-simple, massive cuff and arthroscopic Mason-Allen; DR: double-row fixation	Conditioning elongation, peak-to-peak elongation, ultimate tensile load, and stiffness. Failure type (suture or anchor pull-out) was also reported	No differences were reported for conditioning elongation, stiffness and failure mechanisms among the groups. The mean peak-to-peak elongation was significantly lower for the massive cuff (1.1±0.1 mm) and DR stitches (1.1±0.1 mm) than for the arthro-scopic Mason-Allen stitch (1.5±0.2 mm) ($p < 0.05$) The ultimate tensile load was significantly higher for DR (287±24 N) than for all of the single-row fixations ($p < 0.05$) The massive cuff stitch (250±21 N) was found to have a significantly higher ultimate tensile load than the two-simple (191±18 N) and arthroscopic Mason-Allen (212±21 N) stitches ($p < 0.05$)	Double-row fixation can improve the initial fixation strength
Mahar, 2007 [28]	18 bovine specimens (infra-spinatus)	Group 1:SR with double-loaded suture anchors Group 2: DR with single-loaded medial row and double-loaded lateral row Group 3: DR with single-loaded medial row and single-loaded lateral row	Cyclic elongation, with loads at 3, 5, and 10 mm	No significant differences for peak elongation after cyclic loading and for loads at 3, 5, and 10 mm of elongation among groups	DR does not show a biomechanical advantage compared with single-row repair
Mazzocca, 2005 [33]	20 fresh-frozen cadaveric shoulders (supras-pinatus)	SR and 3 different types of DR: diamond, mattress double anchor (MDA), and modified mattress double anchor (MMDA)	Displacement with cyclic loading and load to failure	No differences in load to failure (>250 N for SR and DR groups) and displacement with cyclic loading between the SR and each DR A significantly greater supraspinatus footprint width was seen with DR compared to SR	Although no biomechanical differences are found, DR techniques provide a larger footprint width

Table 1. Continued

Study (first author)	Specimens (involved tendon)	Technique	Testing methods	Results	Conclusions
Meier, 2006 [34]	7 fresh-frozen shoulders (supraspinatus)	TO; SR: stitch with simple sutures; DR:2 lateral anchors with simple sutures, 2 medial anchors with horizontal mattress sutures	3-dimensional mapping to determine the area of the restored footprint	DR reproduced 100% of the original supraspinatus footprint, SR: 46% and TO: 71% of the insertion site	Footprint area of the DR was significantly larger ($p = 0.05$) than that of the other 2 techniques
Meier, 2006 [19]	30 fresh-frozen cadaveric shoulders (supraspinatus)	Group 1 (TOS): transosseous simple with vertical stitches; group 2 (SRSA): single row with simple vertical stitches; group 3 (DRSA): double row with simple vertical stitches for lateral row and horizontal mattress for medial row	Cyclic load testing until complete failure	Group 1 (TOS) failed at an average of 75.3±22.49 cycles Group 1 (SRSA) at an average of 798.3±73.28 cycles Group 3 (DRSA) had no failures Fixation strength of the DR was significantly greater than SRSA and both SRSA and DRSA were significantly stronger than the TOS group	Suture anchors are superior than transosseous repair and DR is stronger than SR
Milano, 2008 [29]	50 fresh porcine shoulders (infraspinatus)	SR: 2 anchors with simple stitch sutures. DR: 4 anchors, simple stitches for the sutures of the lateral anchors, and mattress stitches for the sutures of the medial anchors Group 1: SR tension-free Group 2: SR tension repair Group 3: DR tension-free repair Group 4: DR tension repair	Cyclic loading test: number of cycles at 5 mm of elongation and at failure, and total elongation	Number of cycles at 5 mm of elongation and at failure: no significant difference between groups 3 and 4, and both of them were significantly greater than Group 1 Total elongation: the difference among groups 1, 3, and 4 was not significant	SR tension repair showed significantly poorest results for all the variables considered DR with and without tension repair are significantly more resistant to cyclic displacement
Nelson, 2008 [30]	6 matched pairs of sheep infraspinatus tendons	DR: 2 single-loaded medial anchors tied in a mattress configuration and 1 single lateral anchor double-loaded with 2 simple suture configurations. SR: 2 double-loaded anchors with modified Mason-Allen sutures	Pressure-sensitive film to measure the surface area of repair. Cyclic loading and loads to failure	DR restored a mean surface area of 258.23±69.7 vs. 148.08±75.5 mm^2 for SR, a 74% increase ($p < 0.025$). No statistically significant differences in peak-to-peak displacement or	DR restores a greater percentage of the anatomic footprint when compared with a SR Mason-Allen technique

Table 1. Continued

Study (first author)	Specimens (involved tendon)	Technique	Testing methods	Results	Conclusions
				elongation during cyclic loading. SR showed a higher (not statistically significant) mean load to failure (110.26±26.4 N) than DR (108.93±21.8 N)	
Smith, 2006 [35]	16 fresh cadaveric shoulders (supra-spinatus)	SR: 2 anchors with simple stitch sutures DR: 2 medial anchors with two mattress sutures and 2 lateral anchors with simple sutures	Gap formation after cycling loading	Gap formation: significantly greater in the SR than in the DR group (mean and SD, 5.0±1.2 mm compared with 3.8±1.4 mm; $p < 0.05$). Cyclic loading: the DR failed at a mean of 320±96.9 N whereas the SR at a mean of 224 ±147.9 N ($p = 0.058$)	Double-row technique demonstrates superior resistance to gap formation under static loads
Tuoheti, et al. 2005 [36]	10 cadaveric shoulders (supra-spinatus)	TO: modified Mason-Allen technique; SR: simple vertical sutures; DR: simple vertical sutures for lateral row anchors and horizontal mattress sutures for the medial row	Contact pressure, contact area, and pressure patterns at the tendon-bone interface	Contact area: DR was 42% greater than TO ($p < 0.0001$) and 60% greater than SR The average pressures of SR and DR were 18% ($p = 0.014$) and 16% ($p = 0.03$) greater, respectively, than that of the TO, but there was no significant difference between SR and DR ($p = 0.915$)	DR produced the greatest contact area and the second-highest contact pressure, whereas the SR created the highest contact pressure and the least contact area
Wellmann, 2009 [37]	10 pairs of human cadaveric shoulders (subs-capularis)	SR: 2 anchors with massive rotator cuff stitch. DR: 2 medial anchors with modified Mason-Allen technique and 2 lateral knotless anchors	Ultimate tensile load, the stiffness and the elongation behaviour	Ultimate load: the DR restored 48% of the intact tendons (332 N), while the SR revealed a significantly lower ultimate load of 244 N ($p = 0.001$) Stiffness: the DR showed a mean stiffness of 81 N/mm which is significantly higher compared to the stiffness of the SR of 55 N/mm ($p = 0.001$)	DR technique has been shown to be stronger and stiffer when compared to a conventional SR

studies demonstrate a superiority of double-row repair compared to single row. Ahmad et al. [32] evaluated 18 human cadaver shoulders, reporting on the gap formation for different rotational positions, showing a better fixation strength for double-row repair. Baums et al. [22, 25, 26] in three biomechanical studies on sheep shoulder specimens compared single and double row both with different suture stitch patterns and different kinds of anchors and sutures. They reported for all the three studies better results in initial fixation strength and ultimate tensile load for double row. Moreover, a study of 2009 [22] evaluated the contact pressure through a pressure-sensitive film system, reporting a higher pressure pattern for double-row repairs. The resulting higher footprint coverage could favour a better healing process of the repaired tendon, and similar results are reported in the studies of Nelson et al. [30] and Touheti et al. [36]. In human shoulder specimens Kim et al. [17], Ma et al. [18] Smith et al. [35] and Wellmann et al. [37] while in porcine models Lorbach et al. [27] and Milano et al. [29] tested variably the gap formation after cycling loading, the ultimate tensile load, stiffness and peak-to-peak elongation. For each variable investigated, the authors reported better outcomes for double-row repair. Meier et al. [34] used a three-dimensional mapping to determine the area of the footprint reproduced by the different repair techniques: the footprint area of tendons repaired by a double-row technique was significantly larger compared to that of the other two techniques (single-row and transosseous repair). Similarly, Touheti et al. [36] analyzed the contact area at the tendon-bone interface, reporting better data for double row and suggesting that it could provide a better environment for tendon healing. Barber et al. [24] compared the biomechanical features of different anchors triply- and doubly-loaded with ultrahigh molecular weight polyethylene-containing sutures placed in single and double rows. A single row of triply-loaded anchors is superior to double-row repair. Mahar et al. [28] in bovine shoulder specimens and Mazzocca et al. [33] in human shoulder specimens compared single and double row reporting no statistically significant differences in load to failure and in peak elongation after cyclic loading. Nevertheless, double-row repairs result in a larger footprint width [33]. Zhang et al. [31] compared the double-row and transtendon single-row suture anchor techniques for repair of grade III partial articular-sided rotator cuff tears. Data from biomechanical analysis showed significantly better results of single-row repair than the double row, relative to gap formation, to the strain over the footprint area, and to the mean ultimate tensile load and stiffness.

Biologic Healing Based on Clinical Studies

Nine studies comparing single row to double row are currently available [15, 38–45]. All these studies evaluated the postsurgical outcomes with common and validated scores (UCLA, Constant, ASES, DASH) (table 2). The results demonstrate a statistically significant improvement of both the techniques from pre- to postoperative evaluation, but no one study demonstrated a significantly better outcome for double-row

Table 2. Clinical studies comparing single-row to double-row repair

Study (first author)	Patients	Follow-up	Involved tendon	Tear size	Technique
Aydin, 2010 [38]	SR: 34 DR: 34	At least 2 years		All lesions <3 cm	SR: 1–3 anchors double-loaded, simple suture stitch DR: 1–2 medial anchors, and 1–3 lateral anchors, creating a suture bridge between the medial and lateral rows
Burks, 2009 [39]	SR: 20 DR: 20	1 year		From 1 to 4.5 cm	SR: double-loaded anchors DR: medial row with a diamond pattern of double-loaded anchors; lateral row in a SR-like fashion
Charousset, 2007 [40]	SR:35 DR: 31	SR: 27.6 months (24–37) DR: 28.7 months (24–40)	Supraspinatus, infraspinatus, subscapularis		SR: Panalok anchors DR: Panalok anchors and cuff tack anchors

Outcome measures	Results	Postoperative diagnostic imaging	Conclusions
Constant score (CS)	Postoperative CS (average): SR: 82.2 DR: 78.8		Difference between the two groups was not significant
UCLA, Constant, WORC, SANE, ASES, ROM internal and external rotation strength	Postoperative values: WORC: SR: 84.8 (18.4) DR: 87.9 (20.0) CS: SR: 77.8 (9.0) DR: 74.4 (18.4) ASES: SR: 85.9 (14.0) DR: 85.5 (20.0) UCLA: SR: 28.6 (3.6) DR: 29.5 (5.6) SANE: SR: 90.9 (11.0) DR: 89.9 (20.0)	MRI measurements of footprint coverage, tendon thickness, and tendon signal: no significant differences between the two repair groups	No significant differences in clinical and MRI outcomes between the two groups
CS	Postoperative CS mean values: SR: 80.7 (62–95) DR: 82.7 (58–94)	CT arthrogram: anatomic and watertight healing: DR:19 SR: 14 Watertight healing with partial defect: DR: 5 SR: 7 Re-tear: DR: 7 SR: 14	No significant differences in clinical results, but tendon healing rates were better with the double-row anchorage

Table 2. Continued

Study (first author)	Patients	Follow-up	Involved tendon	Tear size	Technique
Franceschi, 2007 [41]	SR: 30 DR: 30	22.5 months (18–25)	Supraspinatus, infraspinatus, subscapularis	SR: 18 large (3–5 cm) 8 massive (>5 cm) DR: 21 large and 5 massive	SR: 1 row of double-loaded anchors with mattress fashion sutures DR: lateral row of anchors with simple suture stitch and medial row with mattress suture stitch
Grasso, 2009 [42]	SR:37 DR: 35	24.8 months		SR: mean area, 244.7 mm^2 DR: mean area, 261.9 mm^2	SR: single suture DR: single sutures for lateral row; mattress configuration for medial row
Ji, 2010 [43]	SR: 22 DR: 25	SR: 22 months (18–24) DR: 24 months (22–28)		SR: 3 small (<1 cm), 10 medium (1–3 cm) and 9 large (3–5 cm) DR: 5 small, 12 medium and 8 large	DR: medial row sutured with sutures in a horizontal mattress fashion; lateral row sutured with simple pattern
Park, 2008 [44]	SR: 40; DR:38	25.1 months (22–30)		SR: 25 (62.5%) <3 cm; 15 (37.5%) >3 cm DR: 21 (55.3%) <3 cm; 17 (44.7%) >3 cm	

Outcome measures	Results	Postoperative diagnostic imaging	Conclusions
UCLA and ROM	Postoperative UCLA mean values: SR: 32.9 (29–35) DR: 33.3 (30–35)	MRI: intact tendons: SR: 14 DR: 18 partial-thickness defect: SR: 10 DR:7 full-thickness defect: SR: 2 DR:1	SR and DR provide comparable clinical outcome at 2 years
DASH and Work DASH CS	Postoperative CS mean values: SR: 100.5 (94.8–106.2) DR: 104.9 (97.7–112.1). DASH score: SR: 15.4±15.6; DR: 12.7±10.1 Work DASH: SR: 16.0±22.0; DR: 9.6±13.3		DR showed no significant difference in clinical outcome compared with SR
ASES and UCLA scores	Postoperative mean values: ASES: SR: 87.40 DR: 91.45 UCLA SR: 30.82 DR: 32.40		Although no differences were showed between the ASES and the UCLA scores of the two groups, DR resulted in greater strength compared to SR
ASES, CS and Shoulder Strength Index	Postoperative mean values: ASES: SR: 91.6 DR: 93.0 CS: SR: 76.7 DR: 80.0		No statically significant differences of ASES and CS scores were found between the groups, but when patients were subdivided by the tear's size, large to massive tears (>3 cm) showed better outcomes when repaired with DR

Table 2. Continued

Study (first author)	Patients	Follow-up	Involved tendon	Tear size	Technique
Pennington, 2010 [45]	SR: 78 DR: 54	at least 2 years		All tears were between 1.5 and 4.5 cm SR: mean tear size of 2.7 cm DR: mean tear size of 3.4 cm	
Sugaya, 2005 [15]	SR: 39 DR: 41	35 months (24–60)		SR: 6 small, 17 medium, 14 large, and 2 massive tears DR: 10 small, 17 medium, 11 large, 3 massive	SR: simple sutures DR: simple sutures both in medial and lateral row

repair compared to single row despite the type of stitch configuration, the number of anchors, and the type of sutures. Brady et al. [20] evaluated the residual defect of the rotator cuff intraoperatively. The authors enrolled 26 patients with a full-thickness rotator cuff tear and treated them with a double-row repair. After placing the lateral and the medial row but without tying the suture of this latter, they measured the residual bare footprint, and compared this value after the medial row was secured. While after the completion of the double-row repair there were no remaining residual defects of the cuff footprint, before tying the medial row the mean residual uncovered

Outcome measures	Results	Postoperative diagnostic imaging	Conclusions
UCLA, ASES and VAS	Postoperative mean values: ASES: SR: 86.9 DR: 91.6 UCLA: SR: 29.6 DR: 29.3 VAS: SR: 1.1 DR: 0.4	MRI Sugaya grade: SR (44 patients): grade I: 19 grade II: 13 grade III: 3 grade IV: 6 grade V: 3 DR (37 patients): grade I: 6 grade II: 11 grade III: 8 grade IV: 8 grade V: 4	Clinical results were superior in DR group but not in a statistically significant fashion; dividing patients by tear's size, better results were shown by DR in lesions of 2.5–3.5 cm; MRI showed a statistically significantly improved healing rate with SR repair compared with DR
UCLA and ASES	Postoperative mean values (standard deviation): UCLA: SR: 32.4 (4.7) DR: 3.1 (3.4) ASES: SR: 92.9 (12.1) DR: 94.6 (9.3)	MRI Sugaya grade: SR (39 patients): grade I: 11 (28.2%) grade II: 6 (15.4%) grade III: 12 (30.1%) grade IV: 4 (10.3%) grade V: 6 (15.4%) DR (41 patients): grade I: 22 (53.7%) grade II: 8 (19.5%) grade III: 7 (17.1%) grade IV: 4 (9.8%) grade V: 0 (0.0%)	No statistical difference between the groups in scores outcomes, while a significantly better healing pattern was observed on DR group at MRI

footprint measured was 52.7 ± 9.2%. When patients were stratified for tear size, double-row repair showed better results in patients with greater tears. The first to consider this feature was Park et al. [44], who compared 40 patients treated with single row (25 (62.5%) patients had a tear <3 cm and 15 (37.5%) >3 cm) to 38 treated with double row (21 (55.3%) had a tear <3 cm and 17 (44.7%) >3 cm). Comparing the ASES and the Constant outcomes of patients with large to massive tears (>3 cm), a statistically significant difference was noticed (single row: ASES 89.67 ± 4.45, Constant 72.07 ± 7.4; double row: ASES 93.24 ± 2.08, Constant 79.82 ± 3.34; $p < 0.05$).

Sugaya et al. [15] compared 39 patients treated with single row to 41 patients treated with double-row repair. Besides the clinical assessment with UCLA and ASES scores, the authors developed a magnetic resonance (MRI) classification of postoperative cuff integrity into five categories: from type I (where the rotator cuff has sufficient thickness compared with normal cuff) to type V (where the cuff is likely to have a medium or large full-thickness tear). When the authors compared the MRI results of the two groups (single vs. double row) a statistically significant difference was found with a better healing pattern for the double-row technique. On the contrary, in Burks et al. [39] study comparing 20 patients treated with single row and 20 with double row, the footprint, thickness, or signal content between single- and double-row repair groups at MRI study showed no significant differences. Pennington et al. [45] reported better outcomes of double row in patients with larger tears. They studied the patients with a postoperative MRI according to the criteria of Sugaya et al. [15]. Considering a subset of 43 patients (18 treated with single row and 25 treated with double row) with a tear size of 2.5–3.5 cm, a statistically significant difference in values representing radiological healing was found. Charousset et al. [40] compared 35 patients treated with single row to 31 treated with double row. To evaluate the healing process, the authors used computed tomography (CT) arthrogram after 6 months, classifying the images into three categories: (1) anatomical (no defects and no contrast leakage); (2) healing defect (partially healed tendon), and (3) re-tear. A significant difference between the two techniques for the anatomic healing was found.

Discussion

Single- and double-row repairs are both reliable in the management of full-thickness tears of the rotator cuff. Evidence shows that these two techniques are equivalent in terms of postsurgical outcomes, but several biomechanical studies, with the exception of two studies [28, 33] reporting no statistically significant differences and of two other studies [24, 31] reporting better results from single row, demonstrated that the double-row repair, when compared to single row, leads to: (1) higher initial fixation strength; (2) greater footprint coverage; (3) improved contact area and pressure; (4) decreased gap formation, and (5) higher load to failure. Before supporting the routine use of the double-row technique, it is necessary to investigate whether there are real advantages in clinical outcomes. Do the higher initial fixation strength and the improved contact area and pressure result in better clinical outcomes? Does the wider anatomic reconstruction of the tendon footprint reached through the double row really lead to a better biologic regeneration and healing process? Although all the clinical studies [15, 38–45] comparing single to double row reported no statistically significant differences between the two techniques, there is evidence of superiority of double-row structural healing compared to single row based on MRI [15, 45] and CT arthrogram [40] findings. Interestingly, when considering patients with large and massive tears (≥3 cm) better results were reached with the double-row repair. According to the currently available evidence we suggest that an acute and/or a small to medium lesion (<3 cm), where the tissues are still viable for a sound repair, can be adequately managed with a single-row repair. A chronic and/or a large to massive (>3 cm) lesion may be more likely treated with a double-row repair, but final outcomes do not depend only of tendon to the bone-covered area.

In fact the surgeon has to choose the repair technique on the basis of patient's features, relatively to the quality of the bone and tendon's tissues and to the dimension of the lesion, as well as on their surgical skills. Moreover, the surgeon must take into consideration that the double row is a high cost and a high surgical skill-demanding technique. Franceschi et al. [41] reported a statistically significant difference for the operative time (the mean operative time for single-row repair was 42 ± 18.9 min, while the mean operative time for double-row repair was 65 ± 23.4 min). The longer operative time and the higher cost for placing two rows of anchors make the use of double-row repair, especially for smaller (<3 cm) tears, questionable. Probably, the best cost-effectiveness ratio would be reached using the double row in strictly selected patients. More studies investigating the outcomes in patients with large and massive tears are needed to strengthen the indication to use double-row repair in these patients [46–48].

References

1 Ellman H: Diagnosis and treatment of incomplete rotator cuff tears. Clin Orthop Relat Res 1990;254: 64–74.
2 Macfarlane GJ, Hunt IM, Silman AJ: Predictors of chronic shoulder pain: a population-based prospective study. J Rheumatol 1998;25:1612–1615.
3 Yamamoto A, Takagishi K, Osawa T, et al: Prevalence and risk factors of a rotator cuff tear in the general population. J Shoulder Elbow Surg 2010;19:116–120.
4 Fukuda H: Partial-thickness rotator cuff tears: a modern view on Codman's classic. J Shoulder Elbow Surg 2000;9:163–168.
5 Fukuda H: The management of partial-thickness tears of the rotator cuff. J Bone Joint Surg Br 2003; 85:3–11.
6 Millstein ES, Snyder SJ: Arthroscopic evaluation and management of rotator cuff tears. Orthop Clin North Am 2003;34:507–520.
7 Apreleva M, Ozbaydar M, Fitzgibbons PG, Warner JJ: Rotator cuff tears: the effect of the reconstruction method on three-dimensional repair site area. Arthroscopy 2002;18:519–526.
8 Gazielly DF, Gleyze P, Montagnon C: Functional and anatomical results after rotator cuff repair. Clin Orthop Relat Res 1994;304:43–53.
9 Goutallier D, Postel JM, Bernageau J, et al: Fatty muscle degeneration in cuff ruptures. Pre- and postoperative evaluation by CT scan. Clin Orthop Relat Res 1994;304:78–83.
10 Harryman DT 2nd, Mack LA, Wang KY, et al: Repairs of the rotator cuff. Correlation of functional results with integrity of the cuff. J Bone Joint Surg Am 1991;73:982–989.
11 Boileau P, Brassart N, Watkinson DJ, et al: Arthroscopic repair of full-thickness tears of the supraspinatus: does the tendon really heal? J Bone Joint Surg Am 2005;87:1229–1240.
12 Galatz LM, Ball CM, Teefey SA, et al: The outcome and repair integrity of completely arthroscopically repaired large and massive rotator cuff tears. J Bone Joint Surg Am 2004;86:219–224.
13 Gerber C, Schneeberger AG, Beck M, Schlegel U: Mechanical strength of repairs of the rotator cuff. J Bone Joint Surg Br 1994;76:371–380.

14 Warner JP, Krushell RJ, Masquelet A, Gerber C Anatomy and relationships of the suprascapular nerve: anatomical constraints to mobilization of the supraspinatus and infraspinatus muscles in the management of massive rotator-cuff tears. J Bone Joint Surg Am 1992;74:36–45.

15 Sugaya H, Maeda K, Matsuki K, Moriishi J: Functional and structural outcome after arthroscopic full-thickness rotator cuff repair: single-row versus dual-row fixation. Arthroscopy 2005;21:1307–1316.

16 Lo IK, Burkhart SS: Double-row arthroscopic rotator cuff repair: re-establishing the footprint of the rotator cuff. Arthroscopy 2003;19:1035–1042.

17 Kim DH, Elattrache NS, Tibone JE, et al: Biomechanical comparison of a single-row versus double-row suture anchor technique for rotator cuff repair. Am J Sports Med 2006;34:407–414.

18 Ma CB, Comerford L, Wilson J, et al: Biomechanical evaluation of arthroscopic rotator cuff repairs: double-row compared with single-row fixation. J Bone Joint Surg Am 2006;88:403–410.

19 Meier SW, Meier JD: The effect of double-row fixation on initial repair strength in rotator cuff repair: a biomechanical study. Arthroscopy 2006,22: 1168–1173.

20 Brady PC, Arrigoni P, Burkhart SS: Evaluation of residual rotator cuff defects after in vivo single- versus double-row rotator cuff repairs. Arthroscopy 2006;22:1070–1075.

21 Cofield RH: Rotator cuff disease of the shoulder. J Bone Joint Surg Am 1985;67:974–979.

22 Baums MH, Spahn G, Steckel H, et al: Comparative evaluation of the tendon-bone interface contact pressure in different single- versus double-row suture anchor repair techniques. Knee Surg Sports Traumatol Arthrosc 2009;17:1466–1472.

23 Craft DV, Moseley JB, Cawley PW, Noble PC: Fixation strength of rotator cuff repairs with suture anchors and the transosseous suture technique. J Shoulder Elbow Surg 1996;5:32–40.

24 Barber FA, Herbert MA, Schroeder FA, et al: Biomechanical advantages of triple-loaded suture anchors compared with double-row rotator cuff repairs. Arthroscopy 2010;26:316–323.

25 Baums MH, Buchhorn GH, Gilbert F, et al: Initial load-to-failure and failure analysis in single- and double-row repair techniques for rotator cuff repair. Arch Orthop Trauma Surg 2010;130:1193–1199.

26 Baums MH, Buchhorn GH, Spahn G, et al: Biomechanical characteristics of single-row repair in comparison to double-row repair with consideration of the suture configuration and suture material. Knee Surg Sports Traumatol Arthrosc 2008;16: 1052–1060.

27 Lorbach O, Bachelier F, Vees J, et al: Cyclic loading of rotator cuff reconstructions: single-row repair with modified suture configurations versus double-row repair. Am J Sports Med 2008;36:1504–1510.

28 Mahar A, Tamborlane J, Oka R, et al: Single-row suture anchor repair of the rotator cuff is biomechanically equivalent to double-row repair in a bovine model. Arthroscopy 2007;23:1265–1270.

29 Milano G, Grasso A, Zarelli D, et al: Comparison between single-row and double-row rotator cuff repair: a biomechanical study. Knee Surg Sports Traumatol Arthrosc 2008;16:75–80.

30 Nelson CO, Sileo MJ, Grossman MG, Serra-Hsu F: Single-row modified Mason-Allen versus double-row arthroscopic rotator cuff repair: a biomechanical and surface area comparison. Arthroscopy 2008; 24:941–948.

31 Zhang CG,Wang WM, Ren MF, et al: Biomechanical comparison of double-row versus transtendon single-row suture anchor technique for repair of the grade III partial articular-sided rotator cuff tears. Chin Med J (Engl) 2010;123:3049–3054.

32 Ahmad CS, Kleweno C, Jacir AM, et al: Biomechanical performance of rotator cuff repairs with humeral rotation: a new rotator cuff repair failure model. Am J Sports Med 2008;36:888–892.

33 Mazzocca AD, Millett PJ, Guanche CA, et al: Arthroscopic single-row versus double-row suture anchor rotator cuff repair. Am J Sports Med 2005;33: 1861–1868.

34 Meier SW, Meier JD: Rotator cuff repair: the effect of double-row fixation on three-dimensional repair site. J Shoulder Elbow Surg 2006;15:691–696.

35 Smith CD, Alexander S, Hill AM, et al: A biomechanical comparison of single- and double-row fixation in arthroscopic rotator cuff repair. J Bone Joint Surg Am 2006;88:2425–2431.

36 Tuoheti Y, Itoi E, Yamamoto N, et al: Contact area contact pressure and pressure patterns of the tendon-bone interface after rotator cuff repair. Am J Sports Med 2005;33:1869–1874.

37 Wellmann M, Wiebringhaus P, Lodde I, et al: Biomechanical evaluation of a single-row versus double-row repair for complete subscapularis tears. Knee Surg Sports Traumatol Arthrosc 2009;17: 1477–1484.

38 Aydin N, Kocaoglu B, Guven O: Single-row versus double-row arthroscopic rotator cuff repair in small- to medium-sized tears. J Shoulder Elbow Surg 2010;19:722–725.

39 Burks RT, Crim J, Brown N, et al: A prospective randomized clinical trial comparing arthroscopic single- and double-row rotator cuff repair: magnetic resonance imaging and early clinical evaluation. Am J Sports Med 2009;37:674–682.

40 Charousset C, Grimberg J, Duranthon LD, et al: Can a double-row anchorage technique improve tendon healing in arthroscopic rotator cuff repair? A prospective nonrandomized comparative study of double-row and single-row anchorage techniques with computed tomographic arthrography tendon healing assessment. Am J Sports Med 2007;35: 1247–1253.
41 Franceschi F, Ruzzini L, Longo UG, et al: Equivalent clinical results of arthroscopic single-row and double-row suture anchor repair for rotator cuff tears: a randomized controlled trial. Am J Sports Med 2007;35:1254–1260.
42 Grasso A, Milano G, Salvatore M, et al: Single-row versus double-row arthroscopic rotator cuff repair: a prospective randomized clinical study. Arthroscopy 2009;25:4–12.
43 Ji JH, Shafi M, Kim WY, Kim YY: Clinical outcomes of arthroscopic single- and double-row repair in full-thickness rotator cuff tears. Indian J Orthop 2010;44:308–313.
44 Park JY, Lhee SH, Choi JH, et al: Comparison of the clinical outcomes of single- and double-row repairs in rotator cuff tears. Am J Sports Med 2008;36: 1310–1316.
45 Pennington WT, Gibbons DJ, Bartz BA, et al: Comparative analysis of single-row versus double-row repair of rotator cuff tears. Arthroscopy 2010; 26:1419–1426.
46 Longo UG, Franceschi F, Spiezia F, Marinozzi A, Maffulli N, Denaro V: The low-profile Roman bridge technique for knotless double-row repair of the rotator cuff. Arch Orthop Trauma Surg 2011; 131:357–361.
47 Franceschi F, Longo UG, Ruzzini L, Rizzello G, Maffulli N, Denaro V: Soft tissue tenodesis of the long head of the biceps tendon associated to the Roman Bridge repair. BMC Musculoskelet Disord 2008;9:78.
48 Franceschi F, Longo UG, Ruzzini L, Rizzello G, Maffulli N, Denaro V: The Roman Bridge: a "double pulley – suture bridges" technique for rotator cuff repair. BMC Musculoskelet Disord 2007;8:123.

Nicola Maffulli, MD, MS, PhD, FRCS(Orth)
Centre for Sports and Exercise Medicine
Barts and The London School of Medicine and Dentistry
Mile End Hospital, 275 Bancroft Road, London E1 4DG (UK)
Tel. +44 20 8223 8839, E-Mail n.maffulli@qmul.ac.uk

Maffulli N (ed): Rotator Cuff Tear. Med Sport Sci. Basel, Karger, 2012, vol 57, pp 142–152

Arthroscopic Transosseous Rotator Cuff Repair

Umile Giuseppe Longo[a,b] · Francesco Franceschi[a,b] · Alessandra Berton[a,b] · Nicola Maffulli[c] · Vincenzo Denaro[a,b]

[a]Department of Orthopaedic and Trauma Surgery and [b]Centro Integrato di Ricerca (CIR), Campus Bio-Medico University, Rome, Italy; [c]Centre for Sports and Exercise Medicine, Queen Mary University of London, Barts and The London School of Medicine and Dentistry, Mile End Hospital, London, UK

Abstract

The arthroscopic approach for rotator cuff repair is extensively used worldwide. Different repairing procedures have evolved with the aim of restoring anatomy and function of rotator cuff tendon. Several studies have analyzed biomechanical factors to understand their influence on tendon to bone healing and improve repair configurations. From a biomechanical point of view, single-row anchor techniques are not able to restore all of the original footprint of the rotator cuff, and result in circumferential tension around the tendon. Transosseus simple suture repairs may have greater potential for healing at the tendon-bone interface, because they allow a larger insertion site area and better pressure characteristics. Biomechanically, double-row suture anchor repair increases the area of contact and the initial fixation strength, decreases the load for each suture loop, knot and anchor, and decreases the stress at each suture-cuff contact point. To optimize healing, transosseous-equivalent techniques have been developed. The oblique suture bridges allow greater pressurized contact, low profile, and interconnection between fixation points that permits to shear load. Clinical studies showed equivalent clinical results of single- and double-row suture anchor repair. However, to date, there are no randomized controlled trials on transosseous or transosseous-equivalent techniques for rotator cuff repair. Clearly, studies of higher levels of evidence, including large randomized trials, should be conducted. Future trials should use validated functional and clinical outcomes, adequate methodology, and be sufficiently powered.

Rotator cuff tears are a common cause of shoulder pain and occupational disability [1–4]. More than 50% of individuals older than 60 years have at least a partial-thickness rotator cuff tear [5–7], with significant impact on patients' quality of life, and marked functional impairment [8]. Arthroscopy for rotator cuff repair has become extensively used, as it decreases postoperative morbidity [9–12]. Improvements in surgical techniques, instruments, suture materials and anchor designs [9, 13–17] have been developed to optimize results. Traditional techniques included single-row or transosseous repair, succeeded by double-row and transosseous-equivalent repair. These techniques evolved to restore anatomy and function of rotator cuff tendon providing high fixation strength, stability and minimal gap formation, and enhancing tendon to bone healing [18]. Healing of soft tissue to bone starts with constitution of fibrovascular interposition tissue between the tendon and the bone [19–28], where progressively bone grows and collagen fibres extend [29–31]. Several variables can influence this course, including contact area and pressure [32], tendon-bone interface motion [33], repair strength [34] and tissue quality. Recently, tissue engineering [35], biomaterials [36] and platelet-rich plasma [37] have been proposed to enhance rotator cuff healing.

Numerous studies have analyzed biomechanical factors to understand their influence on tendon to bone healing and improve repair configurations [38–47]. In particular, some studies focused on the anatomical reconstruction of the rotator cuff footprint [48, 49]. It corresponds to the tendon insertion area on the humeral surface. It extends from the lateral ridge of the tuberosity to the articular margin along the anterior 2 cm of the greater tuberosity. Its average width is 14.7 mm, ranging from 12 to 24 mm [50, 51].

These insights and resulting modification of surgical techniques have been developed because of the high persistent tear rate after arthroscopic repair [52–55]. The re-tears rate has been reported to be between 4 and 40% [56–62], reaching the rate of 90% in massive rotator cuff tear [63]. Several factors contribute to these failures, including tendon degeneration, osteoporosis of the humeral head, insufficient fixation of tendon to bone, inadequate contact at tendon-bone interface [18, 64, 65]. The latest techniques, double-row and transosseous-equivalent repair, seem to have the potential to improve this healing rate. Recurrent rotator cuff defects represent the principal postoperative complication requiring revision surgeries [53–55, 64]. Even though arthroscopic suture-bridging repair has better biomechanical properties, a superior clinical outcome has not been confirmed [66].

Biomechanical Studies

The first-generation technique used for rotator cuff repair was a single-row anchor repair. Failure of healing or re-tears, observed on MRI or US [52, 61], seemed to be correlated with the inability to restore anatomic footprint [48] and with little compression between tendon and bone [32]. Single-row anchor suture repair provides only 'point' fixation of the rotator cuff, with a relatively small surface contact area between the tendon and bone, regardless of the type of suture used (simple suture or mattress). The restored area of the original footprint is about 67% [48]. Moreover, it results in circumferential tension around the tendon rather than compression over the tendon on the bony footprint [32]. This determines low fixation and great motion of the tendon relative to the tuberosity [33]. The amount of compression also depends on the depth of anchor placement and thickness of the tendon [67].

Transosseous tunnel repair consists of a bone tunnel where a suture exits at its most medial aspect and then passes through the rotator cuff with 1 cm of tissue bite. Transosseus simple suture repairs may have greater potential for healing at the tendon-bone interface because they allow larger insertion site area, and better pressure characteristics. The restored area of the original footprint is about 85% [48]. Even though it is 15% smaller than the original supraspinatus tendon insertion, it is 20% larger than that provided by suture-anchor simple suture, suture-anchor mattress suture, and transosseous mattress suture [48]. Expansion of the repair site area with a simple stitch occurs thanks to the presence of two fixation points (medial and lateral) in the coronal plane of the humeral head that are spread apart. In addition to a greater major contact area, the transosseous technique provides higher mean footprint pressures. Its compression vector is in the direction of the tendon to bone, allowing broad fixation and limited motion of the repair [32, 33]. The transosseous technique should therefore provide sufficient strength to allow early range of motion [68, 69] when the tendon-bone interface is still weak and complete functional recovery has yet to take place.

Some authors prefer suture anchors for rotator cuff fixation versus transosseous tunnel repair because of lower tendency to bony failure with cyclic loading [45, 70, 71]. Suture-row anchor repair has been improved by adding a second row of sutures. In double-row techniques, two rows of anchors are placed respectively in the medial and lateral aspect of the footprint. The medial anchors are usually fixed with a horizontal mattress stitch, and the lateral anchors with a simple stitch. This produces two spread fixation points that increase the area of contact and the initial fixation strength, decreases the load for each suture loop, knot and anchor, and decreases the stress at each suture-cuff contact point [72]. The higher number of anchor placement and fixation points with the double-row fixation is associated with better initial biomechanical properties than with single-row fixation [67, 73]. Resistance to cyclic elongation, ultimate tensile load to failure and peak-to-peak elongation are better in comparison with single-row fixation. This construct results in reduced failure rates and gap formation [67]. The lateral sutures fail first, protecting the medial row, and consequently prevent re-tears [73].

To optimize healing biology, transosseous-equivalent techniques have been developed. In comparison with double-row repair, which appears to cover the entire footprint but determines pressurized contact only on 39.6% of it, transosseous-equivalent techniques allow greater pressurized contact between tendon and tuberosity. Pressure seems to promote healing [29, 74–81], but further in vivo studies are needed to better understand its benefits and possible disadvantages, such as on vascularity [82]. The favourable pressure properties are attributable to the oblique suture bridges. Suture limbs from the medial mattress sutures traverse a great distance over the tendon, maximizing the utility of the single-row construct. Moreover, it produces a low profile with medial knots flush with the tendon, unlike the double-row repair which leaves four proud knots on top of the repaired tendon. The suture bridge determines edge stability because it flattens the lateral tendon edge preventing contact with the acromion-coracoacromial ligament arch that may cause tears [83]. Another advantage of the transosseous-equivalent technique is that it does not require a suture to pass through the lateral tendon edge, which is often compromised because of the chronicity of the lesion, which makes it fragile and not able to resist tension [54, 84]. By passing through healthy medial tissue, fixation is stronger and healing is favoured [83, 85, 86]. The strength of the repair is also correlated with the interconnection between fixation points, medial to lateral and anterior to posterior. It permits to shear load better than double-row repair, where fixation points are separated [83]. This is particularly evident during rotation, when the supraspinatus force vector produces a relative tension mismatch because it acts on the postero-lateral fixation point [70, 71]. The transosseous-equivalent technique provides significantly more ultimate load-to-failure when compared with double-row repair. Moreover, despite placing suture interference screws distal-laterally, as for transosseous tunnel repair [38], where bone mineral density is lower [87], it can sustain sufficient loads [83]. Another positive consideration about transosseous-equivalent techniques concern the reduced operative time, as they require fewer tendon sutures [82]. Gap formation, strain over the footprint during cyclic testing, stiffness and hysteresis are not statistically different between double-row and transosseous-equivalent techniques [83].

Two novel transosseous-equivalent techniques of suture bridge repair of the rotator cuff include the Roman bridge repair and the low-profile Roman bridge repair.

Roman Bridge Suture Anchor Repair

Two medial row 5.5-mm Bio-Corkscrew suture anchors (Arthrex, Inc., Naples, Fla., USA), double-loaded with No. 2 FiberWire sutures (Arthrex, Inc.), are placed in the medial aspect of the footprint, just lateral to the articular surface of the humeral head [88, 89]. The first anchor is placed in the anteromedial aspect of the footprint. The second anchor is placed approximately 1.5–2 cm posterior to the first anchor. Two suture limbs from a single suture are both passed through a single point in the rotator cuff, producing two points of fixation in the tendon, with a tendon bridge between them. This is performed for both anchors. The medial row sutures are tied using the double-pulley technique. A suture limb is retrieved from each of the medial anchors through the lateral portal, and manually tied as a six-throw surgeon's knot over a metal rod. A tendon grasper introduced through a lateral portal is used to grasp the medial aspect of the rotator cuff tendon, which is pulled laterally toward the bone bed. The two free suture limbs are pulled to transport the knot over the top of the tendon bridge. This technique is called the 'double-pulley' technique, because the eyelets of two suture anchors are used as pulleys to bring the knots down onto the cuff. The two free suture limbs that were used to pull the knot down are then tied as a static, non-sliding knot. This produces a double mattress suture between the two medial anchors. The ends of the sutures are cut. The same double-pulley technique is repeated for the other two suture limbs from the two medial anchors. The other two suture limbs of the same colour from each anchor are sequentially passed through two single points in the rotator cuff, producing two points of fixation in the tendon, with a tendon bridge between them.

The suture limb is retrieved from each of the medial anchors through the lateral portal, and manually tied as a six-throw surgeon's knot over a metal rod. The two free suture limbs are pulled to transport the knot over the top of the tendon bridge. The two free suture limbs are then used to produce suture bridges over the tendon, using a PushLock (Arthrex, Inc.), placed 1 cm distal to the lateral edge of the footprint centred relative to the medially placed suture anchors anterior to posterior. The final result is what we call the Roman bridge – a combination of the double-pulley and suture-bridge techniques.

Low-Profile Roman Bridge Repair

A 5.5-mm Bio-Corkscrew suture anchor, double-loaded with No. 2 FiberWire sutures, is placed in the anteromedial aspect of the footprint, just lateral to the articular surface of the humeral head [90].

Two suture limbs from a single suture are both passed through a single anterior point in the rotator cuff. One suture limb is retrieved from the cannula, and passed through a single posterior point in the rotator cuff, producing two points of fixation in the tendon, with a tendon bridge between them.

A tendon grasper introduced through a lateral portal is used to grasp the medial aspect of the rotator cuff tendon, which is pulled laterally toward the bone bed. The same suture limb is retrieved through the lateral portal, and then inserted into the bone by means of a PushLock placed approximately 1.5–2 cm posterior to the first anchor. The same suture is now passed again in the posterior aspect of the cuff. The first suture limbs are pulled to compress the tendon in the medial aspect of the footprint. This technique is a 'single-pulley' technique, because the eyelet of the anteromedial suture anchor is used as a pulley to bring the suture down onto the cuff. This produces a double mattress suture between the two medial anchors. The two free suture limbs are used to produce suture bridges over the tendon, by means of a PushLock, placed 1 cm distal to the lateral edge of the footprint relative to the medially placed suture anchors anterior to posterior. The final result is the low-profile Roman bridge, a knotless evolution of the Roman bridge repair.

Clinical Studies

To date, controversy exists regarding the optimal fixation technique for rotator cuff repair. Single-row anchor repair has been associated with a high percentage of 'good' results, but on MRI or US a high rates of re-tears has been observed [52, 61]. Significantly lower tear rates have been reported for double-row repair [58, 62]. A comparative study recorded re-tear rates of 40% for single-row and 22.6% for double-row fixation, 6 months postoperatively [57]. Another study calculated the percentage of complete re-tears between 8 and 25.7% for single-row and between 4 and 9.8% for double-row repair, and a rate of partial re-tears between 30.1 and 38% for single-row and between 17.1 and 27% for double-row repairs [58, 62]. A study on 58 patients undergoing double-row technique showed that 89% of patients present an intact rotator cuff at US, at a mean follow-up of 15 months [91]. Nevertheless, the difference in functional outcome between single- and double-row techniques does not seem to be significant [57, 58, 62, 92]. The transosseous-equivalent technique has been associated with a re-tear rate of 11% on MRI evaluation at a median of 14.6 months [93]. Another study reported a similar percentage of re-tears (28.9%) between suture-bridging repair and double-row fixation. The difference between the two studies can be attributed to patient age (57 years [93] vs. 62 years [66]), simultaneous acromioplasty (88 [93] vs. 57% [66]), and number of patients. Thus, these two factors do influence tendon healing. Patients older than 65 are at risk of re-tears [56]. Decompression of the subacromial space is recommended because it promotes healing by favouring stem cells and platelet-derived growth factors migration [66].

Clinical outcomes were comparable between transosseous-equivalent repair and single- or double-row fixation. Functional improvement was independent of the integrity of the supraspinatus tendon. The Constant score ranged between 76.7 and 83.4 points for single-row fixations [57, 61, 92] and between 79.7 and 82.7 points for double-row repairs [57, 59, 60, 92] at a minimum of 22 months of follow-up. Also, shoulder function was not significantly different between single- and double-row techniques. The Constant score for transosseous-equivalent repair increased from preoperative 64%, to 82% at 4 months and 96% at 12 months, but did not change significantly (96%) at 24 months [66]. Similar patterns were found for single parameters of pain relief, activities of daily living, and range of motion [66]. Patient satisfaction was similar for suture-bridging repair and double-row fixation [59]. The observation of independent improvement of functional outcomes has to be explained by the fact that glenohumeral motion is not impaired by supraspinatus tendon lesion [94]. Instead, integrity of infraspinatus tendon is essential for centring mechanism [55, 63, 94, 95].

Conclusions

Arthroscopic rotator cuff repair techniques have been developed to restore tendon footprint and increase pressurized contact at the tendon to bone interface to improve healing [96–99]. To date, there are no randomized controlled trials on transosseous or transosseous-equivalent techniques for rotator cuff repair [100]. Unfortunately the aetiology of rotator cuff tears is still largely unknown [20, 22–25, 35, 36, 58, 88, 89, 101–106], and outcome measures are still not able to detect significant differences [107, 108]. Clearly, studies of higher levels of evidence, including large randomized trials, should be conducted [109–121]. Future trials should use validated functional and clinical outcomes, adequate methodology, and be sufficiently powered.

References

1 Maffulli N, Longo UG, Gougoulias N, Loppini M, Denaro V: Long-term health outcomes of youth sports injuries. Br J Sports Med 2010;44:21–25.

2 Maffulli N, Longo UG, Loppini M, Denaro V: Current treatment options for tendinopathy. Expert Opin Pharmacother 2010;11:2177–2186.

3 Maffulli N, Longo UG, Spiezia F, Denaro V: Sports injuries in young athletes: long-term outcome and prevention strategies. Phys Sportsmed 2010;38:29–34.

4 Maffulli N, Longo UG, Gougoulias N, Caine D, Denaro V: Sport injuries: a review of outcomes. Br Med Bull 2011;97:47–80.

5 Maffulli N, Longo UG, Denaro V: Novel approaches for the management of tendinopathy. J Bone Joint Surg Am 2010;92:2604–2613.

6 Maffulli N, Longo UG, Franceschi F, Rabitti C, Denaro V: Movin and Bonar scores assess the same characteristics of tendon histology. Clin Orthop Relat Res 2008;466:1605–1611.

7 Kibler W, Warme B, Sciascia A, Kuhn J, Wolf B: Nonacute shoulder injuries; in Kibler W (ed): Orthopedic Knowledge Update: Sports Medicine. Rosemont/IL, American Academy of Orthopedic Surgeons, 2009, pp 19–39.

8 Mighell M: Massive irreparable rotator cuff tears; in Frankle M (ed): Rotator Cuff Deficiency of the Shoulder. New York, Thieme Medical, 2008, pp 8–11.

9 Severud EL, Ruotolo C, Abbott DD, Nottage WM: All-arthroscopic versus mini-open rotator cuff repair: a long-term retrospective outcome comparison. Arthroscopy 2003;19:234–238.

10 Tauro JC: Arthroscopic rotator cuff repair: analysis of technique and results at 2- and 3-year follow-up. Arthroscopy 1998;14:45–51.

11 Gartsman GM, Khan M, Hammerman SM: Arthroscopic repair of full-thickness tears of the rotator cuff. J Bone Joint Surg Am 1998;80:832–840.

12 Baker CL, Liu SH: Comparison of open and arthroscopically assisted rotator cuff repairs. Am J Sports Med 1995;23:99–104.

13 Wilson F, Hinov V, Adams G: Arthroscopic repair of full-thickness tears of the rotator cuff: 2- to 14-year follow-up. Arthroscopy 2002;18:136–144.

14 Murray TF Jr, Lajtai G, Mileski RM, Snyder SJ: Arthroscopic repair of medium to large full-thickness rotator cuff tears: outcome at 2- to 6-year follow-up. J Shoulder Elbow Surg 2002;11:19–24.

15 Liu SH, Baker CL: Arthroscopically assisted rotator cuff repair: correlation of functional results with integrity of the cuff. Arthroscopy 1994;10:54–60.

16 Burkhart SS, Danaceau SM, Pearce CE Jr: Arthroscopic rotator cuff repair: analysis of results by tear size and by repair technique-margin convergence versus direct tendon-to-bone repair. Arthroscopy 2001;17:905–912.

17 Yamaguchi K, Levine WN, Marra G, Galatz LM, Klepps S, Flatow EL: Transitioning to arthroscopic rotator cuff repair: the pros and cons. Instr Course Lect 2003;52:81–92.

18 Gerber C, Schneeberger AG, Beck M, Schlegel U: Mechanical strength of repairs of the rotator cuff. J Bone Joint Surg Br 1994;76:371–380.

19 Denaro V, Ruzzini L, Barnaba SA, Longo UG, Campi S, Maffulli N, Sgambato A: Effect of pulsed electromagnetic fields on human tenocyte cultures from supraspinatus and quadriceps tendons. Am J Phys Med Rehabil 2011;90:119–127.

20 Franceschi F, Longo UG, Ruzzini L, Rizzello G, Denaro V: Arthroscopic management of calcific tendinitis of the subscapularis tendon. Knee Surg Sports Traumatol Arthrosc 2007;15:1482–1485.

21 Franceschi F, Longo UG, Ruzzini L, Morini S, Battistoni F, Dicuonzo G, Maffulli N, Denaro V: Circulating substance p levels and shoulder joint contracture after arthroscopic repair of the rotator cuff. Br J Sports Med 2008;42:742–745.

22 Longo UG, Franceschi F, Ruzzini L, Rabitti C, Morini S, Maffulli N, Forriol F, Denaro V: Light microscopic histology of supraspinatus tendon ruptures. Knee Surg Sports Traumatol Arthrosc 2007;15:1390–1394.

23 Longo UG, Franceschi F, Ruzzini L, Rabitti C, Morini S, Maffulli N, Denaro V: Histopathology of the supraspinatus tendon in rotator cuff tears. Am J Sports Med 2008;36:533–538.
24 Longo UG, Oliva F, Denaro V, Maffulli N: Oxygen species and overuse tendinopathy in athletes. Disabil Rehabil 2008;30:1563–1571.
25 Longo UG, Franceschi F, Ruzzini L, Rabitti C, Morini S, Maffulli N, Denaro V: Characteristics at haematoxylin and eosin staining of ruptures of the long head of the biceps tendon. Br J Sports Med 2009;43:603–607.
26 Longo UG, Franceschi F, Ruzzini L, Spiezia F, Maffulli N, Denaro V: Higher fasting plasma glucose levels within the normoglycaemic range and rotator cuff tears. Br J Sports Med 2009;43: 284–287.
27 Longo UG, Forriol F, Campi S, Maffulli N, Denaro V: Animal models for translational research on shoulder pathologies: from bench to bedside. Sports Med Arthrosc 2011 (in press).
28 Longo UG, Berton A, Alexander S, Maffulli N, Wallace AL, Denaro V: Biological resurfacing for early osteoarthritis of the shoulder. Sports Med Arthrosc 2011 (in press).
29 Rodeo SA, Arnoczky SP, Torzilli PA, Hidaka C, Warren RF: Tendon-healing in a bone tunnel. A biomechanical and histological study in the dog. J Bone Joint Surg Am 1993;75:1795–1803.
30 Rodeo SA, Suzuki K, Deng XH, Wozney J, Warren RF: Use of recombinant human bone morphogenetic protein-2 to enhance tendon healing in a bone tunnel. Am J Sports Med 1999;27:476–488.
31 St Pierre P, Olson EJ, Elliott JJ, O'Hair KC, McKinney LA, Ryan J: Tendon-healing to cortical bone compared with healing to a cancellous trough. A biomechanical and histological evaluation in goats. J Bone Joint Surg Am 1995;77:1858–1866.
32 Park MC, Cadet ER, Levine WN, Bigliani LU, Ahmad CS: Tendon-to-bone pressure distributions at a repaired rotator cuff footprint using transosseous suture and suture anchor fixation techniques. Am J Sports Med 2005;33:1154–1159.
33 Ahmad CS, Stewart AM, Izquierdo R, Bigliani LU: Tendon-bone interface motion in transosseous suture and suture anchor rotator cuff repair techniques. Am J Sports Med 2005;33:1667–1671.
34 Kim DH, Elattrache NS, Tibone JE, Jun BJ, DeLaMora SN, Kvitne RS, Lee TQ: Biomechanical comparison of a single-row versus double-row suture anchor technique for rotator cuff repair. Am J Sports Med 2006;34:407–414.
35 Longo UG, Lamberti A, Maffulli N, Denaro V: Tissue engineered biological augmentation for tendon healing: a systematic review. Br Med Bull 2011;98:31–59.
36 Longo UG, Lamberti A, Maffulli N, Denaro V: Tendon augmentation grafts: A systematic review. Br Med Bull 2010;94:165–188.
37 Castricini R, Longo UG, De Benedetto M, Panfoli N, Pirani P, Zini R, Maffulli N, Denaro V: Platelet-rich plasma augmentation for arthroscopic rotator cuff repair: a randomized controlled trial. Am J Sports Med 2011;39:258–265.
38 Caldwell GL, Warner JP, Miller MD, Boardman D, Towers J, Debski R: Strength of fixation with transosseous sutures in rotator cuff repair. J Bone Joint Surg Am 1997;79:1064–1068.
39 Craft DV, Moseley JB, Cawley PW, Noble PC: Fixation strength of rotator cuff repairs with suture anchors and the transosseous suture technique. J Shoulder Elbow Surg 1996;5:32–40.
40 Demirhan M, Atalar AC, Kilicoglu O: Primary fixation strength of rotator cuff repair techniques: a comparative study. Arthroscopy 2003;19:572–576.
41 Goradia VK, Mullen DJ, Boucher HR, Parks BG, O'Donnell JB: Cyclic loading of rotator cuff repairs: a comparison of bioabsorbable tacks with metal suture anchors and transosseous sutures. Arthroscopy 2001;17:360–364.
42 Koh JL, Szomor Z, Murrell GA, Warren RF: Supplementation of rotator cuff repair with a bioresorbable scaffold. Am J Sports Med 2002;30: 410–413.
43 Lee S, Mahar A, Bynum K, Pedowitz R: Biomechanical comparison of bioabsorbable sutureless screw anchor versus suture anchor fixation for rotator cuff repair. Arthroscopy 2005;21:43–47.
44 Ma CB, MacGillivray JD, Clabeaux J, Lee S, Otis JC: Biomechanical evaluation of arthroscopic rotator cuff stitches. J Bone Joint Surg Am 2004;86:1211–1216.
45 Reed SC, Glossop N, Ogilvie-Harris DJ: Full-thickness rotator cuff tears. A biomechanical comparison of suture versus bone anchor techniques. Am J Sports Med 1996;24:46–48.
46 Schneeberger AG, von Roll A, Kalberer F, Jacob HA, Gerber C: Mechanical strength of arthroscopic rotator cuff repair techniques: an in vitro study. J Bone Joint Surg Am 2002;84:2152–2160.
47 Waltrip RL, Zheng N, Dugas JR, Andrews JR: Rotator cuff repair. A biomechanical comparison of three techniques. Am J Sports Med 2003;31: 493–497.
48 Apreleva M, Ozbaydar M, Fitzgibbons PG, Warner JJ: Rotator cuff tears: the effect of the reconstruction method on three-dimensional repair site area. Arthroscopy 2002;18:519–526.
49 Minagawa H, Itoi E, Konno N, Kido T, Sano A, Urayama M, Sato K: Humeral attachment of the supraspinatus and infraspinatus tendons: an anatomic study. Arthroscopy 1998;14:302–306.

50 Meier SW, Meier JD: Rotator cuff repair: the effect of double-row fixation on three-dimensional repair site. J Shoulder Elbow Surg 2006;15:691–696.
51 Dugas JR, Campbell DA, Warren RF, Robie BH, Millett PJ: Anatomy and dimensions of rotator cuff insertions. J Shoulder Elbow Surg 2002;11:498–503.
52 Galatz LM, Ball CM, Teefey SA, Middleton WD, Yamaguchi K: The outcome and repair integrity of completely arthroscopically repaired large and massive rotator cuff tears. J Bone Joint Surg Am 2004; 86:219–224.
53 Gazielly DF, Gleyze P, Montagnon C: Functional and anatomical results after rotator cuff repair. Clin Orthop Relat Res 1994:43–53.
54 Harryman DT 2nd, Mack LA, Wang KY, Jackins SE, Richardson ML, Matsen FA 3rd: Repairs of the rotator cuff. Correlation of functional results with integrity of the cuff. J Bone Joint Surg Am 1991;73: 982–989.
55 Jost B, Pfirrmann CW, Gerber C, Switzerland Z: Clinical outcome after structural failure of rotator cuff repairs. J Bone Joint Surg Am 2000;82: 304–314.
56 Boileau P, Brassart N, Watkinson DJ, Carles M, Hatzidakis AM, Krishnan SG: Arthroscopic repair of full-thickness tears of the supraspinatus: does the tendon really heal? J Bone Joint Surg Am 2005;87: 1229–1240.
57 Charousset C, Grimberg J, Duranthon LD, Bellaiche L, Petrover D: Can a double-row anchorage technique improve tendon healing in arthroscopic rotator cuff repair? A prospective, nonrandomized, comparative study of double-row and single-row anchorage techniques with computed tomographic arthrography tendon healing assessment. Am J Sports Med 2007;35:1247–1253.
58 Franceschi F, Ruzzini L, Longo UG, Martina FM, Zobel BB, Maffulli N, Denaro V: Equivalent clinical results of arthroscopic single-row and double-row suture anchor repair for rotator cuff tears: a randomized controlled trial. Am J Sports Med 2007;35: 1254–1260.
59 Huijsmans PE, Pritchard MP, Berghs BM, van Rooyen KS, Wallace AL, de Beer JF: Arthroscopic rotator cuff repair with double-row fixation. J Bone Joint Surg Am 2007;89:1248–1257.
60 Lafosse L, Brozska R, Toussaint B, Gobezie R: The outcome and structural integrity of arthroscopic rotator cuff repair with use of the double-row suture anchor technique. J Bone Joint Surg Am 2007;89: 1533–1541.
61 Liem D, Lichtenberg S, Magosch P, Habermeyer P: Arthroscopic rotator cuff repair in overhead-throwing athletes. Am J Sports Med 2008;36: 1317–1322.
62 Sugaya H, Maeda K, Matsuki K, Moriishi J: Functional and structural outcome after arthroscopic full-thickness rotator cuff repair: single-row versus dual-row fixation. Arthroscopy 2005;21:1307–1316.
63 Gladstone JN, Bishop JY, Lo IK, Flatow EL: Fatty infiltration and atrophy of the rotator cuff do not improve after rotator cuff repair and correlate with poor functional outcome. Am J Sports Med 2007; 35:719–728.
64 Goutallier D, Postel JM, Bernageau J, Lavau L, Voisin MC: Fatty muscle degeneration in cuff ruptures. Pre- and postoperative evaluation by ct scan. Clin Orthop Relat Res 1994:78–83.
65 Warner JP, Krushell RJ, Masquelet A, Gerber C: Anatomy and relationships of the suprascapular nerve: anatomical constraints to mobilization of the supraspinatus and infraspinatus muscles in the management of massive rotator-cuff tears. J Bone Joint Surg Am 1992;74:36–45.
66 Voigt C, Bosse C, Vosshenrich R, Schulz AP, Lill H: Arthroscopic supraspinatus tendon repair with suture-bridging technique: functional outcome and magnetic resonance imaging. Am J Sports Med 2010;38:983–991.
67 Ma CB, Comerford L, Wilson J, Puttlitz CM: Biomechanical evaluation of arthroscopic rotator cuff repairs: double-row compared with single-row fixation. J Bone Joint Surg Am 2006;88:403–410.
68 Cordasco FA, Bigliani LU: The rotator cuff. Large and massive tears. Technique of open repair. Orthop Clin North Am 1997;28:179–193.
69 McLaughlin HL: Lesions of the musculotendinous cuff of the shoulder. The exposure and treatment of tears with retraction. 1944. Clin Orthop Relat Res 1994;304:3–9.
70 Burkhart SS, Diaz Pagan JL, Wirth MA, Athanasiou KA: Cyclic loading of anchor-based rotator cuff repairs: Confirmation of the tension overload phenomenon and comparison of suture anchor fixation with transosseous fixation. Arthroscopy 1997;13: 720–724.
71 Burkhart SS, Johnson TC, Wirth MA, Athanasiou KA: Cyclic loading of transosseous rotator cuff repairs: tension overload as a possible cause of failure. Arthroscopy 1997;13:172–176.
72 Lo IK, Burkhart SS: Double-row arthroscopic rotator cuff repair: re-establishing the footprint of the rotator cuff. Arthroscopy 2003;19:1035–1042.
73 Smith CD, Alexander S, Hill AM, Huijsmans PE, Bull AM, Amis AA, De Beer JF, Wallace AL: A biomechanical comparison of single- and double-row fixation in arthroscopic rotator cuff repair. J Bone Joint Surg Am 2006;88:2425–2431.

74 Weiler A, Hoffmann RF, Bail HJ, Rehm O, Sudkamp NP: Tendon healing in a bone tunnel. II. Histologic analysis after biodegradable interference fit fixation in a model of anterior cruciate ligament reconstruction in sheep. Arthroscopy 2002;18:124–135.
75 Blickenstaff KR, Grana WA, Egle D: Analysis of a semitendinosus autograft in a rabbit model. Am J Sports Med 1997;25:554–559.
76 Goradia VK, Rochat MC, Kida M, Grana WA: Natural history of a hamstring tendon autograft used for anterior cruciate ligament reconstruction in a sheep model. Am J Sports Med 2000;28:40–46.
77 Grana WA, Egle DM, Mahnken R, Goodhart CW: An analysis of autograft fixation after anterior cruciate ligament reconstruction in a rabbit model. Am J Sports Med 1994;22:344–351.
78 Katsuragi R, Yasuda K, Tsujino J, Keira M, Kaneda K: The effect of nonphysiologically high initial tension on the mechanical properties of in situ frozen anterior cruciate ligament in a canine model. Am J Sports Med 2000;28:47–56.
79 Pinczewski LA, Clingeleffer AJ, Otto DD, Bonar SF, Corry IS: Integration of hamstring tendon graft with bone in reconstruction of the anterior cruciate ligament. Arthroscopy 1997;13:641–643.
80 Yamazaki S, Yasuda K, Tomita F, Minami A, Tohyama H: The effect of graft-tunnel diameter disparity on intraosseous healing of the flexor tendon graft in anterior cruciate ligament reconstruction. Am J Sports Med 2002;30:498–505.
81 Yasuda K, Tsujino J, Tanabe Y, Kaneda K: Effects of initial graft tension on clinical outcome after anterior cruciate ligament reconstruction. Autogenous doubled hamstring tendons connected in series with polyester tapes. Am J Sports Med 1997;25:99–106.
82 Park MC, ElAttrache NS, Tibone JE, Ahmad CS, Jun BJ, Lee TQ: Part I: Footprint contact characteristics for a transosseous-equivalent rotator cuff repair technique compared with a double-row repair technique. J Shoulder Elbow Surg 2007;16:461–468.
83 Park MC, Tibone JE, ElAttrache NS, Ahmad CS, Jun BJ, Lee TQ: Part II: Biomechanical assessment for a footprint-restoring transosseous-equivalent rotator cuff repair technique compared with a double-row repair technique. J Shoulder Elbow Surg 2007;16:469–476.
84 Cofield RH, Parvizi J, Hoffmeyer PJ, Lanzer WL, Ilstrup DM, Rowland CM: Surgical repair of chronic rotator cuff tears. A prospective long-term study. J Bone Joint Surg Am 2001;83:71–77.
85 Burkhart SS: A stepwise approach to arthroscopic rotator cuff repair based on biomechanical principles. Arthroscopy 2000;16:82–90.
86 Burkhart SS, Athanasiou KA, Wirth MA: Margin convergence: a method of reducing strain in massive rotator cuff tears. Arthroscopy 1996;12:335–338.
87 Tingart MJ, Apreleva M, Zurakowski D, Warner JJ: Pullout strength of suture anchors used in rotator cuff repair. J Bone Joint Surg Am 2003;85:2190–2198.
88 Franceschi F, Longo UG, Ruzzini L, Rizzello G, Maffulli N, Denaro V: The Roman bridge: a 'double pulley-suture bridges' technique for rotator cuff repair. BMC Musculoskelet Disord 2007;8:123.
89 Franceschi F, Longo UG, Ruzzini L, Rizzello G, Maffulli N, Denaro V: Soft tissue tenodesis of the long head of the biceps tendon associated to the Roman bridge repair. BMC Musculoskelet Disord 2008;9:78.
90 Longo UG, Franceschi F, Spiezia F, Marinozzi A, Maffulli N, Denaro V: The low-profile Roman bridge technique for knotless double-row repair of the rotator cuff. Arch Orthop Trauma Surg 2011;131:357–361.
91 De Beer J, Berghs B, van Rooyen K: Arthroscopic rotator cuff repair by footprint reconstruction. 19th Annual San Diego Meeting Syllabus, 2002, pp 425–431.
92 Park JY, Lhee SH, Choi JH, Park HK, Yu JW, Seo JB: Comparison of the clinical outcomes of single- and double-row repairs in rotator cuff tears. Am J Sports Med 2008;36:1310–1316.
93 Frank JB, ElAttrache NS, Dines JS, Blackburn A, Crues J, Tibone JE: Repair site integrity after arthroscopic transosseous-equivalent suture-bridge rotator cuff repair. Am J Sports Med 2008;36:1496–1503.
94 Thompson WO, Debski RE, Boardman ND 3rd, Taskiran E, Warner JJ, Fu FH, Woo SL: A biomechanical analysis of rotator cuff deficiency in a cadaveric model. Am J Sports Med 1996;24:286–292.
95 Bellumore Y, Mansat M, Assoun J: Results of the surgical repair of the rotator cuff. Radioclinical correlation (in French). Rev Chir Orthop Reparatrice Appar Mot 1994;80:582–594.
96 Maffulli N, Longo UG: Conservative management for tendinopathy: is there enough scientific evidence? Rheumatology (Oxford) 2008;47:390–391.
97 Maffulli N, Longo UG: How do eccentric exercises work in tendinopathy? Rheumatology (Oxford) 2008;47:1444–1445.
98 Maffulli N, Longo UG, Maffulli GD, Rabitti C, Khanna A, Denaro V: Marked pathological changes proximal and distal to the site of rupture in acute Achilles tendon ruptures. Knee Surg Sports Traumatol Arthrosc 2011;19:680–687.

99 Rizzello G, Franceschi F, Longo UG, Ruzzini L, Meloni MC, Spiezia F, Papalia R, Denaro V: Arthroscopic management of calcific tendinopathy of the shoulder – do we need to remove all the deposit? Bull NYU Hosp Jt Dis 2009;67:330–333.
100 Maffulli N, Franceschi F, Longo UG, Ruzzini L, Denaro V: Clinical evidence for suture anchor repair of rotator cuff tears does add up: some just do not want to see it. Arthroscopy 2010;26:1568–1570.
101 Woodward TW, Best TM: The painful shoulder. Part I. Clinical evaluation. Am Fam Physician 2000; 61:3079–3088.
102 Longo UG, Franceschi F, Spiezia F, Forriol F, Maffulli N, Denaro V: Triglycerides and total serum cholesterol in rotator cuff tears: Do they matter? Br J Sports Med 2010;44:948–951.
103 Tennent TD, Beach WR, Meyers JF: A review of the special tests associated with shoulder examination. Part I: The rotator cuff tests. Am J Sports Med 2003; 31:154–160.
104 Franceschi F, Longo UG, Ruzzini L, Papalia R, Rizzello G, Denaro V: To detach the long head of the biceps tendon after tenodesis or not: outcome analysis at the 4-year follow-up of two different techniques. Int Orthop 2007;31:537–545.
105 Franceschi F, Longo UG, Ruzzini L, Rizzello G, Maffulli N, Denaro V: No advantages in repairing a type ii superior labrum anterior and posterior lesion when associated with rotator cuff repair in patients over age 50: a randomized controlled trial. Am J Sports Med 2008;36:247–253.
106 Lippi G, Longo UG, Maffulli N: Genetics and sports. Br Med Bull 2010;93:27–47.
107 Longo UG, Franceschi F, Loppini M, Maffulli N, Denaro V: Rating systems for evaluation of the elbow. Br Med Bull 2008;87:131–161.
108 Longo UG, Loppini M, Denaro L, Maffulli N, Denaro V: Rating scales for low back pain. Br Med Bull 2010;94:81–144.
109 Maffulli N, Walley G, Sayana MK, Longo UG, Denaro V: Eccentric calf muscle training in athletic patients with Achilles tendinopathy. Disabil Rehabil 2008;30:1677–1684.
110 Longo UG, Rittweger J, Garau G, Radonic B, Gutwasser C, Gilliver SF, Kusy K, Zieliński J, Felsenberg D, Maffulli N: No influence of age, gender, weight, height, and impact profile in achilles tendinopathy in masters track and field athletes. Am J Sports Med 2009;37:1400–1405.
111 Khanna A, Friel M, Gougoulias N, Longo UG, Maffulli N: Prevention of adhesions in surgery of the flexor tendons of the hand: what is the evidence? Br Med Bull 2009;90:85–109.
112 Franceschi F, Longo UG, Ruzzini L, Rizzello G, Maffulli N, Denaro V: Arthroscopic salvage of failed arthroscopic Bankart repair: a prospective study with a minimum follow-up of 4 years. Am J Sports Med 2008;36:1330–1336.
113 Maffulli N, Longo UG, Oliva F, Ronga M, Denaro V: Minimally invasive surgery of the achilles tendon. Orthop Clin North Am 2009;40:491–498.
114 Longo UG, Ronga M, Maffulli N: Acute ruptures of the achilles tendon. Sports Med Arthrosc 2009;17: 127–138.
115 Longo UG, Ronga M, Maffulli N: Achilles tendinopathy. Sports Med Arthros 2009;17:112–126.
116 Maffulli N, Longo UG, Spiezia F, Denaro V: Aetiology and prevention of injuries in elite young athletes. Med Sport Sci 2011;56:187–200.
117 Maffulli N, Longo UG, Gougoulias N, Denaro V: Ipsilateral free semitendinosus tendon graft transfer for reconstruction of chronic tears of the Achilles tendon. BMC Musculoskelet Disord 2008;9:100.
118 Ames PR, Longo UG, Denaro V, Maffulli N: Achilles tendon problems: not just an orthopaedic issue. Disabil Rehabil 2008;30:1646–1650.
119 Franceschi F, Marinozzi A, Papalia R, Longo UG, Gualdi G, Denaro E: Intra- and juxta-articular osteoid osteoma: a diagnostic challenge: misdiagnosis and successful treatment: a report of four cases. Arch Orthop Trauma Surg 2006;126:660–667.
120 Maffulli N, Longo UG, Ronga M, Khanna A, Denaro V: Favorable outcome of percutaneous repair of achilles tendon ruptures in the elderly. Clin Orthop Relat Res 2010;468:1039–1046.
121 Longo UG, King JB, Denaro V, Maffulli N: Double-bundle arthroscopic reconstruction of the anterior cruciate ligament: does the evidence add up? J Bone Joint Surg Br 2008;90:995–999.

Nicola Maffulli, MD, MS, PhD, FRCS(Orth)
Centre for Sports and Exercise Medicine
Barts and The London School of Medicine and Dentistry
Mile End Hospital, 275 Bancroft Road, London E1 4DG (UK)
Tel. +44 20 8223 8839, E-Mail n.maffulli@qmul.ac.uk

Maffulli N (ed): Rotator Cuff Tear. Med Sport Sci. Basel, Karger, 2012, vol 57, pp 153–167

Treatment Options for Chronic Retracted Degenerative Rotator Cuff Tears

Scott J. Deering · Scott D. Mair · Christian Lattermann

Department of Orthopaedic Surgery and Sports Medicine, University of Kentucky, Lexington, Ky., USA

Abstract

Degenerative, retracted, massive rotator cuff tears present surgeons with distinct challenges. Patient selection is key to a successful outcome. Treatment strategies range from non-operative to progressively more complex surgical options, including debridement, partial repair, complete repair utilizing margin convergence and interval slides, tendon transfers, arthrodesis, and arthroplasty. The rationale behind each of these options and more are discussed along with guidance for selecting the appropriate treatment strategy for individual patients. Outcomes of various treatment approaches are discussed as well to facilitate surgeons to successfully manage patients with retracted and degenerative tears of the rotator cuff.

Management of patients who have chronic, retracted, and degenerative rotator cuff tears presents a distinct challenge to orthopedic surgeons. Rotator cuff tears are common in the aging population, with a prevalence of 50% in patients over age 60 and up to 80% of asymptomatic individuals older than 80 [1, 2]. Massive tears represent up to 40% of all rotator cuff tears [3]. Patients with these large lesions are often in significant pain with great limitations in their function. Repair of these tears can be difficult, with a low healing rate from retracted and inelastic tissues, muscle atrophy, and fatty infiltration. Various techniques to improve the success of repairs of massive rotator cuff repairs have been developed and will be discussed in this chapter. Other topics to be reviewed include non-operative management, surgical debridement, partial repair, and salvage options, such as tendon transfers, arthroplasty, and arthrodesis. Biologic and synthetic augmentation of repairs will be discussed in other parts of this text.

Presentation and Diagnosis

Massive rotator cuff tears can induce marked pain and disability to patients. Patients frequently experience pain at night and with activities of daily living [3]. Depending on the ability to compensate and the location and chronicity of the tear, the amount of weakness and the amount of atrophy are variable [3–6]. Functional deficits often correlate with the location of the tear, as posterosuperior tears lead to limitations in motion and weakness with abduction, forward flexion, and active external rotation [3, 4]. Larger tears are associated with external rotation weakness, external rotation lag, and a positive 'hornblower' sign, i.e. an inability to externally rotate the shoulder [3–7]. Anterosuperior deficiency can lead to decreased abduction and forward flexion and subscapularis deficiency can lead to a positive 'lift-off' and 'belly-press' tests with increased passive external rotation [3–7]. The 'bear hug' test is also positive in patients with deficient subscapularis function [3]. Imaging studies can help to confirm the findings of accurate physical examination.

Plain radiographs can be useful to help determine size and reparability of rotator cuff tears. The normal acromiohumeral interval is 7–14 mm [6]. A decrease in the acromiohumeral distance provides evidence of a massive tear [3, 6]. Magnetic resonance imaging (MRI) and ultrasonography are useful adjuncts to plain radiographs to diagnose rotator cuff tears and provide information about the quality and potential reparability of cuff tissues, while also providing information about other structures such as the labrum and biceps [3–6]. The size of the tear alone is not an indication of reparability, as acute massive tears may retain tissue elasticity and thus may be freely mobile [3, 5, 7]. Signs of irreparability include superior migration of the humeral head, a narrowed or absent acromiohumeral interval, and fatty infiltration affecting 50% or more of the rotator cuff musculature [3–7]. MRI follow-up after rotator cuff repair has demonstrated that repair does not halt progression of fatty infiltration, but fatty infiltration progresses faster in tendons that are re-torn [8]. Patients with massive rotator cuff tears may exhibit 'pseudoparalysis' of the shoulder, whereby they are unable to achieve active elevation above 90° in the presence of free passive anterior elevation [9].

Massive rotator cuff tears can occur by a variety of mechanisms in distinctly different patient populations. Young patients usually require a high-energy trauma to suffer from a massive rotator cuff tear. While these injuries are acutely disabling, the patients usually have good quality mobile tissue that is easily reparable. This is in contrast to elderly patients who may have had a chronic asymptomatic tear that often only requires a relatively minor trauma such as a 'far reach' or a sudden movement that subsequently leads to a complete loss of function, pain, and the clinical sign of 'pseudoparalysis'. In this acute on chronic situation, the tissue quality of the remnant rotator cuff is often poor and the cuff tissue may be too stiff and retracted for a formal rotator cuff repair [4–6]. To understand the different treatment options for these patients, a basic understanding of rotator cuff biomechanics is necessary.

Biomechanics

The rotator cuff serves several important biomechanical roles to facilitate function of the shoulder. These roles are relevant to the strategies for treatment, possible repair, reconstruction, or replacement. The rotator cuff serves as a humeral head rotator, humeral head depressor that compresses the humeral head in the glenoid and optimizes deltoid function, and it provides the fulcrum for glenohumeral motion [10]. The deltoid and rotator cuff inferior to the humeral head equator act as a force couple, as do the subscapularis and infraspinatus/teres minor [3]. Patients with supraspinatus tears involving up to half of the infraspinatus can compensate well provided that the anterior and posterior force couples are balanced [3, 7, 11]. This provides a rationale to support the finding that patients in whom a partial repair of the rotator cuff is performed can have good outcomes provided that the construct produced is biomechanically sound [7, 11]. These repairs have been described as anatomically deficient, but biomechanically intact [11]. Evaluation of functional tears has led to the 'suspension bridge' concept of rotator cuff tears that even in the presence of large tears function can be maintained if force couples are intact [4, 6]. Tears of up to 7 cm can be compensated by intact cuff musculature in combination with a fully functional deltoid muscle based on biomechanical studies, but once tears exceed 8 cm in size, supraphysiologic muscle effort is required to compensate [10]. This finding gives evidence to explain why some patients do well after rotator cuff repair even if a re-tear is identifiable on imaging studies, if the re-tear is small and balanced biomechanics are able to be maintained [10]. Partial repairs may also relieve pressure on the suprascapular nerve that is caused by tethering in retracted tissues with massive tears, thus leading to pain relief and improved shoulder function [6].

Non-Operative Management

Some patients with chronic rotator cuff tears do very well with non-operative management of their shoulders. Many patients with cuff tears have little pain and retain adequate shoulder range of motion and function [3]. Patients in whom rotator cuff force couples are maintained may not have impairment in function [3]. Studies have reported that a majority of patients treated non-operatively can show clinical improvement, but symptom duration of longer than 6 months was a negative prognostic factor [3–6]. Non-surgical management involves activity modification, nonsteroidal anti-inflammatory medications, subacromial corticosteroid injections, local therapeutic modalities, and physical therapy [4–7].

Physical therapy should begin by focusing on regaining range of motion, then strengthening internal and external rotators, and scapular stabilization to maximize the function of the remaining musculature, often in conjunction with NSAIDs and steroid injections, to alleviate pain and allow patients' to perform therapeutic exercises [5]. The goal of therapy is to produce a state of biomechanical compensation through muscle substitution [4]. Other goals of therapy include coordination of muscle co-contraction and improvement of proprioception [6]. Physical therapy should focus on re-education of the anterior deltoid to prevent superior migration of the humeral head and to assist in glenohumeral compression [3, 6]. Deltoid strengthening is begun with the patient supine and then progress to anti-gravity exercises [4, 5]. Conservative management may take more than 3 months to prove successful [4].

The ideal patient for non-operative management of a rotator cuff tear is elderly, with low functional demands, tolerable symptoms, and limited pain [12]. Patients with medical comorbidities that preclude surgery may benefit from non-operative measures as well [4]. Non-operative management with therapy, NSAIDs, and injections will not slow the progression of glenohumeral osteoarthritis, superior migration of the humeral head, increase in the size of the tendon tear, or progression of fatty atrophy of rotator cuff musculature, and may limit future treatment options [3, 6, 12]. Humeral head migration is more likely with painful rotator cuff tears and tears that extend into the infraspinatus [13]. These potentially irreversible changes may occur within 4 years, and should be discussed with patients prior to embarking on a course of non-operative management [3, 12].

Debridement

Another option in the treatment of patients with degenerative and retracted rotator cuff tears is surgical debridement. The ideal patient for this method of treatment is generally older, with lower functional demands, preserved function of the arm, and with pain as the main complaint [3–6]. Pain relief with subacromial injections is a good prognostic indicator of success with surgical debridement [3, 4]. At the time of surgery, cuff tendon edges can be debrided, bursal tissue can be excised, and a biceps tenotomy can be performed safely without any significant functional loss [4, 14]. Bony subacromial decompression or reverse decompression of the greater tuberosity, or tuberoplasty, are also surgical options [3–6, 14]. Surgeons should take into consideration maintaining the coracoacromial arch and preserving the coracoacromial ligament to prevent anterosuperior escape [3–6]. Debridement provides good pain relief with improved ASES and Constant scores, but does not prevent the development of glenohumeral arthritis and superior migration of the humeral head, although these changes do not affect clinical outcome [14]. Irreparable tears of the subscapularis or teres minor with superior migration of the humeral head preoperatively are a negative predictor of outcomes for debridement alone [6]. Debridement of chronic massive rotator cuff tears can be effectively performed in the appropriately selected patients with reasonable goals of pain relief and low functional demands.

Rotator Cuff Repair

Repair of the torn rotator cuff tissue can provide a significant benefit to patients with pain and shoulder dysfunction. Massive, chronic, and retracted tears provide challenges for surgeons to perform repairs. Techniques to facilitate a tension-free repair including margin convergence, interval slides, medialization, and augmentation of the repair with biceps tendon can be utilized. Good results have been demonstrated with repair of massive rotator cuff tears, similar to results of smaller tears though with higher re-tear rates [3, 5–7, 11, 15–19]. There is weak evidence that double-row techniques provide better outcomes in repair of massive rotator cuff tears [7, 20, 21]. The following sections discuss techniques for repair of massive, retracted rotator cuff tears.

Margin Convergence

The goal of rotator cuff repair is to facilitate healing of the leading edge of a torn tendon to the humeral head. This is best accomplished if there is a means to provide a tension-free repair. In chronic, massive, and retracted rotator cuff tears, this can be especially challenging. One technique to improve the odds of successful healing is to perform margin convergence. This procedure relies on proper identification of tear patterns, and is most successful in retracted U-shaped tears. Margin convergence converts massive U-shaped tears into more manageable crescent-shaped tears that can be attached to the humerus under lower tension, as seen in figure 1 [22]. In addition to providing a lower tension environment to increase odds of a healed repair, margin convergence decreases the amount of strain on nerve endings in the tendon tissue, which can lead to decreased pain in the repaired tissue [22]. Biomechanical studies of margin convergence have shown that the technique decreases the amount of strain on tendon tissue in addition to decreasing gap size [23]. These benefits in addition to decreasing the distance that the cuff has to be translated to reach the footprint also decrease the amount of tension on the repair, which should increase healing potential [23].

The surgical technique of margin convergence is performed in a stepwise fashion. After performing a diagnostic glenohumeral arthroscopy and addressing any intra-articular pathology, the arthroscope is positioned in the subacromial space. A thorough bursectomy and release of adhesions and scar tissue about the cuff must be performed to allow for adequate visualization and to facilitate passage and management of sutures and anchors. The rotator cuff tear pattern must first be identified. This is easily performed from a mid-lateral portal that gives an overview picture of the entire cuff as seen in figure 2. Once visualization is adequate the pattern of the rotator cuff tear should be identified. Margin convergence is efficacious for U- or L-shaped tears of the supraspinatus. If an appropriate tear pattern is noted, repair begins medially

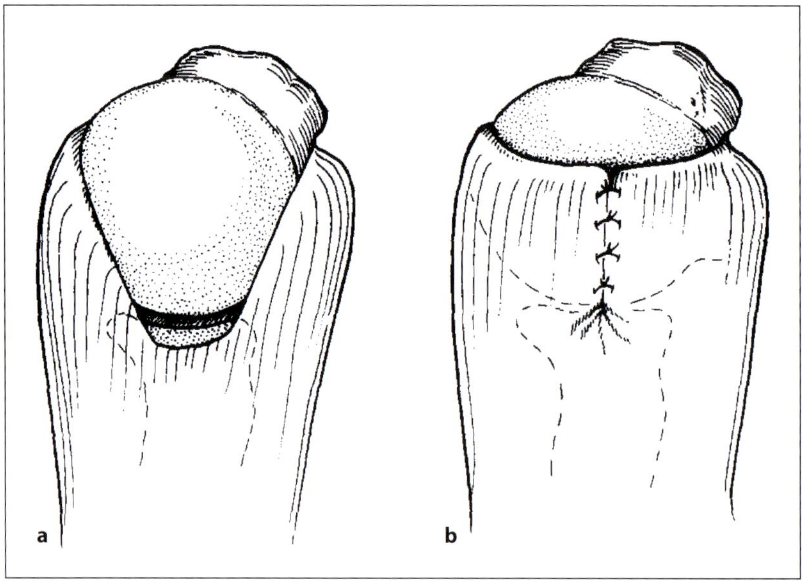

Fig. 1. **a** U-shaped rotator cuff tear viewed from above. **b** Margin convergence sutures placed between the anterior and posterior leaflets of the tear [reprinted from 22, with permission].

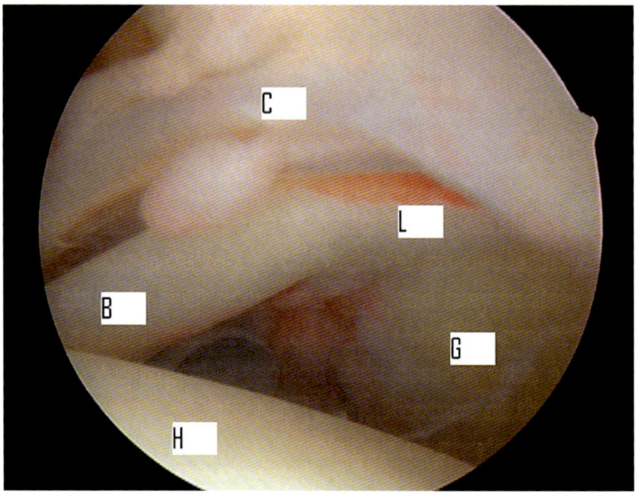

Fig. 2. Overview of a massive rotator cuff tear that is retracted to the edge of the glenoid viewed from the lateral portal. H = Humeral head, G = glenoid, L = labrum, B = long head of biceps tendon, C = free margin of rotator cuff tendon tear.

at the apex of the tear. Care should be taken prior to beginning to pass suture to ensure that the correct orientation of the cuff tissue is established. The goal should be an anatomic repair, similar to reduction of a fracture. Non-absorbable sutures are passed through the anterior and posterior leaflets of the torn tendon and arthroscopic knots are tied in the subacromial space to re-approximate the tendon edges to each other

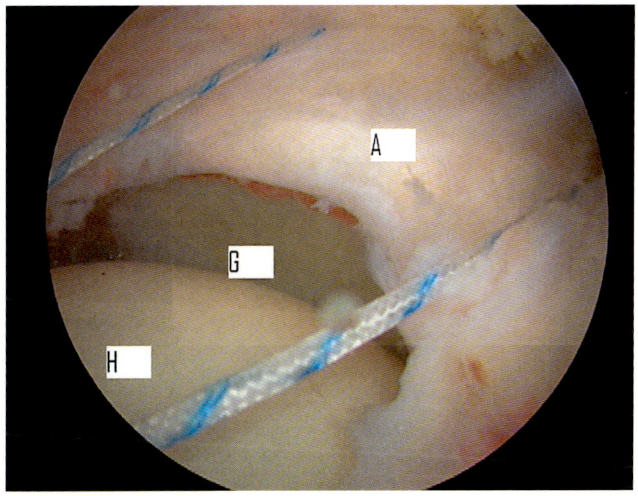

Fig. 3. Initial suture placement for margin convergence. One limb of suture is anterior to the apex of the tear and one limb is posterior. H = Humeral head, G = glenoid, A = apex of U-shaped supraspinatus tear.

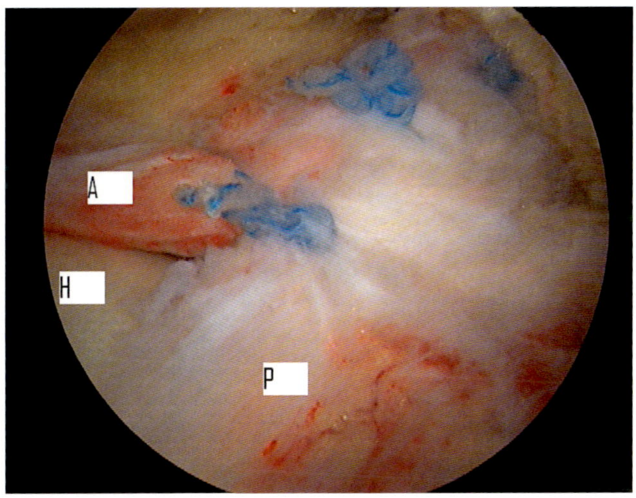

Fig. 4. Completion of margin convergence in a large cuff tear leaves a small lateral defect. H = Humeral head, A = anterior leaflet of rotator cuff tear, P = posterior leaflet.

as seen in figure 3. Repair proceeds sequentially from medial to lateral as the tendon edges are approximated. Each additional suture decreases the size of the remaining gap in the tendon tissue and also decreases the ultimate tension of the final repair. The effect of the first suture is greatest, with each subsequent suture making a similar, but less dramatic difference [23]. Margin convergence repair continues until a small crescent-shaped tear remains, as seen in figure 4. Once the tear has been converted to a small crescent-shaped tear, then the tendon can be repaired to bone using a suture anchor technique. A completed repair is demonstrated in figure 5.

In a report published by Burkhart et al. [19], equivalent outcomes with respect to UCLA scores and time to return to work or activities were achieved in patients in

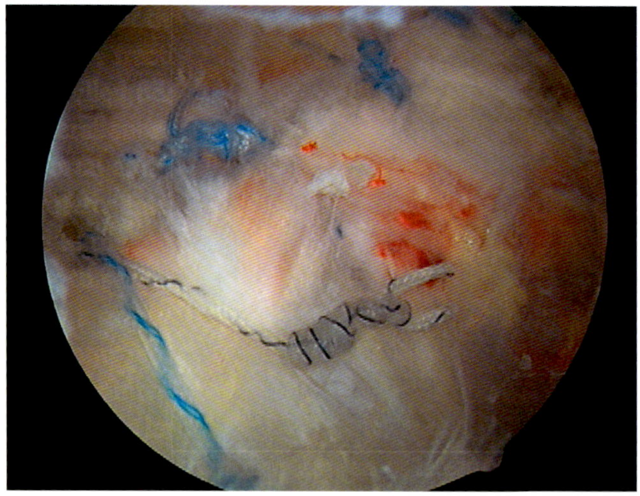

Fig. 5. Completed rotator cuff repair after margin convergence technique viewed from the lateral portal.

whom margin convergence was performed with those in whom direct tendon repair to bone for smaller tears was performed, providing some validation for the efficacy of the technique. Their study demonstrated 95% good to excellent results regardless of tear size [19]. Margin convergence serves as a useful technique for repair of massive U- or L-shaped retracted tears of the rotator cuff.

Releases and Slides

Massive, chronic, and retracted tears of the rotator cuff similar to the ones demonstrated in figure 6 are extremely difficult to mobilize to allow tension-free repair of the tendon to the humeral head. Another method to decrease tension on cuff tissue to increase odds of successful repair is to perform releases of the scarred cuff tissue to facilitate lateral displacement of the tendon tissue. Releases can be performed between the cuff and the capsule, as well as anterior and posterior interval releases to allow complete or partial repair of the torn cuff tissue.

Initial mobilization of retracted tears begins by freeing up adhesions between the retracted tendons and surrounding tissues. The arthroscopic shaver or radiofrequency device can be utilized to develop a plane between the capsule and the undersurface of the tendon, taking care not to damage the glenoid, labrum, and biceps tendon [5, 6, 15, 16]. This technique is then continued in the subacromial space as adhesions between bursal tissue and the retracted tendon are released in a similar manner under direct visualization [3, 5, 6, 15, 16]. Anatomic dissections of the suprascapular nerve have demonstrated that the cuff can be safely mobilized up to 1 cm laterally from its original anatomic position before undue tension is placed on the nerve and with medial detachment of the supra- and infraspinatus with lateral translation and reattachment,

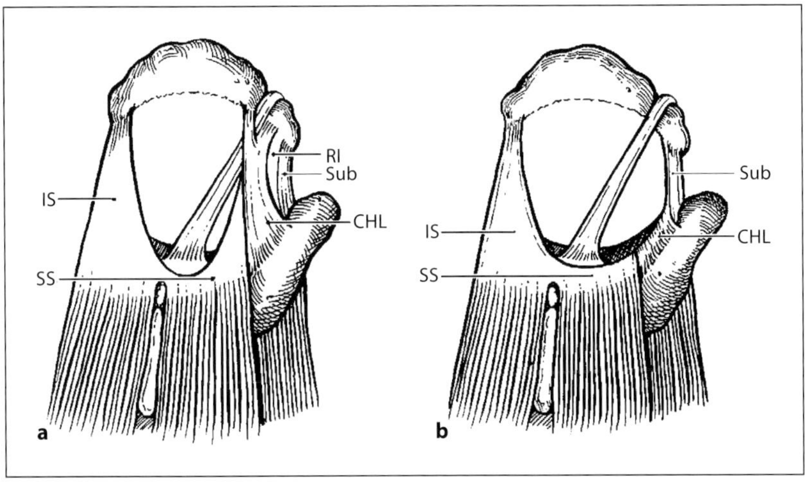

Fig. 6. **a** Superior view of a massive, contracted U-shaped tear of the rotator cuff. **b** Superior view of a massive, contracted crescent-shaped tear of the rotator cuff [reprinted from 17, with permission].

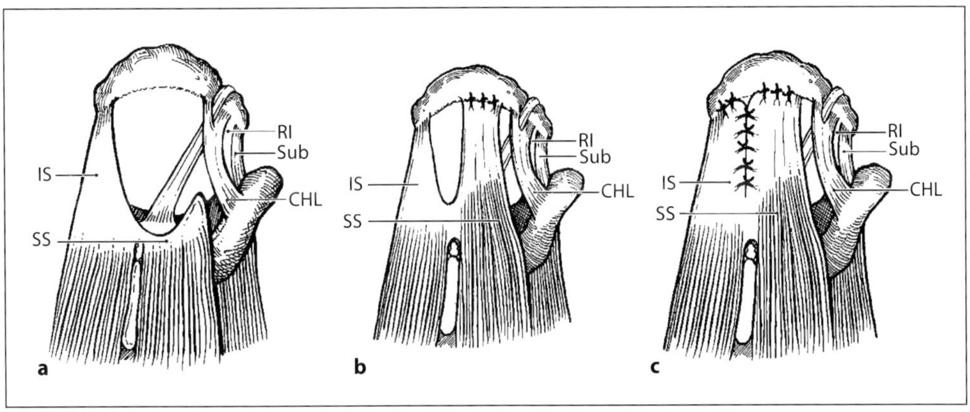

Fig. 7. **a** Anterior interval slide is performed by releasing the interval between the supraspinatus and rotator interval. **b** Improved mobility from the release allows for repair of the supraspinatus to the greater tuberosity. **c** The posterior leaf of the tear is then advanced superiorly and laterally and the residual longitudinal defect is closed by side-to-side sutures [reprinted from 17, with permission].

up to 3 cm of lateral mobility can be achieved [24]. If sufficient mobilization of the tendon is not feasible after these releases are performed, then attention can be turned to anterior and posterior interval slides.

Interval slides allow for increased medial to lateral translation of retracted tendon tissue. The anterior interval slide is performed at the junction of the anterior border of the supraspinatus tendon and the rotator interval tissue as seen in figure 7. The long head of the biceps tendon is the anatomic landmark that facilitates the initiation of the anterior slide [17, 25]. The base of the coracoid is located anteromedial to the root of the biceps tendon [17, 25]. A traction suture is placed at the anterior edge of the supraspinatus tendon and pulled posterolaterally, providing tension [17, 25]. While viewing from a posterolateral subacromial portal, arthroscopic scissors are then brought through a lateral portal and used to separate the anterior edge of the supraspinatus tendon from the rotator interval tissue, including the coracohumeral ligament, which becomes scarred to the torn tendon edge and holds it in a retracted position [17, 18, 25]. Alternatively, this technique can be performed while visualizing from a posterior portal and using a grasper through an accessory lateral portal to maintain tension on the supraspinatus tendon [18]. Care is taken to avoid damage to the biceps tendon while the rotator interval tissue is being divided and dissection proceeds until the tissue is freed up to the level of the base of the coracoid [17, 18, 25]. Anterior interval slide usually provides an additional 1–2 cm of lateral excursion of the supraspinatus tendon [17, 25]. If additional mobilization is required, a posterior slide can be undertaken.

The posterior interval slide develops a plane between the supra- and infraspinatus tendons (fig. 8). Whereas the anatomy of the anterior slide is defined while visualizing from inside the glenohumeral joint, the location for the posterior slide is identified in the subacromial space [17, 25]. The undersurface of the acromion is identified and soft tissue is debrided carefully [17, 25]. Dissection proceeds posteriorly and medially, removing fibrofatty tissue posterior to the acromioclavicular joint to allow for identification of the scapular spine [17, 25]. The scapular spine divides the muscle bellies of the supra- and infraspinatus and serves as the landmark for the posterior slide [17, 25]. Once the spine has been identified, traction sutures are placed at the posterior aspect of the supraspinatus tendon and the anterior aspect of the infraspinatus tendon at the free margin of the rotator cuff tear [17, 25]. Anterior traction is placed on the supraspinatus suture and posterior tension is applied to the infraspinatus suture [17, 25]. While viewing from a lateral portal, arthroscopic scissors are brought in through a posterolateral portal and used to develop the plane between the supra- and infraspinatus tendons [17, 25]. Care is taken to avoid damage to the suprascapular nerve, which is located 2 cm medial to the corner of the glenoid by lifting the blades of the scissors as the dissection is performed [17, 24, 25]. Dissection continues to the level of the scapular spine, facilitating complete separation of the supra- and infraspinatus tendons, and allowing up to an additional 5 cm of lateral translation of the tendon tissue [17, 25]. After the tendons are secured to the humeral head, sutures are placed into the tendinous split to close the gap, similar to a margin convergence repair [17, 25].

Interval slides are useful to increase mobility of massive retracted tears and to decrease tension on repairs. Outcome results of patients who have had repairs performed with interval slides are encouraging, with two-thirds of patients demonstrating a good or excellent result [17, 18]. These techniques are used infrequently and tend to be for chronic retracted tears in older patients, so the results obtained are encouraging.

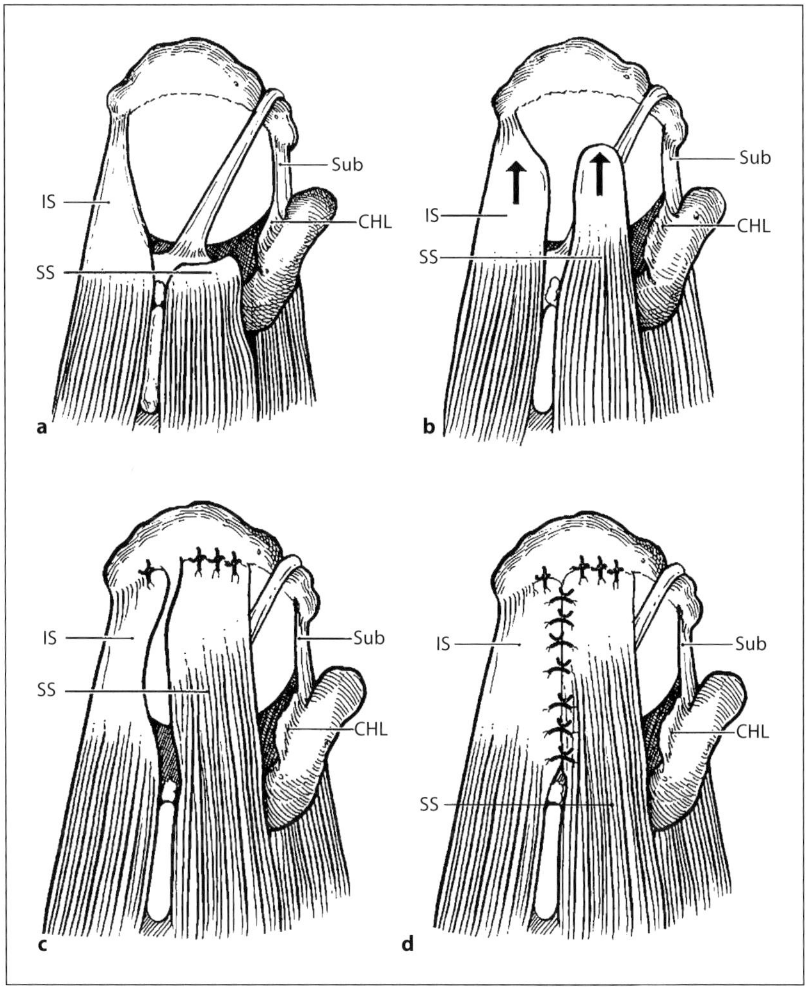

Fig. 8. a Double interval slide is performed by first completing an anterior interval slide and then performing a posterior interval slide between the supra- and infraspinatus tendons. **b** After release, improved mobility of the supra- and infraspinatus tendons is demonstrated. **c** The supraspinatus is repaired to the greater tuberosity in a tension-free manner and the posterior leaf is advanced superiorly and laterally. **d** The residual defect is then closed with side-to-side sutures [reprinted from 17, with permission].

Tendon Transfers

Another option in the management of chronic, retracted, and degenerative rotator cuff tears is transfer of musculotendinous units to compensate for the loss of the native rotator cuff function. This option is most appropriate for younger patients with irreparable tears who have higher functional demands and have a main complaint of weakness without glenohumeral arthritis [3, 4, 6]. Tendon transfers are complex surgical procedures that require extensive rehabilitation for muscular reeducation to deliver favorable results, and are therefore not indicated for older, debilitated patients [4]. Tendon transfers for rotator cuff deficiency were developed from surgical procedures to address brachial plexus birth palsies, and have been modified to address the individual patient's particular functional loss [5, 26]. There have been a multitude of tendon transfers described in the historical literature for rotator cuff deficiency, including the upper third of the subscapularis tendon, teres major, teres minor, split deltoid muscle flap, triceps, trapezius, and lateralization of the supraspinatus muscle in the supraspinatus fossa [4–6]. The most commonly utilized and durable tendons for transfer for rotator cuff deficiency are the latissimus dorsi and pectoralis major [3–6, 26–28].

The latissimus dorsi tendon is useful for reconstruction of posterosuperior defects of the rotator cuff [3–6, 26–28]. The latissimus dorsi tendon is detached from its insertion on the lateral aspect of the bicipital groove of the humerus and tunneled through the plane between the teres major/teres minor/infraspinatus and the deltoid and attached to the greater tuberosity and the stump of remaining rotator cuff tendon tissue, if present [26–28]. Patients are maintained in an abduction brace full time for 5–6 weeks and rehabilitation continues for 9 months postoperatively [26–28]. Patients who had the procedure performed primarily rather than in a revision situation had better outcomes as did patients without subscapularis lesions [26, 27]. Radiographic evidence of osteoarthritis and decreased glenohumeral distance progressed in patients who had the latissimus transfer [26, 27]. Given the disparity in results obtained in patients who had deficiency of subscapularis function, this is now seen as a contraindication to the performance of latissimus dorsi tendon transfer in isolation [26, 27].

Subscapularis deficiency can be addressed through transfer of the pectoralis major to the lesser tuberosity [3, 4, 6, 28]. This tendon can be transferred in its entirety or split, transferring only the sternal head [3, 4, 6]. The transfer can be performed anterior or posterior to the conjoint tendon, but passing the pectoralis tendon below the conjoint allows it to function in a manner that more closely replicates the action of the subscapularis [3, 4, 6]. There is a theoretical concern of increased risk to neurovascular structures with passage of the pectoralis tendon below the conjoint tendon. For patients with combined anterior and posterior deficiencies of the rotator cuff, combined transfers of the latissimus dorsi and pectoralis major can be performed [28]. A series of 11 patients who underwent the combined transfer demonstrated that 5 were significantly improved, 2 improved slightly, and 4 made no improvement [28]. Young patients with irreparable rotator cuff deficiency provide a significant challenge to the surgeon. Tendon transfers are a means to improve function in these patients.

Other Options

In addition to non-operative management, debridement, margin convergence, releases, and tendon transfers, other options exist in the management of patients with chronic, retracted rotator cuff tears. Various other repair techniques as well as more aggressive options such as arthroplasty and arthrodesis have been described. One option that has been explored is medial reattachment of the torn cuff tendon for retracted tears [29]. Good results with maintenance of active forward elevation were demonstrated for repairs up to 13 mm medial to the original cuff insertion point [29, 30]. Another option to augment repair of massive rotator cuff tears is to utilize the tenotomized long head of the biceps tendon to bridge the gap between the torn edge of the cuff and the greater tuberosity [7, 9]. The authors performed a tenotomy and then sewed the biceps to the posterior aspect of the cuff at the greater tuberosity and then performed a side-to-side repair between the cuff and the biceps tendon [9]. This study demonstrated equivalent clinical outcomes with traditional repair techniques [9]. In patients in whom the rotator cuff and deltoid are deficient, glenohumeral arthrodesis is another option for management, especially in shoulders that demonstrate anterosuperior escape of the humeral head [4, 5]. However, achieving a solid fusion can be difficult in osteopenic elderly patients and results of arthroplasty are superior to arthrodesis [4, 5].

Arthroplasty is an attractive option in patients who have glenohumeral arthritis in addition to rotator cuff deficiency. Total shoulder arthroplasty is unsuccessful in rotator cuff deficiency from asymmetric forces on the glenoid component leading to early loosening [3, 5]. This leaves hemiarthroplasty with cuff tear arthropathy heads (so-called mega heads), and reverse total shoulder arthroplasty as options in these patients. In patients who have intact subscapularis function in the setting of a massive irreparable rotator cuff tear, hemiarthroplasty has been proven to be successful in relieving pain and also in improving function to a lesser extent [3]. Anterosuperior escape remains a concern, especially in patients who have previously had a subacromial decompression with a loss of continuity of the coracoacromial arch [3]. Longer term results of patients who have been treated with hemiarthroplasty for cuff tear arthropathy demonstrate persistent pain, possibly from erosion of the glenoid and acromion by the prosthesis [3]. Reverse total shoulder arthroplasty obviates this concern.

Reverse total shoulder arthroplasty is an option for lower demand patients with massive, irreparable tears of the rotator cuff and pseudoparalysis of the shoulder [4]. These prostheses are designed to increase the lever arm of the deltoid by lateralizing the joint, while also medializing the center of rotation [3, 4]. The shear force of the deltoid is converted into a compressive force, increasing the mechanical advantage for shoulder motion [3, 4]. Improved functional results have been demonstrated with reverse prostheses in comparison to hemiarthroplasty in patients with irreparable rotator cuff tears [4]. Reverse shoulder arthroplasty has even been demonstrated to have good results in patients with irreparable rotator cuff deficiency without glenohumeral arthritis [9]. Patients experienced improved outcomes scores and functional parameters with 90.7% implant survivorship at 52 months of average follow-up [9]. Another study demonstrated implant survival of up to 91% at 10 years

[31]. Patients in whom the indication for reverse total shoulder arthroplasty was cuff tear arthropathy perform better, with improved implant survival compared to other operative indications [30 32]. Functional results have been demonstrated to deteriorate after 6 years, though [31]. Reverse arthroplasty of the shoulder is not a benign procedure, however. Complication rates of up to 50% have been reported, including dislocation, infection, glenoid fracture, humeral fracture, persistent pain, radial nerve palsy, glenoid loosening, hematoma, acromial fracture, and scapular notching, with higher rates of complications seen in revision settings [3, 4, 9]. Implant survival rates as low as 30% at 8 years have been reported [3]. Reverse shoulder arthroplasty is a reasonable option in a low-demand patient with a painful pseudoparalytic shoulder with an irreparable rotator cuff tear, though a frank discussion of risk should be held with patients prior to embarking on this treatment strategy.

Conclusion

Patients with retracted and degenerative rotator cuff tears provide a distinct challenge to treating surgeons. Options for management include non-operative management, debridement, partial or complete repair, tendon transfers, arthrodesis, and arthroplasty. Optimum management requires the treating surgeon to match patients and treatment strategies appropriately. Good results can be obtained with careful patient selection, appropriate management, and high-quality rehabilitation in patients with chronic retracted rotator cuff tears.

References

1 Kim HM, Teefey SA, Zelig A, Galatz LM, Keener JD, Yamaguchi K: Shoulder strength in asymptomatic individuals with intact compared with torn rotator cuffs. J Bone Joint Surg Am 2009;91:289–296.
2 Nho SJ, Yadav H, Shindle MK, MacGillivray JD: Rotator cuff degeneration: etiology and pathogenesis. Am J Sports Med 2008;36:987–993.
3 Bedi A, Dines J, Warren RF, Dines DM: Massive tears of the rotator cuff. J Bone Joint Surg Am 2010; 92:1894–1908.
4 Dines DM, Moynihan DP, Dines JS, McCann P: Irreparable Rotator cuff tears: what to do and when to do it; the surgeon's dilemma. J Bone Joint Surg Am 2006;88:2294–2302.
5 Green A: Chronic massive rotator cuff tears: evaluation and management. J Am Acad Orthop Surg 2003;11:321–331.
6 Neri BR, Chan KW, Kwon YK: Management of massive and irreparable rotator cuff tears. J Shoulder Elbow Surg 2009;18:808–818.
7 Nho SJ, Delos D, Yadav H, Pensak M, Romeo AA, Warren RF, MacGillivray JD: Biomechanical and biologic augmentation for the treatment of massive rotator cuff tears. Am J Sports Med 2010;38: 619–629.
8 Gladstone JN, Bishop JY, Lo IKY, Flatow EL: Fatty infiltration and atrophy of the rotator cuff do not improve after rotator cuff repair and correlate with poor functional outcome. Am J Sports Med 2007;35: 719–728.
9 Mulieri P, Dunning P, Klein S, Pupello D, Frankle M: Reverse shoulder arthroplasty for the treatment of irreparable rotator cuff tear without glenohumeral arthritis. J Bone Joint Surg Am 2010;92:2544–2556.
10 Hansen ML, Otis JC, Johnson JS, Cordasco FA, Craig EV, Warren RF: Biomechanics of massive rotator cuff tears: implications for treatment. J Bone Joint Surg Am 2008;90:316–325.

11 Duralde XA, Bair B: Massive rotator cuff tears: the result of partial rotator cuff repair. J Shoulder Elbow Surg 2005;14:121–127.
12 Zingg PO, Jost B, Sukthankar A, Buhler M, Pfirrmann CWA, Gerber C: Clinical and structural outcomes of nonoperative management of massive rotator cuff tears. J Bone Joint Surg Am 2007;89: 1928–1934.
13 Keener JD, Wei AS, Kim M, Steger-May K, Yamaguchi K: Proximal humeral migration in shoulders with symptomatic and asymptomatic rotator cuff tears. J Bone Joint Surg Am 2009;91: 1405–1413.
14 Liem D, Lengers N, Dedy N, Poetzl W, Steinbeck J, Marquardt B: Arthroscopic debridement of massive irreparable rotator cuff tears. Arthroscopy 2008;24: 743–748.
15 Jones CK, Savoie FH III: Arthroscopic Repair of large and massive rotator cuff tears. Arthroscopy 2003;19:564–571.
16 Bittar ES: Arthroscopic management of massive rotator cuff tears. Arthroscopy 2002;18(suppl 2): 104–106.
17 Lo IKY, Burkhart SS: Arthroscopic repair of massive, contracted, immobile rotator cuff tears using single and double interval slides: technique and preliminary results. Arthroscopy 2004;20:22–33.
18 Tauro JC: Arthroscopic repair of large rotator cuff tears using the interval slide technique. Arthroscopy 2004;20:13–21.
19 Burkhart SS, Danaceau SM, Pearce CE Jr: Arthroscopic rotator cuff repair: analysis of results by tear size and by repair technique – margin convergence versus direct tendon-to-bone repair. Arthroscopy 2001;17:905–912.
20 Duquin TR, Buyea C, Bisson LJ: Which method of rotator cuff repair leads to the highest rate of structural healing? A systematic review. Am J Sports Med 2010;38:835–841.
21 Saridakis P, Jones G: Outcomes of single-row and double row arthroscopic rotator cuff repair: a systematic review. J Bone Joint Surg Am 2010;92: 732–742.
22 Burkhart SS, Athanasiou KA, Wirth MA: Margin convergence: a method of reducing strain in massive rotator cuff tears. Arthroscopy 1996;12: 335–338.
23 Mazzocca AD, Bollier M, Fehsenfeld D, Romeo A, Stephens K, Solovyoya O, Obopilwe E, Ciminiello A, Nowak MD, Arciero R: Biomechanical evaluation of margin convergence. arthroscopy. Arthroscopy 2011;27:330–338.
24 Warner JP, Krushell RJ, Masquelet A, Gerber C: Anatomy and relationships of the suprascapular nerve: anatomical constraints to mobilization of the supraspinatus and infraspinatus muscles in the management of massive rotator cuff tears. J Bone Joint Surg Am 1992;74:36–45.
25 Klein JR, Burkhart SS: Identification of essential anatomic landmarks in performing arthroscopic single- and double-interval slides. Arthroscopy 2004; 20:765–770.
26 Irlenbusch U, Bracht M, Gansen H-K, Lorenz U, Thiel J: Latissimus dorsi transfer for irreparable rotator cuff tears: a longitudinal study. J Shoulder Elbow Surg 2008;17:527–534
27 Gerber C, Maquieira G, Espinosa N: Latissimus dorsi transfer for the treatment of irreparable rotator cuff tears. J Bone Joint Surg Am 2006;88: 113–120.
28 Aldridge JM III, Atkinson TS, Mallon WJ: Combined pectoralis major and latissimus dorsi tendon transfer for massive rotator cuff deficiency. J Shoulder Elbow Surg 2004;13:621–629.
29 Takeda H, Urata S, Matsuura M, Nakayama A, Yonemitsu H: The influence of medial reattachment of the torn cuff tendon for retracted rotator cuff tears. J Shoulder Elbow Surg 2007;16:316–320.
30 Cho NS, Yi JW, Rhee YG: Arthroscopic biceps augmentation for avoiding undue tension in repair of massive rotator cuff tears. Arthroscopy 2009;25: 183–191.
31 Guery J, Favard L, Sirveaux F, Oudet D, Mole D, Walch G: Reverse total shoulder arthroplasty; survivorship analysis of eighty replacements followed for five to ten years. J Bone Joint Surg Am 2006;88:-1742–1747.
32 Cuff D, Pupello D, Virani N, Levy J, Frankle M: Reverse shoulder arthroplasty for the treatment of rotator cuff deficiency. J Bone Joint Surg Am 2008; 90:1244–1251.

Christian Lattermann, MD
Center for Cartilage Repair and Restoration
Department of Orthopaedic Surgery and Sports Medicine, University of Kentucky
740 South Limestone St., Kentucky Clinic K401, Lexington, KY 40536 (USA)
Tel. +1 859 218 3065, E-Mail clatt2@uky.edu

Maffulli N (ed): Rotator Cuff Tear. Med Sport Sci. Basel, Karger, 2012, vol 57, pp 168–177

Synthetic Augmentation in Massive Rotator Cuff Tears

Umile Giuseppe Longo[a,b] · Alfredo Lamberti[a,b] · Giacomo Rizzello[a,b] · Nicola Maffulli[c] · Vincenzo Denaro[a,b]

[a]Department of Orthopaedic and Trauma Surgery and [b]Centro Integrato di Ricerca (CIR), Campus Bio-Medico University, Rome, Italy; [c]Centre for Sports and Exercise Medicine, Queen Mary University of London, Barts and The London School of Medicine and Dentistry, Mile End Hospital, London, UK

Abstract

Massive rotator cuff tears represent a great challenge in orthopaedic. They are associated with persistent defects, weakness, and poor outcomes and can cause an uncoupling of forces across the glenohumeral joint, with unstable shoulder kinematics. In the last few years, a notable interest has emerged to develop new treatment strategies that provide effective mechanical reinforcement of rotator cuff repair and stimulate and enhance the patient's intrinsic healing potential. Tissue engineering techniques using novel scaffold materials offer potential alternatives for managing massive irreparable rotator cuff tears. Synthetic scaffolds, manufactured from chemical compounds, have gained much interest to bridge massive rotator cuff tears. Preliminary studies support the idea that synthetic scaffolds can provide an alternative for rotator cuff augmentation with an enormous therapeutic potential. Despite the growing clinical use of synthetic scaffold devices for rotator cuff repair, there are numerous questions related to their indication, surgical application, safety, mechanism of action, and efficacy that remain to be clarified or addressed. We review the current basic science and clinical understanding of synthetic scaffolds for massive rotator cuff repair, reporting the preclinical and clinical studies carried out to date in this field. We underline the benefits and limitations of the available synthetic scaffolds for augmentation of rotator cuff tears, and discuss the implications of these literature data on the future directions for the use of these scaffolds in tendon repair procedures.

Massive tears of rotator cuff have an anterior-posterior dimension >5 cm, and involve at least two tendons [1]. They represent a challenge in orthopaedics because they are difficult to repair, and the failure rate is unacceptably high [2–7]. In primary repairs, re-tear rates up to 90% in large and massive tears have been reported 3–5 years postoperatively [8–11]. These unacceptable failure rates can be attributed to various factors, including the relative hypovascularity of the rotator cuff [12–14], which inherently limits the reparative capacity of the tendon, the microscopic degeneration of the intact portion of the tendon [15–17], and the fact that at times, during the postoperative rehabilitation, forces that exceed the strength of the repair have been applied to the shoulder [18].

Massive tears of the rotator cuff are associated with persistent defects, weakness, and poor outcomes [19], and can cause uncoupling of forces across the glenohumeral joint, greatly altering shoulder kinematics. Current alternatives to repair of massive rotator cuff tears include reverse total shoulder arthroplasty or tendon transfers, which have provided mixed results and are considered invasive procedures [20].

Although considerable effort has been put in developing surgical methods to optimize fixation of tendon to bone to achieve the highest possible initial strength of the repair [21–23], high repair failure rates still persist clinically. Hence, there is a need for new repair strategies that provide effective mechanical reinforcement of rotator cuff repair, and stimulate and enhance the patient's intrinsic healing potential. To decrease structural failure rates of surgically repaired rotator cuff tendons, technological improvements in implant material and structure have been made. A non-resorbable implant similar to those used for vascular reconstructions [24] or hernia repairs [25] provides an appealing approach.

Tissue engineering techniques using novel scaffold materials offer potential alternatives for managing irreparable rotator cuff tears [26]. Tissue engineering strategies to improve rotator cuff repair healing include the use of scaffolds [27, 28], growth factors [29, 30], cell seeding, or a combination of these approaches [26]. Scaffolds have been the most common strategy investigated to date [31]. Rotator cuff repair with devices derived from polylactic acid [32–35], polytetrafluoroethylene [36], extracellular matrix [37–43], chitin [44] and chitosan-hyaluronan [45] has been studied in animal models [46]. The rationale for using a scaffold device for rotator cuff repair may include mechanical augmentation, improving the rate and quality of biologic healing, or both. Scaffolds with robust mechanical and suture retention properties, applied in a surgically appropriate manner, may have the ability to 'off-load' the repair at time zero and for some period of postoperative healing, depending on the rate and extent of scaffold remodelling. Despite the growing clinical use of scaffold devices for rotator cuff repair, there are numerous questions related to their indication, surgical application, safety, mechanism of action, and efficacy that remain to be clarified or addressed.

We review the current basic science and clinical understanding of synthetic scaffolds for massive rotator cuff repair, reporting the preclinical and clinical evidence derived by the studies to date carried out in this field. We will then discuss the implications of these literature data on the future directions for the use of these scaffolds in tendon repair procedures.

Synthetic Scaffolds for Massive Rotator Cuff Tear Augmentation

Synthetic scaffolds are manufactured from chemical compounds. Many materials such polyester, polypropylene, polyacrylamide, Dacron, carbon, silicone and nylon fabric were fabricated into prostheses for tendon or ligament repair [47]. Several animal studies have investigated the benefit of augmenting rotator cuff repair with synthetic scaffolds.

A polyglycolic acid sheet has been used to augment rotator cuff repairs of infraspinatus tendons in Japanese white rabbits [48], showing histological improvement in fibrocartilage layering but only a slight improvement in tensile strength when compared to control tendons augmented with another slowly absorbing synthetic material [48].

Polylactic acid patches have yielded mixed results. In sheep, polylactic acid patches determined a 25% greater strength than the non-augmented repair [34], but no observable differences between the treated and control groups were reported in a similar study in goats [35]. In a canine model, [33] the augmented rotator cuff repair resulted in fewer tendon retractions, greater strength, and increased stiffness when compared to the contralateral untreated rotator cuff repairs. A more recent study demonstrates that the application of the X-Repair device significantly increased the yield load and ultimate load of rotator cuff repairs in a human cadaveric model and altered the failure mode but did not affect initial repair stiffness [49].

Non-woven chitin fabric has been used to regenerate infraspinatus tendons in rabbits [44]. A 10-mm surgical defect was produced at the humeral insertion of the infraspinatus tendon in 21 Japanese white rabbits. In one shoulder, the 10-mm defect was covered with chitin, a biodegradable polymer, sutured into the bone trough and attached to the free end of the infraspinatus tendon. The contralateral shoulder was left untreated as a control. Throughout the experiment, tendon-to-bone junctions covered with chitin fabric demonstrated greater cell number, better collagen fibre alignment, and greater mechanical strength than the tendon-to-bone junctions left free as control [44]. A polyurethane scaffold applied to supply a chronic rupture of rotator cuff in an ovine model resulted in a 74% increase in force at failure relative to the non-augmented surgical control repaired with traditional suture anchor. Apparent increases in stiffness and global displacement at failure were not significant [50]. No inflammatory reaction and a tissue ingrowth of 79.9% were observed in a rat rotator cuff repair model using a polycarbonate polyurethane patch [51].

Polytetrafluoroethylene (PTFE) felt has been applied to reconstruct canine infraspinatus tendon, showing good mechanical recovery and tissue affinity. The ultimate tensile strength was 60.84, 172.88, and 306.51 N immediately after surgery and at 6 and 12 weeks, respectively. The stiffness of the specimens at the PTFE felt-bone interface was 9.61, 64.67, and 135.09 kN/m immediately after surgery and at 6 and 12 weeks, respectively. Histological analysis showed ingrowth of fibrous tissue between the PTFE fibres. Foreign-body reactions were found at the margin of the PTFE-bone interface between 12 and 24 weeks [36].

Some studies have investigated the potential of the application of tissue engineering principle of cells seeding on scaffolds biomechanical properties.

Poly(lactide-co-glycolide) nanofibre-based scaffold has been evaluated for the attachment, alignment, gene expression, and matrix elaboration of human rotator cuff fibroblasts. Rotator cuff fibroblasts cultured on the aligned scaffolds attached along the nanofibre long axis, whereas the cells on the unaligned scaffold were polygonal and randomly oriented. Cell alignment, distribution, and matrix deposition conformed to nanofibre organization. Mechanical properties of the aligned nanofibre scaffolds were significantly higher than those of the unaligned ones [52].

Fibroblast-seeded chitosan-based hyaluronan hybrid scaffold enhances the production of type I collagen, leading to improved mechanical strength in the regenerated tissues of the rotator cuff in rabbits. Significant improvement in tensile strength and tangent modulus was observed from 4 to 12 weeks postoperatively, associated with a significantly greater tangent modulus than did the non-fibroblast-seeded scaffold and the control at 12 weeks [45]. The same encouraging results have also been derived from various clinical studies conducted in the last 25 years.

Ozaki et al. [53] in 1986 presented the first series of clinical cases of massive rotator cuff lesions repaired with synthetic grafts. 25 patients with chronic massive rotator cuff tears, unable to be repaired with McLaughlin's technique, received one of three polyester augmentation grafts (Teflon felt, Teflon fabric and Marlex mesh). Although the results were satisfying, the lack of a standardized scoring system for patient evaluation makes it impossible to compare with alternative treatment options [53].

Carbon fibres are brittle, resulting in the presence of fragments in soft tissues adjacent to the implant site [54, 55] and determining the destruction of synovial joints related to reactive synovitis and catabolic enzyme reactions [56–58]. For these reasons, carbon fibres should not be used as surgical prosthesis in a synovial joint.

A new generation of polyester grafts, able to cause significantly less enzyme and chondrocyte-activating factor production by the synoviocytes, was introduced in 2006 [59]. These grafts have high tensile strength, low friction and excellent tissue reactions when used as a surgical prosthesis [53, 60], no mechanical degradation and the ability to support early collagenous ingrowth, organized in the direction of loading, in the implant, even in the mid-joint space [61].

The Leeds-Keio artificial ligament, so called because it was developed by the University of Leeds and the Keio University, is made of polyester (ethylene terephthalate) [47]. Initially designed for ACL reconstruction [62], it has also been used to augment subscapularis transposition on patients with rheumatoid arthritis undergoing total shoulder arthroplasty, showing superior clinical scores, compared to those of 19 shoulders with cuff repair by subscapularis transposition alone and similar to those of 22 shoulders with intact rotator cuffs. Clinical scores continued to improve after the first postoperative year [63].

A polyester fibre mesh (Dacron) ligament has been recently used by Nada et al. [64] to augment chronic massive tears of the rotator cuff in 21 symptomatic patients. All the patients remained pain-free, with improvement in function and range of movement. The mean pre- and postoperative Constant scores were respectively 46.7

and 85.4. The mean patient satisfaction score was 90%. Two failures are reported, one from a ruptured ligament after 1 year, and the other a deep-seated infection. The MR scan at the final follow-up confirmed intact and thickened bands in 15 of 17 patients.

The Gore-Tex soft tissue patch, which gained popularity for its use in thoracoabdominal surgery, has been associated with a low infection rate, few adhesions, and good mechanical strength and suture retention [31]. A Gore-Tex patch was used to repair rotator cuff tears irreparable by direct suture in 27 patients. No difference appeared in the improvement in score between shoulders treated with small (<2 cm) and those treated with large (>2 cm) patches. Good clinical results, especially pain relief, could be achieved with this procedure in both the small- and the large-patch groups, but good abduction strength was obtained only in the small-patch group [65].

Discussion

The ideal scaffold for rotator cuff tendon repair must be able to meet the physiologic demand of the native tendon by matching its mechanical properties, and it should promote host cell-mediated healing by mimicking the ultrastructural organization of the native tendon. In addition, the scaffold should be biodegradable to allow new tissue to be replaced gradually while physiologically relevant mechanical properties are maintained. Finally, the scaffold must be able to integrate with the host tendon and surrounding bone tissue [66].

Tissue induction ability of synthetic scaffold is scanty, probably because of the fact that they do not possess a surface chemistry that is familiar to host tissue. The interaction between scaffold surface and host cells is a key aspect of the use of scaffolds for tendon reconstruction. In the first phase of cellular ingrowth, multiple attachment points are established by the cells through the interaction between transmembrane proteins and proteins at the scaffold surface [47], later strengthened by accumulating integrin receptors, eventually forming a focal adhesion which acts as a connection between the actin cytoskeleton of the cell and the surface [47]. The cell proliferation cycle and cell migration start after the formation of focal adhesions and spreading of cells on the surface [47]. Cell attachment, proliferation and migration are facilitated by the porosity of scaffolds [67]. The surfaces of synthetic scaffold are composed of macromolecules from random coils and lacking the well-defined structure that allows host cells to perform a strong binding point and start growing.

However, synthetic ligaments and tendons have excellent mechanical characteristics, because they permit better control of the chemical and physical properties, leading to strong mechanical strength and consistency in quality [47].

An important reason of concern is the poor biocompatibility of synthetic scaffolds, as they can cause numerous long-term complications such as implant degeneration, decreased stability, device failure, severe synovitis, osteolysis and osteoarthritis from a florid inflammation response associated with foreign body reaction [68–71]. They can never be absorbed or integrated into host tissue, and high incidences of postoperative infection and chronic immune response have been reported with the use of such materials [47]. Perhaps acid by-products during synthetic scaffold degradation can alter the local environment and disrupt the proliferation of host tissue and cells, thus compromising the induction ability of synthetic scaffold. On the other hand, there is no risk of disease transmission using synthetic scaffolds.

Another limitation is that available scaffolds are produced to mimic the tendon extracellular microenvironment to stimulate cell proliferation and tissue ingrowth, largely ignoring the healing process at the enthesis. The repair procedure often involves reconstruction of the osteo-tendinous junction, and failure of surgery could be caused by osteolysis and scaffold pullout. Further investigations are required to better understand how to promote the healing of bone-tendon junction.

Even though synthetic scaffolds are becoming more popular, well-conducted clinical studies in humans are lacking, and little data describing the complications or adverse events associated with the use of these products are available. Tissue engineering application to synthetic scaffolds may increase their mechanical properties, such as synthetic scaffolds seeded with bone marrow stem cells or tenocytes. However, clinical evidence in this field is scanty [27, 28, 46, 72–86].

Conclusions

Preliminary studies support the idea that synthetic scaffolds can provide an alternative for rotator cuff augmentation with an enormous therapeutic potential [87]. However, available data are lacking to allow definitive conclusion on the use of these scaffold for cuff augmentation [81, 88–90]. Rather than providing strong evidence for or against the use of these scaffolds for tendon augmentation, this study instead generates potential areas for additional prospective investigation [91–104]. Further investigations are required to evaluate the role of synthetic scaffolds in the clinical practice.

References

1 Cofield RH: Rotator cuff disease of the shoulder. J Bone Joint Surg Am 1985;67:974–979.

2 Longo UG, Franceschi F, Spiezia F, Marinozzi A, Maffulli N, Denaro V: The low-profile Roman bridge technique for knotless double-row repair of the rotator cuff. Arch Orthop Trauma Surg 2011;131:357–361.

3 Franceschi F, Ruzzini L, Longo UG, Martina FM, Zobel BB, Maffulli N, Denaro V: Equivalent clinical results of arthroscopic single-row and double-row suture anchor repair for rotator cuff tears: a randomized controlled trial. Am J Sports Med 2007;35:1254–1260.

4 Franceschi F, Longo UG, Ruzzini L, Rizzello G, Maffulli N, Denaro V: No advantages in repairing a type II superior labrum anterior and posterior lesion when associated with rotator cuff repair in patients over age 50: a randomized controlled trial. Am J Sports Med 2008;36:247–253.
5 Franceschi F, Longo UG, Ruzzini L, Rizzello G, Maffulli N, Denaro V: Soft tissue tenodesis of the long head of the biceps tendon associated to the Roman bridge repair. BMC Musculoskelet Disord 2008;9:78.
6 Franceschi F, Longo UG, Ruzzini L, Rizzello G, Maffulli N, Denaro V: The Roman bridge: a 'double pulley-suture bridges' technique for rotator cuff repair. BMC Musculoskelet Disord 2007;8:123.
7 Franceschi F, Longo UG, Ruzzini L, Papalia R, Rizzello G, Denaro V: To detach the long head of the biceps tendon after tenodesis or not: outcome analysis at the 4-year follow-up of two different techniques. Int Orthop 2007;31:537–545.
8 Cofield RH, Briggs BT: Glenohumeral arthrodesis. Operative and long-term functional results. J Bone Joint Surg Am 1979;61:668–677.
9 Halverson PB, Cheung HS, McCarty DJ, Garancis J, Mandel N: 'Milwaukee shoulder' – association of microspheroids containing hydroxyapatite crystals, active collagenase, and neutral protease with rotator cuff defects. II. Synovial fluid studies. Arthritis Rheum 1981;24:474–483.
10 Neer CS 2nd, Craig EV, Fukuda H: Cuff-tear arthropathy. J Bone Joint Surg Am 1983;65:1232–1244.
11 Sarris IK, Papadimitriou NG, Sotereanos DG: Bipolar hemiarthroplasty for chronic rotator cuff tear arthropathy. J Arthroplasty 2003;18:169–173.
12 Arntz CT, Matsen FA 3rd, Jackins S: Surgical management of complex irreparable rotator cuff deficiency. J Arthroplasty 1991;6:363–370.
13 Boileau P, Watkinson DJ, Hatzidakis AM, Balg F: Grammont reverse prosthesis: design, rationale, and biomechanics. J Shoulder Elbow Surg 2005;14:147S-161S.
14 Nyffeler RW, Werner CM, Gerber C: Biomechanical relevance of glenoid component positioning in the reverse delta III total shoulder prosthesis. J Shoulder Elbow Surg 2005;14:524–528.
15 Maffulli N, Longo UG, Franceschi F, Rabitti C, Denaro V: Movin and Bonar scores assess the same characteristics of tendon histology. Clin Orthop Relat Res 2008;466:1605–1611.
16 Longo UG, Franceschi F, Ruzzini L, Rabitti C, Morini S, Maffulli N, Denaro V: Histopathology of the supraspinatus tendon in rotator cuff tears. Am J Sports Med 2008;36:533–538.
17 Longo UG, Franceschi F, Ruzzini L, Rabitti C, Morini S, Maffulli N, Forriol F, Denaro V: Light microscopic histology of supraspinatus tendon ruptures. Knee Surg Sports Traumatol Arthrosc 2007;15:1390–1394.
18 Maffulli N, Longo UG, Denaro V: Novel approaches for the management of tendinopathy. J Bone Joint Surg 2010;92:2604–2613.
19 Harryman DT 2nd, Mack LA, Wang KY, Jackins SE, Richardson ML, Matsen FA 3rd: Repairs of the rotator cuff. Correlation of functional results with integrity of the cuff. J Bone Joint Surg Am 1991;73:982–989.
20 Khan WS, Longo UG, Ahrens PM, Denaro V, Maffulli N: A systematic review of the reverse shoulder replacement in rotator cuff arthropathy, rotator cuff tears and rheumatoid arthritis. Sports Med Arthrosc 2011 (in press).
21 Domb BG, Glousman RE, Brooks A, Hansen M, Lee TQ, ElAttrache NS: High-tension double-row footprint repair compared with reduced-tension single-row repair for massive rotator cuff tears. J Bone Joint Surg Am 2008;90(suppl 4):35–39.
22 Nelson CO, Sileo MJ, Grossman MG, Serra-Hsu F: Single-row modified Mason-Allen versus double-row arthroscopic rotator cuff repair: a biomechanical and surface area comparison. Arthroscopy 2008;24:941–948.
23 Tocci SL, Tashjian RZ, Leventhal E, Spenciner DB, Green A, Fleming BC: Biomechanical comparison of single-row arthroscopic rotator cuff repair technique versus transosseous repair technique. J Shoulder Elbow Surg 2008;17:808–814.
24 Puskas JE, Chen Y: Biomedical application of commercial polymers and novel polyisobutylene-based thermoplastic elastomers for soft tissue replacement. Biomacromolecules 2004;5:1141–1154.
25 Iannitti DA, Hope WW, Norton HJ, Lincourt AE, Millikan K, Fenoglio ME, Moskowitz M: Technique and outcomes of abdominal incisional hernia repair using a synthetic composite mesh: a report of 455 cases. J Am Coll Surg 2008;206:83–88.
26 Longo UG, Lamberti A, Maffulli N, Denaro V: Tissue engineered biological augmentation for tendon healing: a systematic review. Br Med Bull 2011;98:31–59.
27 Longo UG, Lamberti A, Khan WS, Maffulli N, Denaro V: Synthetic augmentation for massive rotator cuff tears. Sports Med Arthrosc 2011 (in press).
28 Longo UG, Berton A, Alexander S, Maffulli N, Wallace AL, Denaro V: Biological resurfacing for early osteoarthritis of the shoulder. Sports Med Arthrosc 2011 (in press).

29 Castricini R, Longo UG, De Benedetto M, Panfoli N, Pirani P, Zini R, Maffulli N, Denaro V: Platelet-rich plasma augmentation for arthroscopic rotator cuff repair: a randomized controlled trial. Am J Sports Med 2011;39:258–265.
30 Forriol F, Longo UG, Concejo C, Ripalda P, Maffulli N, Denaro V: Platelet-rich plasma, rhOP-1 (rhBMP-7) and frozen rib allograft for the reconstruction of bony mandibular defects in sheep. A pilot experimental study. Injury 2009;40(suppl 3):S44–S49.
31 Longo UG, Lamberti A, Maffulli N, Denaro V: Tendon augmentation grafts: a systematic review. Br Med Bull 2010;94:165–188.
32 Aoki M, Miyamoto S, Okamura K, Yamashita T, Ikada Y, Matsuda S: Tensile properties and biological response of poly(L-lactic acid) felt graft: an experimental trial for rotator-cuff reconstruction. J Biomed Mater Res B Appl Biomater 2004;71:252–259.
33 Derwin KA, Codsi MJ, Milks RA, Baker AR, McCarron JA, Iannotti JP: Rotator cuff repair augmentation in a canine model with use of a woven poly-L-lactide device. J Bone Joint Surg Am 2009;91:1159–1171.
34 Koh JL, Szomor Z, Murrell GA, Warren RF: Supplementation of rotator cuff repair with a bioresorbable scaffold. Am J Sports Med 2002;30:410–413.
35 MacGillivray JD, Fealy S, Terry MA, Koh JL, Nixon AJ, Warren RF: Biomechanical evaluation of a rotator cuff defect model augmented with a bioresorbable scaffold in goats. J Shoulder Elbow Surg 2006;15:639–644.
36 Kimura A, Aoki M, Fukushima S, Ishii S, Yamakoshi K: Reconstruction of a defect of the rotator cuff with polytetrafluoroethylene felt graft. Recovery of tensile strength and histocompatibility in an animal model. J Bone Joint Surg Br 2003;85:282–287.
37 Dejardin LM, Arnoczky SP, Ewers BJ, Haut RC, Clarke RB: Tissue-engineered rotator cuff tendon using porcine small intestine submucosa. Histologic and mechanical evaluation in dogs. Am J Sports Med 2001;29:175–184.
38 McDevitt CA, Wildey GM, Cutrone RM: Transforming growth factor-β_1 in a sterilized tissue derived from the pig small intestine submucosa. J Biomed Mater Res A 2003;67:637–640.
39 Nicholson GP, Breur GJ, Van Sickle D, Yao JQ, Kim J, Blanchard CR: Evaluation of a cross-linked acellular porcine dermal patch for rotator cuff repair augmentation in an ovine model. J Shoulder Elbow Surg 2007;16:S184–S190.
40 Sano H, Kumagai J, Sawai T: Experimental fascial autografting for the supraspinatus tendon defect: remodeling process of the grafted fascia and the insertion into bone. J Shoulder Elbow Surg 2002;11:166–173.
41 Schlegel TF, Hawkins RJ, Lewis CW, Motta T, Turner AS: The effects of augmentation with swine small intestine submucosa on tendon healing under tension: histologic and mechanical evaluations in sheep. Am J Sports Med 2006;34:275–280.
42 Zalavras CG, Gardocki R, Huang E, Stevanovic M, Hedman T, Tibone J: Reconstruction of large rotator cuff tendon defects with porcine small intestinal submucosa in an animal model. J Shoulder Elbow Surg 2006;15:224–231.
43 Zheng MH, Chen J, Kirilak Y, Willers C, Xu J, Wood D: Porcine small intestine submucosa is not an acellular collagenous matrix and contains porcine DNA: possible implications in human implantation. J Biomed Mater Res B Appl Biomater 2005;73:61–67.
44 Funakoshi T, Majima T, Suenaga N, Iwasaki N, Yamane S, Minami A: Rotator cuff regeneration using chitin fabric as an acellular matrix. J Shoulder Elbow Surg 2006;15:112–118.
45 Funakoshi T, Majima T, Iwasaki N, Suenaga N, Sawaguchi N, Shimode K, Minami A, Harada K, Nishimura S: Application of tissue engineering techniques for rotator cuff regeneration using a chitosan-based hyaluronan hybrid fiber scaffold. Am J Sports Med 2005;33:1193–1201.
46 Longo UG, Forriol F, Campi S, Maffulli N, Denaro V: Animal models for translational research on shoulder pathologies: from bench to bedside. Sports Med Arthrosc 2011 (in press).
47 Chen J, Xu J, Wang A, Zheng M: Scaffolds for tendon and ligament repair: review of the efficacy of commercial products. Expert Rev Med Devices 2009;6:61–73.
48 Yokoya S, Mochizuki Y, Nagata Y, Deie M, Ochi M: Tendon-bone insertion repair and regeneration using polyglycolic acid sheet in the rabbit rotator cuff injury model. Am J Sports Med 2008;36:1298–1309.
49 McCarron JA, Milks RA, Chen X, Iannotti JP, Derwin KA: Improved time-zero biomechanical properties using poly-L-lactic acid graft augmentation in a cadaveric rotator cuff repair model. J Shoulder Elbow Surg 2010;19:688–696.
50 Santoni BG, McGilvray KC, Lyons AS, Bansal M, Turner AS, Macgillivray JD, Coleman SH, Puttlitz CM: Biomechanical analysis of an ovine rotator cuff repair via porous patch augmentation in a chronic rupture model. Am J Sports Med 2010;38:679–686.
51 Cole BJ, Gomoll AH, Yanke A, Pylawka T, Lewis P, Macgillivray JD, Williams JM: Biocompatibility of a polymer patch for rotator cuff repair. Knee Surg Sports Traumatol Arthrosc 2007;15:632–637.
52 Moffat KL, Kwei AS, Spalazzi JP, Doty SB, Levine WN, Lu HH: Novel nanofiber-based scaffold for rotator cuff repair and augmentation. Tissue Eng Part A 2009;15:115–126.

53 Ozaki J, Fujimoto S, Masuhara K, Tamai S, Yoshimoto S: Reconstruction of chronic massive rotator cuff tears with synthetic materials. Clin Orthop Relat Res 1986;202:173–183.
54 Post M: Rotator cuff repair with carbon filament. A preliminary report of five cases. Clin Orthop Relat Res 1985;196:154–158.
55 Visuri T, Kiviluoto O, Eskelin M: Carbon fiber for repair of the rotator cuff. A 4-year follow-up of 14 cases. Acta Orthop Scand 1991;62:356–359.
56 Hehl G, Kinzl L, Reichel R: Carbon-fiber implants for knee ligament reconstruction. 10-year results (in German). Chirurg 1997;68:1119–1125.
57 Olson EJ, Kang JD, Fu FH, Georgescu HI, Mason GC, Evans CH: The biochemical and histological effects of artificial ligament wear particles: in vitro and in vivo studies. Am J Sports Med 1988;16:558–570.
58 Parsons JR, Bhayani S, Alexander H, Weiss AB: Carbon fiber debris within the synovial joint. A time-dependent mechanical and histologic study. Clin Orthop Relat Res 1985;196:69–76.
59 Audenaert E, Van Nuffel J, Schepens A, Verhelst M, Verdonk R: Reconstruction of massive rotator cuff lesions with a synthetic interposition graft: a prospective study of 41 patients. Knee Surg Sports Traumatol Arthrosc 2006;14:360–364.
60 Karas SE, Giachello TL: Subscapularis transfer for reconstruction of massive tears of the rotator cuff. J Bone Joint Surg Am 1996;78:239–245.
61 Amis AA, Camburn M, Kempson SA, Radford WJ, Stead AC: Anterior cruciate ligament replacement with polyester fibre. A long-term study of tissue reactions and joint stability in sheep. J Bone Joint Surg Br 1992;74:605–613.
62 Matsumoto H, Fujikawa K: Leeds-Keio artificial ligament: a new concept for the anterior cruciate ligament reconstruction of the knee. Keio J Med 2001;50:161–166.
63 Tanaka N, Sakahashi H, Hirose K, Ishima T, Ishii S: Augmented subscapularis muscle transposition for rotator cuff repair during shoulder arthroplasty in patients with rheumatoid arthritis. J Shoulder Elbow Surg 2006;15:2–6.
64 Nada AN, Debnath UK, Robinson DA, Jordan C: Treatment of massive rotator-cuff tears with a polyester ligament (Dacron) augmentation: clinical outcome. J Bone Joint Surg Br 2010;92:1397–1402.
65 Hirooka A, Yoneda M, Wakaitani S, Isaka Y, Hayashida K, Fukushima S, Okamura K: Augmentation with a Gore-Tex patch for repair of large rotator cuff tears that cannot be sutured. J Orthop Sci 2002;7:451–456.
66 Valentin JE, Badylak JS, McCabe GP, Badylak SF: Extracellular matrix bioscaffolds for orthopaedic applications. A comparative histologic study. J Bone Joint Surg Am 2006;88:2673–2686.
67 Hutmacher DW: Scaffolds in tissue engineering bone and cartilage. Biomaterials 2000;21:2529–2543.
68 Fukubayashi T, Ikeda K: Follow-up study of Gore-Tex artificial ligament – special emphasis on tunnel osteolysis. J Long Term Eff Med Implants 2000;10: 267–277.
69 Miller MD, Peters CL, Allen B: Early aseptic loosening of a total knee arthroplasty due to Gore-Tex particle-induced osteolysis. J Arthroplasty 2006;21: 765–770.
70 Muren O, Dahlstedt L, Brosjö E, Dahlborn M, Dalén N: Gross osteolytic tibia tunnel widening with the use of Gore-Tex anterior cruciate ligament prosthesis: a radiological, arthrometric and clinical evaluation of 17 patients 13–15 years after surgery. Acta Orthop 2005;76:270–274.
71 Macnicol MF, Penny ID, Sheppard L: Early results of the Leeds-Keio anterior cruciate ligament replacement. J Bone Joint Surg Br 1991;73:377–380.
72 Maffulli N, Longo UG, Loppini M, Denaro V: Current treatment options for tendinopathy. Expert Opin Pharmacother 2010;11:2177–2186.
73 Khanna A, Friel M, Gougoulias N, Longo UG, Maffulli N: Prevention of adhesions in surgery of the flexor tendons of the hand: what is the evidence? Br Med Bull 2009;90:85–109.
74 Lippi G, Longo UG, Maffulli N: Genetics and sports. Br Med Bull 2010;93:27–47.
75 Longo UG, Franceschi F, Ruzzini L, Rabitti C, Morini S, Maffulli N, Denaro V: Characteristics at haematoxylin and eosin staining of ruptures of the long head of the biceps tendon. Br J Sports Med 2009;43:603–607.
76 Longo UG, Franceschi F, Ruzzini L, Spiezia F, Maffulli N, Denaro V: Higher fasting plasma glucose levels within the normoglycaemic range and rotator cuff tears. Br J Sports Med 2009;43:284–287.
77 Longo UG, Franceschi F, Spiezia F, Forriol F, Maffulli N, Denaro V: Triglycerides and total serum cholesterol in rotator cuff tears: do they matter? Br J Sports Med 2010;44:948–951.
78 Longo UG, Garau G, Denaro V, Maffulli N: Surgical management of tendinopathy of biceps femoris tendon in athletes. Disabil Rehabil 2008;30:1602–1607.
79 Longo UG, Rittweger J, Garau G, Radonic B, Gutwasser C, Gilliver SF, Kusy K, Zielinski J, Felsenberg D, Maffulli N: No influence of age, gender, weight, height, and impact profile in Achilles tendinopathy in masters track and field athletes. Am J Sport Med 2009;37:1400–1405.

80 Longo UG, Rittweger J, Garau G, Radonic B, Gutwasser C, Gilliver SF, Kusy K, Zielinski J, Felsenberg D, Maffulli N: Patellar tendinopathy in master track and field athletes: influence of impact profile, weight, height, age and gender. Knee Surg Sports Traumatol Arthrosc 2011;19:508–512.
81 Maffulli N, Longo UG, Spiezia F, Denaro V: Sports injuries in young athletes: long-term outcome and prevention strategies. Phys Sportsmed 2010;38:29–34.
82 Longo UG, Buchmann S, Berton A, Maffulli N, Denaro V: Arthroscopic knots and strength sutures for rotator cuff repair. Sports Med Arthrosc 2011 (in press).
83 Longo UG, Berton A, Khan WS, Maffulli N, Denaro V: Histopathology of rotator cuff tears. Sports Med Arthrosc 2011 (in press).
84 Longo UG, Vasta S, Maffulli N, Denaro V: Scoring systems for the functional assessment of patients with rotator cuff pathology. Sports Med Arthrosc 2011 (in press).
85 Denaro V, Ruzzini L, Longo UG, Franceschi F, De Paola B, Cittadini A, Maffulli N, Sgambato A: Effect of dihydrotestosterone on cultured human tenocytes from intact supraspinatus tendon. Knee Surg Sports Traumatol Arthrosc 2010;18:971–976.
86 Denaro V, Ruzzini L, Barnaba SA, Longo UG, Campi S, Maffulli N, Sgambato A: Effect of pulsed electromagnetic fields on human tenocyte cultures from supraspinatus and quadriceps tendons. Am J Phys Med Rehabil 2011;90:119–127.
87 Maffulli N, Franceschi F, Longo UG, Ruzzini L, Denaro V: Clinical evidence for suture anchor repair of rotator cuff tears does add up: some just do not want to see it. Arthroscopy 2010;26:1568–1570.
88 Maffulli N, Longo UG, Gougoulias N, Caine D, Denaro V: Sport injuries: a review of outcomes. Br Med Bull 2011;97:47–80.
89 Maffulli N, Longo UG, Spiezia F, Denaro V: Aetiology and prevention of injuries in elite young athletes. Med Sport Sci 2011;56:187–200.
90 Maffulli N, Longo UG, Berton A, Loppini M, Denaro V: Biological factors in rotator cuff tears. Sports Med Arthrosc 2011 (in press).
91 Longo UG, Ramamurthy C, Denaro V, Maffulli N: Minimally invasive stripping for chronic Achilles tendinopathy. Disabil Rehabil 2008;30:1709–1713.
92 Longo UG, Ronga M, Maffulli N: Achilles tendinopathy. Sports Med Arthrosc 2009;17:112–126.
93 Longo UG, Oliva F, Denaro V, Maffulli N: Oxygen species and overuse tendinopathy in athletes. Disabil Rehabil 2008;30:1563–1571.
94 Ames PR, Longo UG, Denaro V, Maffulli N: Achilles tendon problems: not just an orthopaedic issue. Disabil Rehabil 2008;30:1646–1650.
95 Franceschi F, Marinozzi A, Papalia R, Longo UG, Gualdi G, Denaro E: Intra- and juxta-articular osteoid osteoma: a diagnostic challenge: misdiagnosis and successful treatment: a report of four cases. Arch Orthop Trauma Surg 2006;126:660–667.
96 Maffulli N, Longo UG, Gougoulias N, Denaro V: Ipsilateral free semitendinosus tendon graft transfer for reconstruction of chronic tears of the Achilles tendon. BMC Musculoskelet Disord 2008;9:100.
97 Maffulli N, Walley G, Sayana MK, Longo UG, Denaro V: Eccentric calf muscle training in athletic patients with Achilles tendinopathy. Disabil Rehabil 2008;30:1677–1684.
98 Longo UG, Ronga M, Maffulli N: Acute ruptures of the achilles tendon. Sports Med Arthrosc 2009;17:127–138.
99 Maffulli N, Longo UG: Conservative management for tendinopathy: is there enough scientific evidence? Rheumatology 2008;47:390–391.
100 Maffulli N, Longo UG: How do eccentric exercises work in tendinopathy? Rheumatology 2008;47:1444–1445.
101 Franceschi F, Longo UG, Ruzzini L, Rizzello G, Denaro V: Arthroscopic management of calcific tendinitis of the subscapularis tendon. Knee Surg Sports Traumatol Arthrosc 2007;15:1482–1485.
102 Maffulli N, Longo UG, Ronga M, Khanna A, Denaro V: Favorable outcome of percutaneous repair of achilles tendon ruptures in the elderly. Clin Orthop Relat Res 2010;468:1039–1046.
103 Maffulli N, Longo UG, Gougoulias N, Loppini M, Denaro V: Long-term health outcomes of youth sports injuries. Br J Sports Med 2010;44:21–25.
104 Longo UG, King JB, Denaro V, Maffulli N: Double-bundle arthroscopic reconstruction of the anterior cruciate ligament: does the evidence add up? J Bone Joint Surg Br 2008;90:995–999.

Nicola Maffulli, MD, MS, PhD, FRCS(Orth)
Centre for Sports and Exercise Medicine
Barts and The London School of Medicine and Dentistry
Mile End Hospital, 275 Bancroft Road, London E1 4DG (UK)
Tel. +44 20 8223 8839, E-Mail n.maffulli@qmul.ac.uk

Maffulli N (ed): Rotator Cuff Tear. Med Sport Sci. Basel, Karger, 2012, vol 57, pp 178–183

Understanding and Preventing Complications in Repairing Rotator Cuff Tears

Leonardo Osti[a] · Rocco Papalia[b,c] · Angelo Del Buono[b,c] · Vincenzo Denaro[b,c] · Nicola Maffulli[d]

[a]Unit of Arthroscopy and Sports Medicine, Hesperia Hospital, Modena, [b]Department of Orthopaedic and Trauma Surgery and [c]Centro Integrato di Ricerca (CIR), Campus Bio-Medico University, Rome, Italy; [d]Centre for Sports and Exercise Medicine, Barts and The London School of Medicine and Dentistry, Mile End Hospital, London, UK

Abstract

Repair of rotator cuff tears is a common procedure. Prior to approaching this surgery, it should be realized that each surgical step can lead to complications, including those related to positioning and anaesthesia. Stiffness, infection and failure of repair are the more frequent complications reported.

Overall, complications of arthroscopic rotator cuff surgery are more common than the ones occurring in knee arthroscopy [1, 2]. A lack of consensus has been observed in defining the list of complications in this field, but stiffness and failure of the repair are the ones most commonly recognized [1, 3]. Complications of arthroscopic rotator cuff repair are similar to those reported for open repair [4].

Complications can be classified as general and specific. General complications are those described for any type of arthroscopic surgery and include, for example, cerebral ischaemia and pulmonary events [2, 3].

Among the general complications, the risk of deep vein thrombosis has recently been outlined even in patients without apparent specific risk factors. Polzhofer et al. [5] reported a patient with a thromboembolic complication following shoulder arthroscopy without any risk factors. Garofalo et al. [6] reported 2 patients of a cohort of 10,400 shoulder arthroscopies, with 1 of these 2 patients developing bilateral pulmonary microembolism. A national survey of 9,500 shoulder arthroscopies reported 6 patients affected by thromboembolic complications. Of these 6 patients, 4 had undergone an uncomplicated rotator cuff repair [7]. Bongiovanni et al. [8]

reported 3 cases with thromboembolic complication following arthroscopic rotator cuff repair in patients with previously undetected hereditary thrombophilia. Recently, Kim et al. [9] reported a fatal thromboembolism of the contralateral axillary vein in a 45-year-old woman without any haematologic risk factor identified. At present, there are no guidelines specific for preventing deep vein thrombosis in shoulder arthroscopic procedures [6, 7].

Positioning and Anaesthesia

Patient positioning and set-up are essential to prevent general complications. The beach chair or the lateral position can be used, with no clear superiority of one over the other in terms of set-up, surgical visualization, portals placement and patients risk [10]. However, patients undergoing shoulder surgery with interscalene block presented a much higher incidence of cerebral desaturation-related effects when the beach chair was used in comparison with the lateral position [11].

Phol et al. [12] and Dippmann et al. [13] confirmed the risk of severe cerebral desaturation, which can lead to ischaemic complication specifically related to the position of the head. Papadonikolakis et al. [14] recommend blood pressure monitoring at the contralateral arm kept at the heart level to avoid errors in pressure measurement producing possible devastating complications such as stroke and death. General anaesthesia complications ranging from pulmonary oedema and fatal ischaemic cerebral events outlined the potential risk of arthroscopic rotator cuff repair not related solely to the procedure itself [3].

Neurological Complications

A consistent risk for neurological damage has been reported, up to 30% in older series, with a major component of transient neurapraxia [1, 15]. Segmüller et al. [16] reported an overall nerve injury rate of 7% in patients undergoing shoulder arthroscopy, with most involving the cutaneous branch of the axillary nerve.

Neurological damage can be related to the use of arm traction. Klein et al. [17], analyzing the use of arm traction and its negative impact on the brachial plexus, reported an increased stress from increased extension and decreased abduction. Low weight traction, limited length of the procedure and accurate patient positioning are recommended to prevent neurological complications to the brachial plexus from traction [18]. Permanent nerve damages are uncommon, but some have been reported from excessive traction, swelling and limb wrapping [19]. Lo et al. [20], in a cadaveric study, showed the close relationship between the coracoid area and the axillary and musculocutaneous nerve (28–33 mm), warning the surgeon for both portals and subacromial space procedures [4]. Cogan et al. [21] reported neurapraxia of the

9th, 10th and 12th cranial nerves, possibly from general anaesthesia intubation and beach-chair positioning.

Proper positioning of the head and neck, avoiding heavy prolonged traction on the arm, reducing the strain on brachial plexus, are recommended to prevent neurological complications of the procedure [1, 3].

Fluid Extravasation

Fluid extravasation should be limited to prevent complications related to pathological pulmonary complications which can lead to tracheal obstruction [22, 23] and skin necrosis [24].

Surgically Related Complications

Each step of the repair can lead to surgical complications according to the technique used for the repair [19]. The most common mode of failure was pulling of the tendon at the suture junction, accounting for 19 of 22 failures [25]. Anchor pull-out is one of the more worrying surgical complications reported [3, 19], resulting from both improper anchor insertion and osteoporotic bone [19]. Benson et al. [26] analyzed the early metallic pull-out in 269 with 550 metallic suture anchors implanted reported: there was an early pull-out rate of 2.4%, with an increased risk in patients presenting larger tear, with 89% of the failure site at the posterior aspect of the greater tuberosity.

Anchor pull-out is clinically difficult to be differentiated from postoperative symptoms, and radiographs can easily locate the metallic anchor, with indirect signs such as bone erosion at the footprint for the radiotransparent bioabsorbable anchors [19, 27].

Stiffness

Shoulder stiffness is a common event following shoulder surgery, especially rotator cuff repair [1]. Brislin et al. [4], evaluating retrospectively the overall complication rate of rotator cuff repair, reported that the major postoperative complications related to rotator cuff tears repair are stiffness, infection and failure of the repair, defining stiffness as patients having external rotation <10° and forward elevation >100°.

Postoperative stiffness is greatly related to the preoperative degree of limitation of range of motion. Hatch et al. [28], studying patients who developed this complication, classify them in four categories: (1) stiffness without a tear; (2) stiffness with a tear; (3) stiffness with untreated osteoarthritis, and (4) stiffness with nerve or deltoid injury. In most patients, a modified rehabilitation program is effective [1, 4, 28], and in the patients refractory to such a rehabilitation regimen an arthroscopic capsular release should be considered, excluding patients in categories 3 and 4 [28].

In patients undergoing rotator cuff repair with identified risk factors for stiffness, such as PASTA lesion, single tendon tear, and previous adhesive capsulitis, Koo et al. [29] evaluated the benefit of an early close chain exercise regimen with good results.

Infection

Infection is uncommon following repair of a rotator cuff tear, with a lower rate in arthroscopic reports compared to the open and mini-open ones. McFarland et al. [2], in a review of arthroscopic RC repair complications, reported a rate of 0.04–0.23. An early diagnosis and aggressive treatment are considered the key to eradicate the infection [4, 28, 29].

Brislin et al. [4] reported one deep infection in 263 operated shoulders, Herrera et al. [30] reported 7 in 360 arthroscopic and mini-open rotator cuff repairs. *Staphylococcus aureus* and *Propionibacterium* acnes are the most common bacteria involved [31]. Athwal et al. [32] reported 39 deep infections following rotator cuff repair, emphasizing the attention in recognizing the *Propionibacterium* acne which needs at least a 1-week culture to be indentified, with early diagnosis and aggressive treatment the key to eradicate the infection [4, 30–32].

Failure of Rotator Cuff Repair

Failure of the repair is possible regardless of whether the proper technique had been used: patients factors associated with failed rotator cuff tears repair are age, gender, smoking, size of the tear, and poor tendon quality [2, 3, 33, 34]. Errors in diagnosis for associated pathologies such as cervical radiculopathy or spinoglenoid notch cyst can lead to poor outcomes of rotator cuff repair given the unrecognized and untreated pathology [35]. Each failure should be properly addressed and appropriately managed, as should lesions of the long head of the biceps tendon and SLAP lesions [35, 36]. In patients undergoing rotator cuff repair, better results were evident in the patients in whom a biceps tenotomy was performed compared with those in whom only the SLAP tear was addressed [37].

Imaging and Clinical Failure

Often there is no correlation between the imaging results and the clinical picture. A study of 169 patients demonstrated that the healing rate is affected both by age and tear size, regardless of the technique used. In the patients presenting fatty degeneration above grade 2, the repair was more likely to fail and the re-tear was usually less symptomatic than the original tear [38]. Indeed, satisfactory clinical results can be obtained in patients undergoing a new rotator cuff repair with MRI evidence of a re-tear even though they may have a lower Constant score. Also, a re-tear after rotator cuff repair can be asymptomatic [39, 40].

Conclusions

Complications of surgical management of rotator cuff tears are not uncommon, and should be managed on a patient-to-patient basis. It should be kept in mind that failure at imaging does not necessarily correspond to clinical failure, and therefore accurate physical examination should be performed to prevent unnecessary surgery.

References

1 Nottage WM: How to avoid and manage complications in arthroscopic rotator cuff repair; in Abrams JS, Bell RH (eds): Arthroscopic Rotator Cuff Surgery. Berlin, Springer, 2008, pp 363–373.

2 McFarland E, O'Neil O, Hsu C: Complications of shoulder arthroscopy. J South Orthop Assoc 1997; 6:190–196.

3 Tasto JP, Noud PH: Complications in shoulder arthroscopy; in Angelo RL, Esch JC, Ryu RK (eds): AANA Advanced Arthroscopy: The Shoulder. Philadelphia, Saunders Elsevier, 2010, pp 304–312.

4 Brislin KJ, Field LD, Savoie FH 3rd: Complications after arthroscopic rotator cuff repair. Arthroscopy 2007;232:124–128.

5 Polzhofer GK, Petersen W, Hassenpflug J: Thromboembolic complication after arthroscopic shoulder surgery. Arthroscopy 2003;199:E129–E132.

6 Garofalo R, Notarnicola A, Moretti L, Moretti B, Marini S, Castagna A: Deep vein thromboembolism after arthroscopy of the shoulder: two case reports and a review of the literature. BMC Musculoskelet Disord 2010;11:65.

7 Randelli P, Castagna A, Cabitza F, Cabitza P, Arrigoni P, Denti M: Infectious and thromboembolic complications of arthroscopic shoulder surgery. J Shoulder Elbow Surg 2010;19:97–101.

8 Bongiovanni SL, Ranalletta M, Guala A, Maignon GD: Case reports: heritable thrombophilia associated with deep venous thrombosis after shoulder arthroscopy. Clin Orthop Relat Res 2009;467:2196–2199.

9 Kim SJ, Yoo KY, Lee HG, Kim WM, Jeong CW, Lee HJ: Fatal pulmonary embolism caused by thrombosis of contralateral axillary vein after arthroscopic right rotator cuff repair. A case report. Korean J Anesthesiol 2010;59(suppl):S172–S175.

10 Peruto CM, Ciccotti MG, Cohen SB: Shoulder arthroscopy positioning: lateral decubitus versus beach chair. Arthroscopy 2009;25:891–896.

11 Murphy GS, Szokol JW, Marymont JH, Greenberg SB, Avram MJ, Vender JS, Vaughn J, Nisman M: Cerebral oxygen desaturation events assessed by near-infrared spectroscopy during shoulder arthroscopy in the beach chair and lateral decubitus positions. Anesth Analg 2010;111:496–505.

12 Pohl A, Cullen DJ: Cerebral ischemia during shoulder surgery in the upright position: a case series. J Clin Anesth 2005;17:463–469.

13 Dippmann C, Winge S, Nielsen HB: Severe cerebral desaturation during shoulder arthroscopy in the beach-chair position. Arthroscopy 2010;26(suppl): S148–S150.

14 Papadonikolakis A, Wiesler ER, Olympio MA, Poehling GG: Avoiding catastrophic complications of stroke and death related to shoulder surgery in the sitting position. Arthroscopy 2008;24:481–482.

15 Rodeo S, Forster R, Weiland A: Neurological complications due to arthroscopy. J Bone Joint Surg Am 1993;75:917–926.

16 Segmüller HE, Alfred SP, Zilio G, Saies AD, Hayes MG: Cutaneous nerve lesions of the shoulder and arm after arthroscopic shoulder surgery. J Shoulder Elbow Surg 1995;4:254–258.

17 Klein AH, France JC, Mutschler TA, et al: Measurement of brachial plexus strain in arthroscopy of the shoulder. Arthroscopy 1987;3:45–52.
18 Stanish WD, Peterson DC: Shoulder arthroscopy and nerve injury: pitfalls and prevention. Arthroscopy 1995;11:458–466.
19 Trantalis J, Lo IKL: Avoiding and managing rotator cuff complications of arthroscopic rotator cuff repair; in Meislin RJ, Albrecht J (eds): Complications of Knee and Shoulder Surgery. Berlin, Springer, 2009, pp 225–244.
20 Lo I, Burkhart S, Parten P: Surgery about the coracoid: neurovascular structures at risk. Arthroscopy 2004;20:591–595.
21 Cogan A, Boyer P, Soubeyrand M, Hamida FB, Vannier JL, Massin P: Cranial nerves neuropraxia after shoulder arthroscopy in beach chair position. Orthop Traumatol Surg Res 2011;97:345–348.
22 Venkat G, Moon YL, Na WC, So KY: Upper airway compromise by extravasated fluid: a rare complication after arthroscopic repair of atrophic cuff tear. Orthopedics 2009;32:pii.
23 Saeki N, Kawamoto M: Tracheal obstruction caused by fluid extravasation during shoulder arthroscopy. Anaesth Intensive Care 2011;39:317–318.
24 Mohammed KD, Hayes MG, Saies AD: Unusual complications of shoulder arthroscopy. J Shoulder Elbow Surg 2000;9:350–352.
25 Cummins CA, Murrel GA: Mode of failure for rotator cuff repair with suture anchors identifies at revision surgery. J Shoulder Elbow Surg 2003;12: 128–133.
26 Benson EC, MacDermid JC, Drosdowech DS, Athwal GS: The incidence of early metallic suture anchor pullout after arthroscopic rotator cuff repair. Arthroscopy 2010;26:310–315.
27 Endrizzi DP: Failure of arthroscopic rotator cuff repair; in Duralde XA (ed): Complications in Orthopaedics. Shoulder Arthroscopy. AAOS Bone and Joint Decade, 2008, pp 27–36.
28 Hatch RGF, Gobetzie R, Miller PJ: Stiffness after rotator cuff repair; in Green A (ed): Complications in Orthopaedics. AAOS Rotator Cuff Surgery, 2006, pp 13–29.
29 Koo SS, Parsley BK, Burkhart SS, Schoolfield JD: Reduction of postoperative stiffness after arthroscopic rotator cuff repair: results of a customized physical therapy regimen based on risk factors for stiffness. Arthroscopy 2011;27:155–160.
30 Herrera M, Bauer G, Reynolds F, et al: Infections after mini-open rotator cuff repair. J Shoulder Elbow Surg 2002;11:605–608.
31 Kwon Y, Kalainov D, Rose H, et al: Management of deep infection after rotator cuff repair surgery. J Shoulder Elbow Surg 2005;14:1–5.
32 Athwal GS, Sperling JW, Rispoli DM, Cofield R: Deep infection after rotator cuff repair. J Shoulder Elbow Surg 2007;16:306–311.
33 Mallon W, Misamore G, Snead G, et al: The impact of preoperative smoking habits on the results of rotator cuff repair. J Shoulder Elbow Surg 2004; 13:129–132.
34 Romeo A, Hang D, Bach B, et al: Repair of full thickness rotator cuff tears. Gender, age and other factors affecting outcome. Clin Orthop Relat Res 1999; 367:243–255.
35 Brems JJ: Errors in diagnosis; in Green A (ed): Complications in orthopaedics – rotator cuff surgery. AAOS Bone and Joint Decade, 2006, pp 12–21.
36 Pai V, Larson D: Rotator cuff repair in a district hospital setting: outocmes and analysis of prognostic factors. J Shoulder Elbow Surg 2001;10:236–241.
37 Franceschi F, Longo UG, Ruzzini L, Rizzello G, Maffulli N, Denaro V: No advantages in repairing a type II superior labrum anterior and posterior (SLAP) lesion when associated with rotator cuff repair in patients over age 50: a randomized controlled trial. Am J Sports Med 2008;36:247–253.
38 Cho NS, Yi JW, Lee BG, et al: Re-tear pattern after arthroscopic rotator cuff repair: single row vs. suture bridge technique. Am J Sports Med 2010; 38:664–671.
39 Demirors H, Circi E, Akgun RC, Tarhan NC, Cetin N, Akpinar S, Tuncay IC: Correlations of isokinetic measurements with tendon healing following open repair of rotator cuff tears. Int Orthop 2010;34: 531–536.
40 Spielmann AL, Forster BB, Kokan P, et al: Shoulder after rotator cuff repair: MR imaging findings in asymptomatic individuals. Radiology 1999;213: 705–708.

Leonardo Osti, MD
Unit of Arthroscopy and Sports Medicine
Hesperia Hospital I Modena
Via Arqua 80/B, IT–40125 Modena (Italy)
Tel. +39 0 59 393101, E-Mail n.maffulli@qmul.ac.uk

Subject Index